Fitting and Dispensing
Hearing Aids

Brad A. Stach, Ph.D.
Editor-in-Chief for Audiology

Fitting and Dispensing Hearing Aids

Brian Taylor
H. Gustav Mueller

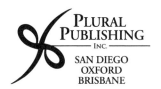

PLURAL
PUBLISHING
INC.

SAN DIEGO
OXFORD
BRISBANE

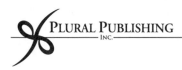

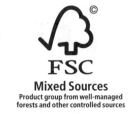

5521 Ruffin Road
San Diego, CA 92123

e-mail: info@pluralpublishing.com
Web site: http://www.pluralpublishing.com

49 Bath Street
Abingdon, Oxfordshire OX14 1EA
United Kingdom

FSC
Mixed Sources
Product group from well-managed
forests and other controlled sources

Cert no. SW-COC-002283
www.fsc.org
© 1996 Forest Stewardship Council

Library of Congress Cataloging-in-Publication Data

Taylor, Brian, 1966-
  Fitting and dispensing hearing aids / Brian Taylor, H. Gustav Mueller.
      p. ; cm.
  Includes bibliographical references and index.
  ISBN-13: 978-1-59756-347-5 (alk. paper)
  ISBN-10: 1-59756-347-1 (alk. paper)
  1. Hearing aids. I. Mueller, H. Gustav. II. Title.
  [DNLM: 1. Hearing Aids. WV 274]
  RF300.T39 2010
  617.8'9—dc22
                        2010054530

Contents

Preface   *vii*

1 Basic Psychology of Hearing Loss in Adults   1

2 Acoustics at the Speed of Sound   17

3 Basic Anatomy and Physiology of the Ear   45

4 Measurement of Hearing   71

5 Hearing Disorders and Audiogram Interpretation   109

6 The Hearing Aid Selection Process   137

7 All About Style: Hearing Aids and Earmolds   169

8 Hearing Aids: How They Work!   201

9 Advanced Hearing Aid Features   231

10 Hearing Aid Fitting Procedures   277

11 Outcome Assessments and Postfitting Issues   329

12 "Selling" Hearing Aids: It's Not a Bad Thing!   375

Appendix   *417*
References   *421*
Index   *423*

Preface

The exact beginning of our collaboration on this textbook is debatable. It was either during a visit to a pub on the outskirts of Manchester, United Kingdom, in May, 2007, or while enjoying an aperitif at a café in Milan, Italy, in the autumn of that same year that we began work on this project. Regardless of its origins, the writing of this book has been a memorable journey with many twists and turns. Whenever you decide to pick it up and begin reading it—regardless of your background—we hope you find the content both helpful and engaging.

This textbook is intended *primarily* for nonaudiologists or undergraduate students who have yet to fit their first pair of hearing aids. Prospective hearing instrument specialists, audiology assistants, speech pathologists, and other professionals aspiring to fit hearing aids, or those who simply want a better understanding of hearing aids, will find the content especially helpful. This book is also perfectly suited for the individual who has just joined the hearing aid industry workforce, and does not have an audiology background. With all that said, in the second half of the book we included considerable practical information about hearing aid features, selection, and fitting procedures that is not so basic; even the savvy, seasoned dispenser will find these chapters useful. From soup to nuts, we have included a broad range of subject matter that you need to know related to the process of actually selecting and fitting hearing aids (and selling them too!). Portions of the book contain the information that you need to know for obtaining your hearing instrument dispensing license.

Because we used a "something for everybody" approach when thinking of our target audience, you'll see that we struggled with deciding what to call you, the reader. You'll see terms such as audiologist, clinician, professional, dispenser, and instrument specialist. As much as we're not fond of the term "hearing health care provider" that probably slipped in a few times too. Regardless, you know who you are, and hopefully there is something here for everyone. When it comes to the actual art and science of fitting hearing aids, there probably are more similarities among groups than differences. We consistently called patients "patients," although some of you may think of them as clients, or maybe even customers.

You'll notice that the 12 chapters of this book are sequenced to match the necessary steps that you need to complete when dispensing hearing aids, including conducting basic audiometry, determining hearing aid candidacy, understanding hearing aid features, selecting and fitting hearing aids, and finally, verifying and validating your recommendation. The first three chapters provide the reader with some essential prerequisite information about the psychology of hearing loss, anatomy and physiology of the ear and basic acoustics. Beginning with Chapter 4, even if you're a beginner, we provide you with the information that will give you the skills to actually perform all the necessary tasks and procedures needed for selecting and fitting hearing aids on adults — with of course some guidance and supervision from an experienced audiologist or hearing instrument specialist.

Although we provide a lot of essential information, this book, of course, is not intended to replace university-level coursework or direct supervision from an experienced clinician. Rather, we provide you with just enough information to get you started on your career journey. It's our hope that the style and content of this book may inspire some of you to obtain your hearing aid dispensing license or doctorate in audiology. Or, if you already have this achievement, we hope you find some useful tidbits to assist you in improving patient benefit and satisfaction with amplification.

Budweiser likes to say that its beer has a "drinkability" advantage, and we like to think our book has a lot of "readability." Introductory textbooks devoted to basic concepts and core knowledge are sometimes known by students to be mundane, tedious, boring, and somewhat unreadable. In order to overcome the effects of dullness, we have "themed" each chapter to add some entertainment value and make the material a little more fun and perhaps more readable. If you happen to be a person who is not enthralled by rudimentary coursework devoted to ear anatomy, physics of sound, or audio-gram interpretation, you may find our themes entertaining enough to help you get through the chapter. For example, you may find the psychology of hearing loss uninteresting, but when country music vignettes are interwoven throughout this chapter, it just might inspire you to more readily absorb the material. (We're not quite sure what will happen if you don't enjoy country music.) Sports fans, pop culture enthusiasts, lovers of old movies, and wine aficionados — who also happen to want to learn a little something about hearing aids — might find entertainment value in our themed approach. After all, hearing aid fitting is fun, so reading about it should be, too.

Although the book might have shreds of entertainment value, we also believe it provides timely, accurate, and cutting-edge information on many of the "best practices" needed to fit modern hearing aids. Included in the book are several prefitting, day-of-the-fitting, and follow-up procedures that must be properly completed in order to optimize patient satisfaction and ensure your business is successful. For these reasons, we think this book is a valuable addition to any professional library, as you are likely to find an informative tidbit or two on the use of speech-in-noise testing during the prefitting appointment, a succinct review of cutting-edge advanced hearing aid features, or how to administer self-reports of hearing aid outcome. Because most readers of this book are likely to just be getting started, it's important to instill the importance of conducting tests and completing clinical procedures that are supported by scientific principles. This book aims to provide that information in an easy-to-read format.

Lastly, this book has "accessibility." We have written this book knowing students and clinicians have nearly instant access to the Web. Today, you can be reading a book in one hand, surf the Internet with the other, and still drink your favorite morning beverage. We take advantage of this reality by listing many Web sites throughout this book. In every chapter, there are several sidebars that refer to Web sites where more detailed information, animations, or videos may be downloaded to further enhance learning.

Regardless of your background or training, we hope you enjoy reading our 12-chapter journey as much as we enjoyed writing it.

Brian Taylor, AuD
Holcombe, WI

H. Gustav Mueller, PhD
Ryder, ND

1

Basic Psychology of Hearing Loss in Adults

> *How country music and working with hearing-impaired adults are alike.*

Nearly every patient seeking your services exhibits some of the qualities outlined in this chapter. In order to provide the best care and service to your patients it is critical for you to understand, from the patient's perspective, why they are acting in such a way. This chapter will help you do this. Once you have read it, you will be more familiar with some of the behaviors associated with acquired hearing loss in adults. You also will have a better understanding of why hearing-impaired people have many of these behaviors and personality traits. Last, it will help you develop insight as to how you can interact with your patients in an understanding and upbeat manner—and of course, your hearing aid fitting will go more smoothly.

The Honky-Tonk Message

Many of you have probably been in Nashville, and if you're like us, it's hard not to stop by Tootsies, one of the top honky-tonks in the United States. Most all country and western ballads have a message, and here's a line from one of our favorites:

> *What drives you insane about me is the very thing keeping me from losing my mind.*

This phrase, taken from the perspective of a hearing care professional, simply means that our adult hearing-impaired patients sometimes have behaviors that are hard for us to understand. These often challenging behaviors and personality traits, when put in the context of a lifelong hearing impairment, are normal. The good news is you don't have to own a guitar, carry a tune, or even appreciate country and western music to understand the personality of the typical hearing-impaired adult.

For the person who experiences hearing difficulties, hearing loss is usually just the beginning of a series of social obstacles. In most cases, hearing loss is a communication disorder of gradual onset. This means that the hearing loss occurs slowly over many years. Typically, the hearing loss comes on so slowly that the individual is not even aware of the change as it occurs. In fact, there are some data to suggest that it takes the average person with hearing loss 7 to 10 years after they first notice the problem to come to an office for a hearing test. Unlike many other health problems, hearing loss is not physically noticeable, and it does not hurt. Usually, it is a workplace associate, spouse, friend, or other loved one who notices the hearing loss first. All of us know someone who has trouble with hearing conversations, especially when background noise is present. Many times we notice that they are having difficulties before they even admit they have a problem. As you will learn later in this chapter, this is completely normal behavior.

Developing a relationship with your hearing-impaired patient ultimately will increase your chance to successfully help this person do something about his communication deficit. In addition, his ability to adapt to using hearing aids may be enhanced as a result of your ability to diagnose his hearing loss and understand his personality traits associated with it. As a hearing care professional, you have an opportunity to have a profound and lasting influence on his life that goes beyond simply fitting him with hearing aids. We know that people successfully fitted with hearing aids have improved socialization, family life, and even increased income—more on all this later.

Understanding the Problem

As Waylon Jennings said in his 1993 song "Dirt," "Dirt is quiet, it don't make noise, it's fun to play in, especially for boys."

Unfortunately, much of the surroundings where we work and play is not as quiet as dirt. It is not easy to communicate and function comfortably in many of today's noisy listening environments even with normal hearing. Take a moment and think about the last time you were in a popular, crowded restaurant on a Saturday night: It takes a lot of concentration to follow the conversation of the person sitting next to you. It is even more difficult, sometimes impossible, to hear in these important situations when you have a hearing loss. It's no wonder people with hearing loss are withdrawn, embarrassed or agitated about this "hidden handicap."

Over 32 million Americans, adults as well as children, suffer some degree of hearing loss. The most common type is sensorineural hearing loss (predominantly cochlear etiology—more on this in Chapter 3). The encouraging fact is that people with this type of hearing loss can be helped with hearing aids. Given these facts, it might seem logical that adults with hearing loss readily seek treatment for it. Unfortunately, this is seldom the case as there is a strong stigma associated with adult hearing loss. Because hearing loss is so strongly related to old age, and aging is often not a positive attribute in Western culture, the stigma can be quite powerful. This stigma has been called the "Hearing Aid Effect" and it is present among both professionals and patients of all ages and all walks of life. Studies have shown that a substantial number of hearing-impaired patients refuse to wear hearing aids—even those with the latest modern digital technology—because they believe that hearing aids appear to make them look old or handicapped. As a professional you will encounter this stigma often. When you are interested in learning more about the detrimental effects of acquired untreated hearing loss and the stigma commonly associated with it check out this Web site: http://www.betterhearing.org

Audiologic Variables

There are some common ways to categorize the adult hearing-impaired population. Knowing something about these classifications, will help you appreciate some of the differences in behavior you may observe. It stands to reason that the more you know about these variables, and some of their associated behaviors, the more likely you will not take things personally when one of your patients appears to be acting out of the ordinary.

Late Versus Early Onset

Hearing loss can occur before or during the development of language, or after language has already developed. The dividing line between hearing loss of late and early onset is considered to be adolescence. Adults who have early onset hearing loss usually have come to incorporate the hearing loss into their personalities. Because the loss occurred at a younger age, the hearing loss becomes part of their identity. As a result, they have developed ways to cope with and manage hearing loss in their daily lives. The situation can be very different for adults who acquire hearing loss later in life. These individuals have developed a personally that does not include coping with a hearing

loss. They have jobs, families, and hobbies that have nothing to do with dealing with a hearing loss. When a hearing loss does occur it is normal for it to be a disorienting, even traumatic experience.

Gradual Versus Rapid

The vast majority of the patients that you will see will have a hearing loss that developed gradually over many years. Hearing loss that occurs rapidly due to an underlying medical condition, however, is considered the most disorienting. Rapid onset typically means that a person experiences a sudden change in hearing within a few weeks, or even within a few hours. They may go to bed with normal hearing, and wake up with a significant hearing loss. It is not unusual for adults experiencing a hearing loss of rapid onset to be in a "near panic" mode. Of course, your primary responsibility with any patient, but particularly those presenting to you with a hearing loss of rapid onset, is to refer them to a physician for a medical examination, prior to discussing any treatment options.

Common Behaviors Associated with Hearing Loss

It was Hank Williams who penned the line, "I bowed my head in grief and shame as I felt the teardrops start, but as the organ played, we stood there and prayed, just me and my broken heart."

You certainly don't have to be a down-on-your-luck songwriter to appreciate the fact that the grieving process can be a difficult ordeal for many patients with acquired hearing loss.

It is a commonly held belief that adults with acquired hearing loss of late onset go through Kübler-Ross's five stages of grief: denial, anger, bargaining, depression, and acceptance (Table 1–1). As a professional, you need to try to gain an understanding of which stage each patient falls into when he or she seeks your services. It is always a good idea to involve family members and other significant others as you guide patients through these five stages. When it comes to understanding the psychology of hearing loss, your main task is to be a tolerant and nonjudgmental listener, helping each patient adjust on their own terms to their acquired hearing loss.

Denial and anger are easy to observe in many patients ("I can hear just fine, my husband mumbles"). Bargaining frequently takes the form of comparing or devaluing ("Who cares that I can't hear?" "I can't hear, but at least I still have my health."). Depression can manifest itself in sudden changes of behavior. Finally, acceptance takes many forms, but it could simply mean that the patient is more accepting of your recommendations, is wearing his hearing aids more often, or has positive comments concerning hearing aid use. Although most hearing care professionals do not need to be experts on psychological issues surrounding hearing loss, some insights into how the five stages of grieving manifest themselves in daily practice will help you do a better job and make the task of working with some of these issues less stressful.

All of us would like to think of ourselves as leading healthy and productive lifestyles. Our self-esteem is strongly related to our health and general well-

Table 1–1. The Elisabeth Kübler Ross Five Psychological Stages of Grieving, Applied to Hearing Loss.

Stage	What the Patient Might Say
Denial	"I don't have a hearing problem; other people mumble. I hear everything I need to hear."
Anger	To their friends: "Are you purposely talking behind my back?" To the professional: "Are you sure you did the testing correctly?"
Bargaining	"Okay, maybe I just wasn't listening, I'll pay more attention." "Let's see if I'm still having problems next year."
Depression	"Maybe my family avoids me because of my hearing loss." "There are things I'll probably never hear again." "I'm getting old."
Acceptance	"My quality of life will probably improve with the use of hearing aids." "A lot of people my age have worse health problems than hearing loss."

being. For example, when someone first becomes aware they are missing out on conversation it is normal behavior to deny there is a problem. Acquiring a hearing loss goes against our perception of reality. It is not part of our own self-image to have a deficit like this. Think about how you felt the last time you were at a noisy social gathering and someone told a funny story, and you missed the punch line. Did you pretend you heard what was said and laugh like everyone else? Or, did you ask the person to repeat the part you missed? Most people just laugh and go along with the group, not wanting to draw attention to themselves, but probably consider it a somewhat uncomfortable situation. Now, think about the hearing-impaired person having to go through this many times a day. Imagine how they must feel. It's no wonder hearing loss is associated with emotions like embarrassment, frustration, and even anger.

It's easy to generalize and say that all hearing-impaired individuals have similar personality traits. This assumption is certainly false, however, given the nature of their impairment there are some commonalties among the adult hearing-aid population that are worthy of further discussion. Let's examine four common characteristics associated with adult hearing loss of gradual onset, and how you—the professional—may assist the individual in overcoming these negative self images. Not every hearing-impaired person exhibits all of these traits, but if you have a busy practice, chances are good that you will observe at least some of these on a daily basis. As we said earlier, country music and working with adults with hearing loss have some similarities. For each of the four characteristics discussed below we draw from the rich lyrical tradition of country music to illustrate our point.

TAKE FIVE:
Hands-On Exercise

Find out what it is like to have a hearing impairment. For an entire day wear earplugs. Go about your daily routine and make a record of your reactions and emotions surround-ing your temporary hearing loss. The next time you encounter a hearing-impaired person acting in a negative way, think about what it is like to live with a hearing loss every minute of the day. In a hundred words or so, on a separate sheet of paper, write about your experiences with a temporary hearing loss.

Denial

This ole boy stood up in the aisle
Said he'd been living a life of denial
And he cried as he talked about wasted years
I couldn't believe what I heard.

Kenny Chesney

When something bad happens to us, it is normal behavior to deny the problem exists. Denial has an important function: It allows us to recover from the shock of a painful or negative experience. For the person experiencing a hearing loss for the first time, or being told by a professional that they have a hearing loss for the first time, it is easy to simply ignore the problem. Fortunately, most patients do not strongly deny their hearing loss. They will acknowledge the existence of the problem, but the other behaviors stemming from the initial denial can cause a great deal of emotional pain and stress. Simply stated, ignoring the hearing loss often times leads to some of the other behaviors we'll talk about shortly.

Probably the single most common response that hearing care professionals hear from their patients, once the presence of hearing loss is explained is this emphatic question: "Is my hearing loss bad enough that I need hearing aids?" This question might show that the patient recognizes the presence of hearing loss but is trying to find a reason not to do anything about it. One of your greatest professional challenges will be to recognize when someone is in denial and not ready to acknowledge their hearing impairment. No amount of convincing, cajoling, or explaining will make the hearing-impaired patient solve the problem. Allowing a patient to accept his or her hearing loss and take the necessary steps to fix the problem is a skill that takes time and effort to develop.

Withdrawal and Avoidance

Please, say it's not too late,
So I can stop while there's still time,
An' avoid me some small bit of ache.

Dwight Yoakam

The easiest way to deal with the psychological hurt of hearing loss is simply not to expose ourselves to situations in which we continue to be vulnerable. The hearing-impaired person, therefore, might begin to withdraw from society, even situations that previously may have been the focal point of his social interaction. For example, an individual who has been an active, participating lodge or club member may find it increasingly difficult to communicate at meetings. People with hearing loss gradually begin to attend meetings less frequently, eventually not at all.

As you begin your case history with a patient, note that there generally is a direct correlation between the length of time the individual has withdrawn from social situations and the length of time the person has noticed a hearing loss. Unfortunately, the hearing-impaired individual does not always associate this withdrawal to their hearing problem, but often to other external influences. This individual may even develop a false sense of wanting to be alone.

As the hearing-impaired person becomes more and more withdrawn from the world around him he begins to avoid situations he once loved to enjoyed. Unable to hear and being isolated is a terribly lonely way to live. The longer people with hearing loss avoid seeking professional help, the more they become entrenched with a hearing loss that rules their life. Once people who have lived with hearing loss for many years finally make the choice to seek help from you it is common for them to show feelings of anger and hostility.

Hostility and Anger

I know that sometimes my temper
*   ain't so good*
Cause things haven't worked out the way
*   we thought they would*
But let's don't give in to our doubts and
*   our fears*

*Let's try to put an end to our anger and
tears.*

Mel McDaniel

Family members often notice personality changes in the hearing impaired individual. Family members may comment that this person is "grouchy," or has become "difficult to live with." Hostility develops. This is normal behavior for some adults with acquired hearing loss.

The hearing-impaired person may become less tolerant of others as a result of hearing these kinds of comments over and over again. Imagine you have a hearing problem. Every time you have to ask someone to repeat themselves, it's a reminder to you that you have a hearing loss. Eventually, you become resentful and angry at others over your own need to have things repeated. You already know you have a hearing problem and you don't want to be constantly reminded of it. This is an emotionally painful experience. To compound the problem, your family and friends feel you are being stubborn and are resistance to help. This sets up a vicious cycle of events in which your family and friends become angry at you because they think you are being stubborn, and you are angry with them because they keep reminding you about your "problem." This cycle of anger and hostility can be wearing on relationships, and has been known to end some.

TIPS and TRICKS: Case Study

Mrs. Johnson, age 85, has just ordered a pair of $6,000 hearing aids. She was brought to the office by a family member. You are told by the family that Mrs. Johnson is in the early stages of Alzheimer disease. Although she seems a little quiet, Mrs. Johnson is a very nice lady. After a complete evaluation, it has been determined that she is a good candidate for hearing aids. Mrs. Johnson easily agrees with your recommendations and orders a pair of $6,000 hearing aids that are very appropriate for her hearing loss. A few days later, you get a call from Mrs. Johnson daughter, who tells you Mrs. Johnson has lost all the information you have given her, including the bill of sale/contract for the hearing aids. The family is upset because Mrs. Johnson already has an older pair of hearing aids, and wants to know why she needs new ones. The family wants to cancel the order, even though they admit Mrs. Johnson really does need new hearing aids.

After you have patiently explained the results and agreed to send them a report, the family reschedules an appointment for a hearing aid fitting in two weeks.

The very next day Mrs. Johnson shows up with her daughter unannounced in the office demanding to be seen that very day for hearing aids. The office manager tries to schedule an appointment with you, but you are busy. The patient gets even more angry and decides to cancel her order for the second time.

What common behaviors associated with acquired hearing loss are being exhibited in this case study? What if anything could you do differently to prevent this from occurring?

Selfishness and Suspicion

I'd like to take away the suspicion that I know clouds your world at times. By giving you some faith to hold on to, honey whenever your hand is not in mine.

Conway Twitty

Living with someone who refuses to get the necessary help for his hearing impairment is a challenge. Because the development of hearing loss typically is a slow process, getting the courage to even make an appointment to get a hearing test is often times a terrifying experience. The hearing-impaired person's unwillingness to help himself may be seen as a selfish act. Many persons with hearing loss come to expect all their daily interactions with others to be arranged around their hearing loss. This is, no doubt, a selfish act. Unable to trust his own ability to hear and understand what is being said the hearing-impaired person may become suspicious of others. The individual who is suspicious of others may believe that people are talking about him. Because of his inability to hear conversations clearly, this person finds it harder to depend on information as accurate. The suspicious hearing-impaired person who has lived with slowly degenerating hearing is slow to develop trust.

The Two Types of Counseling

"Counseling" is the type of word that means different things to different people. When it comes to dispensing hearing aids, there are really two different types of counseling. There are many books devoted to both types of counseling, some of which are listed at the end of this chapter.

Informational counseling provides the patient with all the relevant information needed to understand the type and degree of hearing loss as well as how to manage it. When you are explaining test results or offering a hearing aid recommendation, that is informational counseling. Many of us are most comfortable with this type of counseling, and often use this counseling, approach too much, at the expense of more appropriate counseling.

TIPS and TRICKS: Effective Informational Counseling

You probably have realized by now that you will be working with a lot of elderly people, many of whom may have some trouble remembering things. Well, it's not just the elderly who have memory trouble. It has been documented that patients forget between 40 to 80% of what we tell them.

Fortunately, there are some things you can do to help patients remember more of what we say. You need to speak clearly and use relatively simple sentences. Also, make sure you present information in a relaxed manner. If you are nervous and uptight, chances are your patient will be as well. Last, you also should supplement your verbal presentation with written or graphic material. Supplying the patient with some simple written explanations to take home with them can be very helpful for their use after they leave your office, and they start to think of questions.

Personal adjustment counseling is the process of guiding the patient and family in coping with the emotional impact of hearing loss. Personal adjustment counseling requires that the hearing care provider and the patient form a relationship focused on trust. Rather than taking the point of view that the problem can be solved, personal adjustment counseling requires the hearing care provider to look at the patient in a holistic manner. The cornerstone of this relationship-centered approach is your ability to see the patient's perspective. By creating a dialogue based on mutual trust, rather than being the expert, professionals can facilitate the acceptance process. This approach implies that you trust the patient's ability to articulate their problem, then determine their goals and how they want to reach them.

Given the fact that there are many emotional issues surrounding hearing loss, we will spend some time on strategies geared to help you with personal adjustment counseling.

Practical Counseling Strategies

Because hearing loss manifests itself in so many negative behaviors and emotions it is absolutely critical to your success as a professional to try to gain a better understanding of these behaviors and their interactions. Trying to understand the emotional consequences of hearing loss requires a lifetime of study and experience. It is beyond the scope of this text to delve into detail; nevertheless, let your journey begin now. Here are a few events that occur every day in hearing aid dispensing offices around the country.

Because so many people with hearing loss experience feelings of denial, it is a profound step for them to even be in your office for a hearing test. Realize that it may be a really big deal for this person to acknowledge that they might have a problem. Although these patients might react to you in a hostile or suspicious manner, it is your professional duty to first acknowledge the courage it took this person to arrive at your doorstep.

A patient must first accept ownership of the office visit before disclosing his communication difficulties. You probably have already encountered patients who are accompanied by a spouse at the initial consultation. Many times these patients will say that their spouse made them come in to see you for the hearing test. This patient does not own the visit. Ownership of the visit refers to the fact that the patient acknowledges he has a problem and is willing to talk about it. Until ownership of the visit occurs, it will be difficult for you to assess the impact a potential hearing loss has on this person. As a professional you must ask open-ended questions that allow the patient to take ownership. For example, a patient will not accept your recommendation to buy hearing aids until he believes he has been profoundly understood. This is the very reason why understanding the emotional consequences are so important. After a patient has taken ownership of the office visit, the next step is to connect with this patient on an emotional level. This requires two things on your part:

1. Courage. You must be courageous enough to ask the patient thought provoking, open-ended questions, and

2. Curiosity. You must be curious enough about the patient's life

experiences to listen intently to his answers. When patients feel emotionally connected to you, they are more likely to accept your recommendation of better hearing.

For the most part, hearing aids are effective, but some of the emotional consequences of hearing loss will still remain. Even after you have successfully fit someone with hearing aids, they still may struggle from time to time with the emotional consequences of the hearing loss. One of your duties as a professional is to establish long lasting relationships with your patients who wear hearing aids. No hearing aid, no matter how sophisticated, will completely solve all the difficulties associated with communicating in various environments. You must be there when called upon by your patients to offer emotional support and guidance.

TIPS and TRICKS: Asking Good Questions

One of the hallmarks of a successful clinician is the ability to ask good, open-ended questions. Here are six questions you should consider asking every new hearing aid patient you see. Remember, once you have asked the question, you need to sit back and quietly listen to the response.

- Tell me what brought you into the office.
- How long have you been noticing difficulty with communication?
- Do other people notice you are having difficulty with communication?
- Tell me about the areas you are having difficulty with communication.
- Would you be willing to accept help or assistance with the difficulties you are having?
- On a scale of 1 to 10, 1 being I don't need help and 10 being I need help right away, how would you rate your ability to communicate?

TAKE FIVE: Hearing Ability and Purchase Decision

Recently published research from audiologist Catherine Palmer and colleagues reveals that there is a direct relationship between the patient's rating of his or her hearing ability (on a 1–10 scale, "1" being the worst) and his or her subsequent decision to purchase hearing aids. This also can be used in conjunction with the 1–10 scale we discussed of "Do I need help?". The following chart is the probability of hearing aid purchase related to patient rating of hearing ability, developed using the data of Palmer and colleagues:

Rating (1–10)	Probability of Purchase
1	98%
2	96%
3	92%
4	83%
5	73%
6	58%
7	37%
8	20%
9	10%
10	6%

Motivational Interviewing

Professionals working with individuals with hearing loss must be aware of both the audiologic and psychological variables associated with hearing loss. When working with hearing impaired people it is important to establish a dialogue that invites information about social and emotional nature of the hearing loss. Part of the conversation you have with any patient not only needs to include the time of onset and degree of hearing loss, but also how the patient might be feeling about the onset of hearing loss. In practical terms this means professionals must relinquish control of the visit, always attempting to dispense advice, and allow the patient to take ownership of their hearing loss.

One tactic that has been proven to successfully address the psychological nature of acquired hearing and allow the patient to take ownership of the hearing loss is called Motivational Interviewing. As discussed by Michael Harvey, Ph.D. in numerous articles, there are four components of motivational interviewing that professionals can use when conducting an initial interview or case history with a patient.

1. **Problem Recognition**—This is the initial phase of the interview process in which the patient is able to recognize a hearing problem. A question you would typically ask the patient during this problem recognition phase would be: "Do you think you have a hearing loss?"
2. **Elicit Expression of Concern** —During this phase of the interview, the professional is attempting to generate any responses that show the patient is feeling upset or concerned about their hearing loss. One example of a question designed to elicit expressions of concern would be: "What worries you the most about your hearing loss?"
3. **Intention to Change**—This is the part in which the professional is trying to understand if the patient is ready to accept help for their hearing problems. For example, you could ask a patient during this phase, "What makes you think you actually need to obtain hearing aids now?"
4. **Self-Efficacy**—This is the part of the interview when you are determining if the patient has the ability to make a long term commitment to change. In other words, you could ask the patient during this phase, "What is keeping you from getting help?"

Getting From Point A to Point B

Imagine a man walks into your office and says he wants to discuss hearing aids with you. You can tell from his body language and vocal inflections that he is full of fear and apprehension. He appears to be a little hostile. He even sounds agitated. Indeed, it has taken many years of consternation to get the courage for him to even get into his car and drive to your office. It is monumental that this man is now speaking with you face to face.

This person proceeds to tell you he has suffered with hearing loss for more than 10 years. He knows he needs hearing aids, but they cost too much. He

---

TAKE FIVE: The Many Shapes of Hearing Impairment

The Ida Institute has created a handy set of tools to help clinicians more effectively persuade their patients to take action on their hearing impairment. The tools are referred to as the "Line," the "Box," and the "Circle." The "Circle" describes the different stages of behavior a patient with hearing loss goes through as they contemplate getting help or guidance from professional. These stages are very similar to the Kubler-Ross stages we described earlier in this chapter.

The "Box" and "Line" are used to help make the patient aware of his or her positive and negative thoughts regarding hearing loss, and allows the patient to assess their motivation for receiving help. To obtain your own pencil and paper version of these tools, go to http://www.idainstitute.com

---

also has several friends, relatives, and acquaintances all of whom have spent thousands of dollars on devices that sit in the drawer. He doesn't want to waste his money. He tells you he's been to every office in the area shopping around. He wants to know what makes your product different. He refuses to fill out any preliminary paperwork. He just wants a few minutes of your time. You assume from his mannerisms that he is beyond help. He's just another angry, agitated consumer who is not motivated to get the necessary help he needs. What can we do to reverse this trend?

Innovative hearing aid technology breakthroughs simply will not address the underlying emotional issues that have plagued this gentleman for the better part of a generation. Addressing this patient's emotional needs falls squarely on the shoulders of the hearing care professional. Indeed, this task must be accomplished before any remediation of the hearing loss can occur. Using information covered in this section, here are five practical pointers to help you better manage these challenging situations.

1. Shifting to a Learning Stance

Almost without exception, hearing care professionals want to tell, educate, and advise the patient. This thought process has been ingrained in us from the beginning stages of our professional education. We are the "professional," therefore, we have all the answers. We are trained to deliver a technical message. We have to ask ourselves, is our message being heard? Unfortunately, all too often this mindset creates a passive and disconnected patient. Have you noticed that when you are able to tell someone your story, and that person listens without judgment, you feel that you have been heard on a deeper level? These circumstances are the bonds of intimacy and often they are the missing link in our practice.

As a helping professional, the first step is addressing the emotional needs of the patient. This requires a shift from being a message deliverer to one of learning all you can about the emotional needs of the individual in front of you. Indeed, our message of improved communication will never be embraced until the patient's emotional needs have been addressed. Addressing the emotional needs of any patient requires we shift to a Learning Stance.

In order for this patient to open up to you, it is critical for you to be yourself. Being yourself means to be authentic. Authenticity requires that you are sincere about your actions. It's important for you to get at the heart of what brought the patient into your clinic after many years of anger, denial, and frustration.

The case history is the ideal time to adapt this Learning Stance. Shifting from certainty to curiosity, from debate to exploration, enables you to fully engage the patient. When you are able to emotionally connect with the patient you can begin to problem-solve together.

2. Establishing a Flow of Communication from Patient to Professional

Once you have tapped into the emotional needs, a flow of communication can take place between you and the patient with the flow of communication going from the patient to you. All clinicians have experienced the following: You are taking the case history on a reluctant patient who has been dragged to your office by a concerned loved one. Initially, this patient does not want to discuss a hearing deficit. However, as you doggedly continue to ask questions you stumble upon one that triggers an emotional response. This patient starts to open up, and talk about the years of frustration and anger associated with the hearing loss. Too often, we interrupt this flow of communication to complete

the hearing test. This behavior on our part is logical. We have been trained to do this. It is our comfort zone to complete the hearing test during the initial stages of the visit. Next time you find yourself in this situation resist all temptation to do the test. Sit back, take a deep breath, pause, and ask the patient a thoughtful question about how they're feeling.

Establishing a flow of communication from the patient to you allows the professional to more deeply explore the emotional consequences of the hearing loss of the person sitting knee-to-knee with you. It is this flow of communication that helps bond you to your patient, and helps define your role as a true "helping professional." The flow of communication allows you to transition from the case history to the hearing test. In most cases you know you have established a strong flow of communication when you have completed the needs assessment part of the appointment before placing the earphones on the patient.

3. Shifting from a Learning Stance to a Teaching Stance

Once the needs assessment and hearing test are completed, you can shift from a Learning Stance to a Teaching Stance. One of the hallmarks of any exceptional teacher is an ability to communicate in language everyone can understand. This means adapting your message to the level of your audience. As helping professionals we all are teachers on some level. After the hearing test we typically explain the results of the exam to the patient. This is the first of many opportunities to start teaching your patient the importance of improved hearing.

All of us have had memorable teachers. They are motivating and inspiring. We often connect with them on an emotional level. The explanation of results phase of your appointment with the patient is the ideal time to strive to be a memorable teacher. The use of colorful metaphors and visual props to describe the hearing loss are two possible ways to become more memorable and effective. Instead of giving a long explanation of the importance of bilateral hearing, give the patient a demonstration of why two ears are better than one.

The part of the appointment customarily reserved for you to explain the test results is an ideal time to adapt a Teaching Stance. Challenge yourself to come up with metaphors and props describing the hearing loss and effectiveness of amplification.

4. The Power of an Informed Buying Decision

The consequence of adapting a teaching stance is that it leads directly to an informed buying decision. This requires navigating the patient through the vast array of technology choices. This is a daunting task. The number of amplification options is truly mind numbing, and it is easy to overwhelm the patient with too many choices. When it comes to making a buying decision, customers want a small number of choices.

5. The Assumptive Conclusion

The power of the informed decision cannot be underestimated. The informed decision leads directly to an assump-

tive consequence of the patient accepting your recommendation. If you have first adapted a learning stance, then transitioned to a teaching stance and followed that with one or two thoughtful choices, the natural culmination in this series of events is the assumptive conclusion. Too often, the hearing care professional focuses on trying to talk the patient into accepting his recommendations for hearing aids.

Once the patient feels they have been profoundly heard, only then can you deliver your message of better hearing through amplification. The patient will embrace your message of hope and you can allow them to make an informed decision. Simply stated, the reluctant patient does not have the language of healing. If they did they would walk in and say, "I need hearing aids." To make this point further; we go to see counselors when we are struggling with major life issues. Why would we pay a stranger several hundred dollars an hour over a period of weeks or months to help us solve our most personal problems? The answer is that we do not possess the language that it takes for us to deal effectively with our own issues. We need to be guided in our thinking and self-discovery. That is exactly what must happen in the hearing professional's office. Before the patient will embrace our message we must address the emotional needs of this person. We must first listen to the feelings behind the words, and then acknowledge the feelings. We cannot assume we know what this patient is feeling. Even though we have observed these emotions hundreds of times in countless other patients, we must sit back and allow this patient to express their feelings, and listen for the feelings behind the words. As the lyrics go:

It makes no sense to waste these words and twenty-five cents on a losing game.

In Closing

The purpose of this chapter was to provide you with insights about how the typical adult with acquired hearing loss "ticks." Many hearing care professionals believe that effective counseling skills, like the ones mentioned here, take a lifetime to master. Taking the time to learn the psychological underpinnings of acquired adult hearing loss will allow you not only to take better care of your patients, but to work with less stress. After all, remember what we learned at the honky-tonk:

What might be driving you insane about your patient is probably keeping them from going insane.

Fortunately, with a better understanding of this psychological process, life can be a little easier for both of you. Now you know how country music and the adult with hearing loss are alike.

2

Acoustics at the Speed of Sound

How Acoustics and Old War Movies Are Alike

This is the end—beautiful friend
This is the end—my only friend
No safety, no surprise—the end
Opening Scene, *Apocalypse Now*, The Doors

Don't be too alarmed by our opening quote—We just wanted to get your attention, as this is an area that requires some concentration. It's really not the end, but rather the beginning of some interesting areas of physics, and we'll tell you how *Apocalypse Now* and other old war movies fit in shortly.

Understanding how humans hear is a complex subject involving the fields of physiology, psychology, and acoustics. In this chapter, we focus on the acoustics of hearing (the branch of physics pertaining to sound). Before you fit your first pair of hearing aids you will need to acquire a basic understanding of the acoustical properties of sound and become familiar with some basic terms and concepts.

For many who are just beginning to dispense hearing aids, learning the essential physics underlying the dynamics of sound can be a daunting, almost terrifying challenge. We are here to say that you cannot allow the science to get the best of you.

As Colonel Kurtz in the epic war movie Apocalypse Now *said, "If you cannot make a friend of mortal terror, then it is an enemy to be feared."*

That might sound a little ominous, and unfortunately our experiences tell us that there are more than a few students out there who have not made acoustics their friend. But let's change that!

The basic acoustics of fitting hearing aids need to be fully embraced if you are to be a successful professional. This chapter presents the essential information in an uncomplicated and painless manner. We begin our epic journey through the maze of acoustics.

The Traveling Sound Wave

Like a platoon heading into battle there is no randomness to the sound wave. Both the platoon and the sound wave travel in lock step, following the orders of their originator.

Sound is part of our everyday sensory experience. The basis for understanding sound and hearing is the physics of waves. Sound is a wave that is created by vibrating objects and then propagated through a medium from one location to another.

To begin, let's consider the primordial question that you no doubt have heard before, "If a tree falls in the forest, and there is no one there to hear it, does it make a sound?" This question is not just a rhetorical one but a query regarding the nature of basic acoustics. Acoustics is that branch of physics pertaining to sound. As you will soon discover, the answer to the "falling tree" question can be found in the four elements required for sound to "take place."

What is a Wave

A wave may be described as a force or disturbance that travels through a medium transporting energy from one place to another. The medium is simply the material through which the disturbance moves and can be thought of as a series of interacting particles. For example, when our "tree in the forest" falls, a disturbance is created. Neighboring trees are shaken or moved. The ground quakes and the surrounding air vibrates, as each displaced particle acts to displace an adjacent particle; subsequently, this disturbance will travel through the entire forest. As the disturbance moves from tree to tree, along the ground and through the air, the energy that was originally introduced by the falling tree is transported along each medium from one location to another. The bigger the tree and the harder it falls, the larger the disturbance. The larger the disturbance, the greater the

impact it will have. However, independent of the impact our falling tree has no audience, and is it actually *sound* as no human ear is available to hear it?

Four Critical Elements

By definition, sound is only considered to be sound when each of these four very important elements are in place:

1. An Energy Source (falling tree, electrical current, air from the lungs, a striking hammer),
2. A Vibrating Body (ground, diaphragm of a speaker, vocal chords, a tuning fork, or a violin string),
3. A Medium (air, solid, liquid or gas), and
4. A Receiver (human ear).

In our earlier question about the tree, there is no Element #4, and if we subscribe to this definition, then the sound was never heard, and logically if sound is not heard then it cannot be considered sound. You might guess of course, that even if no humans were present, there probably were a few animals around the forest to hear the sound. So, we can assume a sound was produced. Now, an engineer might say that if he set up a sound level recording device in the forest and it recorded sound, then there was sound. We'll let you take up that discussion with your engineer friends over a late night cup of coffee.

To actually see how the four elements we have discussed interact to create sound, go to this Web site: http://www.physicsclassroom.com/Class/sound/soundtoc.html

You can also refer to this Web site for animations and graphic displays of the concepts reviewed in this chapter.

Compression and Rarefaction

This is war, Peacock. Casualties are inevitable. You can't make an omelet without breaking some eggs, every cook will tell you that.

Colonel Mustard (played by
Martin Mull), *Clue* (1985)

Now it's time to start breaking some eggs and getting into the knitty gritty of physics. Sound pressure waves travel through a medium displacing particles, pushing and bumping and moving each other, coming together in tight groups, and then dispersing in a series of what is known as compressions (or condensations) and rarefactions. When the molecules are close together you have compressions and when they spread apart it is called rarefaction.

One completed cycle of a single condensation and rarefaction occurring over one second in time can be drawn as a sine wave as shown in Figure 2–1, and expressed as 1 cycle per second (cps) or 1 Hz. We always measure pitch or frequency in cycles per second, so when you see "Hz," think cycles per second.

Like dB, the term Hertz is for both singular and plural—you don't say dBs or Hertzs! The latter term is named after the German physicist Heinrich Rudolf Hertz, who made important scientific contributions to electromagnetism. The name was established in the 1930s and replaced "cps" in most areas of audiology in the 1960s. Take a close look at Figure 2–2. When the sound wave is in the condensation mode the air molecules are densely packed together, and when they are in the rarefaction mode, the air molecules are farther apart from each other.

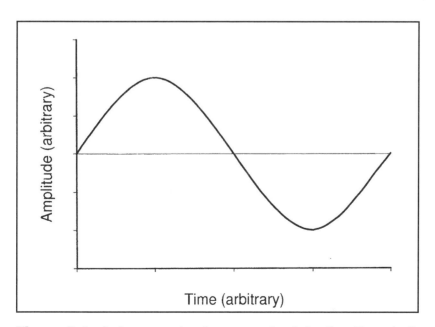

Figure 2–1. A sine wave showing one cycle of vibration. From *Audiology: Science to Practice* by Steven Kramer. Copyright © 2008, Plural Publishing Inc. All rights reserved. Used with permission, p. 40.

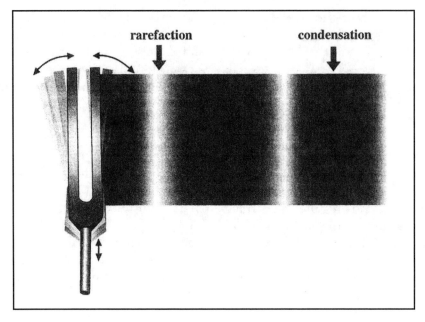

Figure 2–2. A vibrating tuning fork illustrates alternating areas of rarefaction and condensation (compression) of air molecules. From *Audiology: Science to Practice* by Steven Kramer. Copyright © 2008, Plural Publishing Inc. All rights reserved. Used with permission, p. 37.

Phase

When discussing condensation and rarefaction patterns of sound waves the term phase is bound to come up. *Starting phase* refers to where the wave's cycle of vibration begins. Phase is expressed in degrees relative to the angle around a circle. The waveform shown in Figure 2–1 starts at zero degrees. Waveforms can begin at any point and go in the direction of condensation or rarefaction. Another important point to remember about phase is that our ears are not sensitive to the starting point of a sound wave. However, when two or more sounds interact with each other phase can have an impact on how the ear hears them. This concept is commonly used in modern hearing aids to reduce that annoying whistling sound called feedback—we discuss feedback reduction using phase cancellation in Chapter 8. Figure 2–3 illustrates the concept. In this example, two tones of the same frequency have opposite starting phases. In other words, they are 180° out of phase with each other. Notice that no sound is generated because the two waves cancel themselves out.

Also, it's important to remember that sound waves travel in expanding spherical patterns in all directions, and depending on the medium, at different speeds.

When Lightning Strikes

As a child, you may have played the game of guessing how far away the lightning is striking in a thunderstorm,

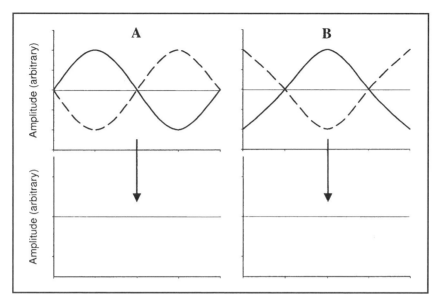

Figure 2–3. An example of how two pure tones of the same frequency that are 180° out of phase from each other will cancel each other out. In (**A**) the solid line represents a sound with a 0° starting point and the dashed line represents a sound with a staring phase of 180°. In (**B**) the solid line represents a sound with 270° starting phase, and the dashed line represents a sound with a 90° starting phase. From *Audiology: Science to Practice* by Steven Kramer. Copyright © 2008, Plural Publishing Inc. All rights reserved. Used with permission, p. 45.

but counting the seconds between the *sight* of the lightning and the *sound* of the thunder (the two events occur at the same time). If you only count to one, you might be in trouble, and here is why: The speed of sound through average air is 700 miles per hour (1,100 feet per second or 340 meters per second). The denser the medium, the faster the sound will travel. Sound travels four times faster through water, and 14 times faster through steel. So, if we do some simple math, we know that if you're standing outside on an average day (not underwater) and you count to five after the lightning (before you hear thunder), the lightning strike is about one mile away (5,500 feet).

TAKE FIVE: Careful Listening

Think of a time when you heard a familiar sound farther away than you normally would hear it. What was the sound? Low pitch? High pitch? A train, a coyote, a bell ringing, people talking? What was the listening condition? A summer night? A winter day? Across a lake? Believe it or not, the air temperature and humidity level play a significant role in the sounds that you hear.

Reflection and Absorption

Two key factors affect how sound eventually reaches the ear, reflection and absorption. Both of these are important regarding hearing aid benefit and how you counsel your patients regarding hearing aid use.

Reflection

Reflection of sound waves off of surfaces can lead to one of two phenomena—an echo or a reverberation. While sounding similar, these events can be viewed separately.

Reverberation

A noticeable reverberation often occurs in a small room with height, width, and length dimensions of approximately 17 meters or less. Perhaps you have observed reverberations when talking in an empty room or honking the horn while driving through a highway tunnel or underpass. These reverberations can mask other sounds, especially those having higher frequencies. In auditoriums and concert halls, reverberations occasionally occur and can lead to a displeasing garbling of a sound or music. Reflection of sound waves in auditoriums and concert halls, or even in your own home, however, do not always lead to displeasing results, especially if the reflections are controlled by being *purposefully built into the design.* Smooth walls have a tendency to direct sound waves in a specific direction. Rough walls tend to diffuse sound, reflecting it in a variety of directions. For this reason, auditorium and concert hall designers prefer construction materials that are rough rather than smooth.

In the field of audiology, many of the leading universities have large rooms constructed in their research laboratories called "anechoic chambers." These rooms are essentially free of any reverberation. Although this type of room is good for acoustic research, the absence of reverberation makes speech and especially music sound unusual.

TIPS and TRICKS:
Testing Hearing Aids

As you might guess, the performance of hearing aids easily is affected by reflections and reverberation. For this reason, when standard hearing aid testing is conducted by the manufacturer, it is performed in a "test box," which is mostly anechoic. Conducting quality control by testing hearing aids in a test box will be part of your test protocol too!

Echoes

Reflection of sound waves also leads to echoes. Echoes are different from reverberations. Echoes are reflected sound, heard later enough than the original sound to be perceived separately. Echoes typically are heard when the reflected sound reaches the ear more than a tenth of a second after the original sound was produced. An acoustically corrected room may, *by design,* eliminate these echoes and the loss of intelligibility they cause.

Echoes occur any time sound travels and bounces off a surface. That means that echoes can occur virtually anywhere. Probably the most common place to hear the best echoes is inside a large train station. Large train stations have hard reflective surfaces, and there is a lot of noise from the trains and crowds of people. Granted, there are a lot more train stations in Europe than North America, but next time you are inside one, pay attention to the great echoes you are hearing. Many small town U.S. train stations have been turned into microbreweries or restaurants, but yes, the echoes remain and often make communication difficult.

Absorption

Absorption is the opposite of reflection. Certain materials can absorb sound: rubber, cork, and acoustic tiles, for example. Sound-absorbing materials have high absorption coefficients. Soft, pliable items such as draperies, upholstered furniture, and carpeting help absorb sound and improve the listening environment for hearing-impaired people who experience more auditory distortion in the presence of reflection or reverberation than those of us with normal hearing. The absorption of sound is greater in warm rather than in cold, and in moist conditions rather than dry. Knowing which materials absorb sound and which reflect it is very important in acoustical engineering projects, such as the design of concert halls built to minimize unwanted effects.

TAKE FIVE: A Busted Myth about Echoes

There is an urban legend that says a duck's quack doesn't echo. No one knows where this myth got started; perhaps it's related to the relatively short duration of a quack. After reading this chapter, you should know enough about the physics of sound to quickly disprove this bit of folklore. If you're still not convinced that a duck's quack echoes, the Discovery Channel's Mythbusters bust the myth on Episode 8 in 2003.

Diffraction and Refraction

Like any wave, a sound wave doesn't just *stop* when it reaches the end of the medium or when it encounters an obstacle in its path. Rather, a sound wave will undergo certain behaviors when it encounters the end of the medium or an obstacle.

Sound Diffraction

The diffraction of sound involves a directional "about-face" of waves as they pass through an opening or around a barrier in any medium. The wavelength of a wave is the distance that a disturbance travels along the medium in one complete wave cycle. The amount of diffraction (the sharpness of the change in direction) increases with increasing wavelength (low-pitched sounds) and decreases with decreasing wavelength (high-pitched sounds). In fact, when the wavelength of the waves is smaller than the obstacle or opening, no noticeable diffraction occurs.

Diffraction is a commonly observed phenomenon. In our homes, sound literally bends around corners or slips through door openings allowing us to hear other voices from other rooms. In nature, owls communicate across long distances because their low-pitched long-wavelength hoots are able to diffract around forest trees and carry farther than the high-pitched short-wavelength tweets of songbirds. (Low-pitched sounds always carry farther and are more bendable than high-pitched sounds.)

Sound Refraction

Refraction involves a change in the direction of waves as they pass from one medium to another. Refraction is accompanied by a change in speed and wavelength (frequency) of the waves. Likewise, if there is a change in the medium (and its properties), the speed of the waves is changed.

Refraction of sound waves is most evident in situations in which the sound wave passes through a medium with gradually varying properties. For example, sound waves commonly refract when traveling over water. Since water has a moderating effect on the temperature of air, the air directly above the water tends to be cooler than the air far above the water. As sound waves travel more slowly in cooler air than they do in warmer air, that portion of the wavefront directly above the water is slowed down, while the portion of the wavefronts far above the water speeds ahead. Subsequently, the direction of the wave changes, refracting downward toward the water.

More on Reverberation

It is well to dream of glorious war in a snug armchair at home, but it is a very different thing to see it first hand.

Narrator (Michael Hordern)
Barry Lyndon (1975)

Now that we've introduced several terms regarding sound transmission, let's talk about some real-world issues regarding reverberation—how you will "see it firsthand" when you are dispensing hearing aids. *Reverberation* is a term with real-world importance, and one that you will spend a lot of time discussing with your hearing aid users. As you begin to fit hearing aids you will see first hand how reverberation can affect hearing aid performance and benefit. Therefore, as they suggest in the movie *Barry Lyndon*, it might be a good idea to get off your armchair and spend some time learning about reverberation. In practical terms, it's the echo you hear when you talk in a large room. Of course, it's much more complicated than that. Sound is reflected and absorbed by the walls, ceiling, and floor. You can think of reverberation as the combined effects of reflection, absorption, diffraction, and retraction. The amount of reverberation is largely a byproduct of the type of material found on the room surfaces, and the distance the sound has to travel to be heard by the listener.

There are actually two types of reverberation; early and late. Early reverberation is the sound that reaches the listener after a small number of reflections, and it actually enhances comprehension when listening with two ears. On the other hand, late reverberation, which is the sound reaching the listener after several reflections, has many negative effects. Late reverberation often sounds like noise and it interferes with comprehension, even with hearing aids in many cases.

One aspect of reverberation that you frequently will discuss with your hearing aid patients is the difference between the "near listening field" and

TIPS and TRICKS: Directional Microphones

As you'll learn in Chapter 8, directional microphone technology works very well with hearing aids, and can significantly improve the signal to noise ratio. **BUT**, when the listener is listening in background noise in a reverberant room and in the "late reverberation" area, the benefits of directional technology are significantly reduced. Listening in a place of worship is a typical example.

the "far listening field," as illustrated in Figure 2–4. To optimize the signal to noise ratio, we want our hearing aid users to be in the "near field." The listener is in the near field when the direct sound from the talker is more intense than the reflected sounds. In the far field, the reflected sounds are equal to or greater than the direct sound path from the talker. The distance that determines the near field varies as a function of the reverberation of the room, in a highly reverberant room it could be six feet or less.

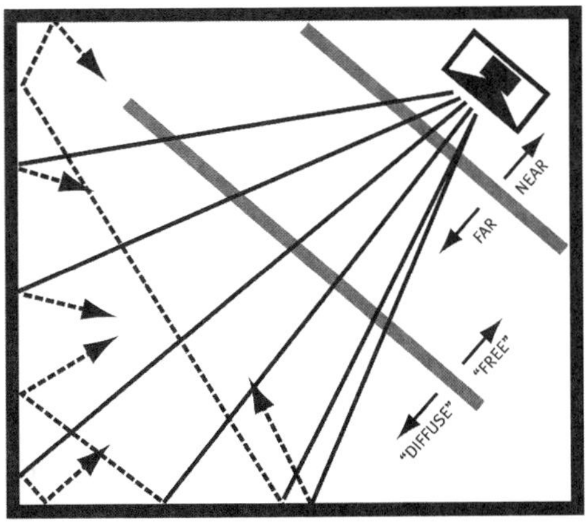

TAKE FIVE

Hearing scientist Dr. Arthur Boothroyd has put together an effective classroom reverberation computer simulation. You can download this program by going to http://www.ArthurBoothroyd.com and clicking on the Files Download link.

Frequency

As you already know, nearly all objects, whether hit, struck, strummed, or somehow disturbed, will vibrate. If you drop a pencil on the floor, it will begin to vibrate. If you pluck a guitar string, it will begin to vibrate. If you blow over the top of a pop bottle, the air inside will vibrate. When each of these objects vibrates, they tend to vibrate at a particular frequency or a set of frequencies. The frequency of a disturbance refers to how often the particles of the medium vibrate when a sound wave passes through the medium.

The frequency or frequencies, at which an object tends to vibrate when hit, struck, strummed, or somehow disturbed is known as the natural frequency of the object. If the size or

Figure 2–4. Near versus far sound field in reference to the loud speaker in the top right corner. The dotted lines illustrate the path of reflected sound. Notice that in the "diffuse field," reflected sound is essentially equal to direct sand. Modified from Hirsch, *The Measurement of Hearing*, 1952, McGraw-Hill Co., out of print.

amplitude of the vibration is large enough, and if the natural frequency is within the range of human hearing (20 to 20,000 Hz), then the object will produce sound waves that can be interpreted by the human ear. Any sound with a frequency below the audible range of human hearing (i.e., less than 20 Hz) is known as an infrasound and any sound with a frequency above the audible range of hearing (i.e., more than 20,000 Hz) is known as an ultrasound.

All objects have a natural frequency or set of frequencies at which they vibrate. Some objects tend to vibrate at a single frequency and they are often said to produce a pure tone. A flute tends to vibrate at a single frequency, and in the hands of a trained flutist, it will produce a very pure tone (e.g., 200 Hz). Figure 2–5 shows two pure tones with two difference frequencies. The frequency of pure tone A vibrations is slower than pure tone B vibrations

Other vibrating objects produce more complex waves with a set of frequencies that have a mathematical relationship between them; these are said to produce a rich sound. A tuba tends to vibrate at a set of frequencies that form simple mathematical patterns; it produces a rich tone.

Still other objects will vibrate at a set of multiple frequencies that have no identifiable mathematical patterns between them. These objects are not musical and the sounds that they create are best described as *noise*. Noise is erratic, intermittent, or statistically random sound. When a pencil is dropped from a distance on a hard cement floor, it vibrates with a number of unrelated frequencies, producing a complex sound wave that is considered to be *noisy*.

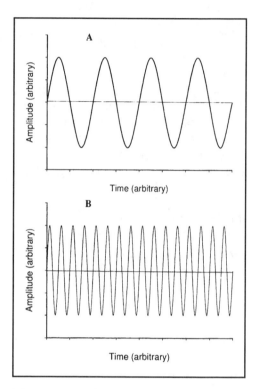

Figure 2–5. A comparison of two different pure tone vibrations. Because (**B**) has more cycles per second, it's a higher frequency tone than (**A**). From *Audiology: Science to Practice* by Steven Kramer. Copyright © 2008, Plural Publishing Inc. All rights reserved. Used with permission, p. 41.

Figure 2–6 compares the frequency of three different types of sounds.

Fundamental Frequency, First Harmonic and Timbre

Each natural frequency produced by an object or instrument has its own characteristic vibrational mode. This is also referred to as a standing wave pattern. These patterns only occur within

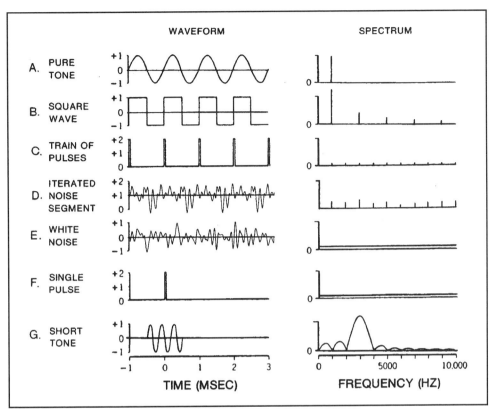

Figure 2–6. A comparison of three different sound waves. From *Audiology: Science to Practice* by Steven Kramer. Copyright © 2008, Plural Publishing Inc. All rights reserved. Used with permission, p. 61.

the object or instrument at specific frequencies of vibration; these frequencies are known as harmonic frequencies, or harmonics. The lowest frequency produced by any vibrating body is known as the fundamental frequency. Each time a frequency doubles it is called an octave. The fundamental frequency is alternatively called the first harmonic (F_1). The frequency of the second harmonic (F_2) is two times the frequency of the first harmonic. The frequency of the third harmonic (F_3) is three times the frequency of the first harmonic. For example, a vibrating body with a fundamental frequency of 400 Hz would have a 2nd har-

monic at 800 Hz and a 3rd harmonic at 1200 Hz. A 4th harmonic would be found at 1600 Hz, a 5th would be at 2000 Hz, and so forth. Of these, the harmonic at 800 Hz is one octave above the fundamental frequency, whereas the harmonic at 1600 Hz is two octaves above the fundamental frequency (Figure 2–7).

We promised that this was going to be fun and easy, but here is something that you'll have to think about. As the frequency of each harmonic increases the wavelength decreases. This is what is called an inverse relationship. For example, the wavelength of (F_2) is one-half (1/2) the wavelength of the first

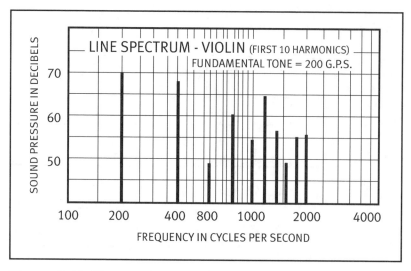

Figure 2–7. The sound spectrum for a violin. The fundamental frequency is 200 Hz. Notice that the second and sixth harmonics are the strongest: Traveling Waves and Wilburys. Modified from Hirsch, *The Measurement of Hearing*, 1952, McGraw-Hill Co., out of print.

harmonic. The wavelength of (F$_3$) is one-third (1/3) the wavelength of the first harmonic.

The number of harmonics that are present impact on our perception of a sound. When the guitar is played, the string, sound box, and surrounding air vibrate at a set of frequencies to produce a wave with a mixture of harmonics. The exact composition of that mixture determines the timbre or quality of sound that is heard. In other words, the quality or timbre of the sound produced by a vibrating object is dependent on the natural frequencies of the sound waves produced by the objects. If there is only a single harmonic sounding out in the mixture (in which case, it wouldn't be a mixture), then the sound is rather pure sounding. On the other hand, if there are a variety of frequencies sounding out in the mixture, then the timbre of the sound is rather rich in quality.

TAKE FIVE: Traveling Waves and Wilburys

When you watch American Idol you might notice two relatively competent singers can hit all the notes correctly, but one singer might sound much more pleasant than the other. The difference, assuming the notes are sung correctly is the timbre. All of us who watch American Idol know: When someone sings off key it sounds terrible. Timbre explains why you may adore Frank Sinatra's voice, but can't stand to listen to any of the Traveling Wilburys (not to be confused with the Traveling Sound Waves).

Resonance

Let's go back to our guitar example. Pick up an acoustic guitar and pluck one of the strings. The sound fills the entire cavity behind the hole and resonates. Now, cover the hole behind the strings and strike the same note. Notice the difference. This time the sound just quickly dies off. It does not resonate, and it doesn't sound as rich. Any time sound fills an open cavity, like the open body of an acoustic guitar or ear canal, it will vibrate in a certain way. The way a sound resonates depends on factors such as the size of the cavity, the composition of the medium it is traveling through, and the barriers or walls it encounters along the way.

You will encounter acoustic resonators every day in clinical practice. For example, the ear canal, because it is a open cavity enclosed on one end (by the tympanic membrane), it is a specific type of resonator, called a Helmholz resonator. Earmolds, earmold tubing, the hook of the hearing aid, and other parts of the instrument also contain many types of resonators. If we simply think of the resonance of tubes or cylinders that are closed on one end, like an empty plastic water bottle or the ear canal, we also know that reducing the size by one-half will cause a one octave increase in the resonant frequency. The inverse also would be true, doubling the size would lower the resonant frequency by one-half. If you are one of those people who are talented enough to create a resonant tone by blowing across the opening of a water bottle (or beer bottle if this is your preference), you can test this out during a boring evening at home. At this stage of your training we are not yet recommending that you blow into ear canals! Maybe when you finish the book.

TIPS and TRICKS: Ear Canal Resonance

Within the human ear small differences like the length, diameter, thickness of the skin lining the ear canal, the shape of the ear canal, and the sensitivity of the eardrum can greatly affect how sound resonates. It's important to know that the human ear resonates somewhere between 2000 and 3000 Hz for most persons. The average resonating frequency is about 2700 Hz. As you will learn later, this has several significant implications when fitting and dispensing hearing aids, and selecting earmold plumbing.

Frequency Versus Pitch

The relationship *between* frequency and pitch is similar to the relationship between intensity and loudness (we will discuss those concepts later in this chapter). Pitch is the psychological interpretation or perception of frequency. Two people listening to the same mid-frequency sound (e.g., 1000 Hz) may perceive and then describe its pitch differently. One person may perceive and describe it as a high-pitched sound whereas the other may perceive and describe it as a mid-range sound, being neither high pitched nor low pitched.

For a sound to have pitch it must have a number of successive cycles of the same frequency. These successive cycles being repeated make the sound periodic. Periodic sounds have a definite pitch.

The pitch scale is presented in units called mels. The mel scale assigns a standard reference value of 1000 mels to the pitch associated with 1000 Hz. As someone who fits hearing aids, you won't spend any time thinking about mels, so we won't mention them again. Just remember that pitch changes with intensity. In general, increasing intensity results in an increased pitch for the lower frequencies, and a decreased pitch for lower frequencies. These changes in pitch are relatively small and generally not noticeable except in controlled laboratory conditions.

TIPS AND TRICKS:
Pitch for Counseling

As a "professional," you'll be working alot with the term "frequency"—test frequencies of the audiometer, the frequency response of the hearing aid, and so forth. But don't forget that your patients are more familiar with the word "pitch." For counseling purposes, therefore, it's okay to use the term "pitch" now and then if it helps get your message across: *"Your hearing loss is primarily in high pitches, the frequencies important for understanding speech."*

Nonperiodic
Sounds and Noise

Many of the sounds we encounter in the real world are nonperiodic in nature.

Because these sounds do not have a repeatable number of cycles, we classify many of them as "noise." Although you probably simply think of noise as those sounds that are naturally occurring in your everyday life, noise can also be generated and shaped containing a different mix of many frequencies. This type of noise often is used for testing different types of equipment and amplification systems. The type of noise being generated depends on the way it is shaped or filtered.

The Color of Noise

From the 1930 epic All Quiet on the Western Front *to the 2010 Oscar-winning picture,* The Hurt Locker, *sound effects have played a crucial role in bringing the film to life. A huge part of the special effects of war movies is the recreation of sounds from the battle field. Special effects engineers have a keen knowledge of acoustics in order to make the effects seem realistic. Although we are not exactly talking about special effects here, it's important to know there are many types of noises that can "color" the way we hear something.*

The type of noise we are going to discuss next is typically not found in a crowded restaurant or on the set of your favorite old war movie. There are a few different types of specific generated noises that you need to know about, mainly because they are used for conducting certain kinds of tests and for calibration of equipment. Don't worry, you will probably never have to conduct an exhaustive calibration, but it's good to know what the technician is doing when he arrives at your office each year to perform these tasks, especially as you will be paying him for the work! Fortunately, digital electronics allows us to use these calibrated noises easily. Let's just say, a lot of math is going on behind the scenes; you only need to know a few basics.

White Noise

Noise that is generated to have equal energy per cycle across a wide range of frequencies is called white noise. You hear white noise when no signal is broadcast over a television channel or radio station. Although most of us think of it as an annoying, unpleasant sound, some people use it to sleep better by running a fan or using a "noise machine" during the night. This works because this steady sound at all frequencies can mask all kinds of other noises that might disturb a light sleeper.

Although white noise is a good starting point and an important noise to know about, it is usually not used in the hearing aid clinic for a couple of reasons. First, the equal energy distribution of white noise is not representative of noise found in the real world, and therefore it is not a very realistic masker for test signals. Second, most hearing-impaired people have more hearing loss in the higher frequencies; therefore, they are more likely to hear white noise at reduced levels relative to speech. In general, white noise is ineffective for audiologic and hearing aid testing purposes.

Pink Noise

Noise that is generated with equal energy at each octave is called pink noise. Because each octave has half the power of the octaves before it, pink noise rolls off at 3 dB per octave. Pink noise gives more weight to the lower frequencies to compensate for the increased number of frequencies of each higher octave. Pink noise is sometimes used for calibrating our equipment, and as in input signal for testing hearing aids—more on that in Chapter 8. Fortunately, we have other types of noises that are more useful. In fact, you will be relying on these noises virtually every day during routine hearing testing.

Narrowband Noise

Narrowband noise has its energy distributed over a relatively small section of the audible range. Because the energy is confined to a specific auditory area it is an efficient type of noise for masking. Masking is sometimes necessary when hearing testing is conducted to assure that the desired ear is responding to the test signal. Masking is something you need to learn how to do well if you want to complete an accurate hearing test; we'll work through that in Chapter 4.

Speech-Shaped Noise

The final type of noise we mention (believe it or not, there are many other types of noises we *aren't* mentioning) is called speech-shaped noise. Speech-shaped noise is generated to match the frequency distribution of typical speech. Because it is shaped like real speech it is good masker when you are conducting speech testing. It also has good functionality and face validity as a signal for testing the performance of hearing aids.

TIPS and TRICKS: Troubleshooting

When you fit someone with a hearing instruments you are not only providing amplification (making sounds louder), you are creating a whole new listening environment for that individual. In an ongoing effort to maintain the optimum listening environment for each patient you will have to make occasional adjustments to both the intensity and frequency of their hearing instruments. Being knowledgeable about subjec-

tive differences in each individual's ability to perceive and describe what and how they hear with their hearing instruments will ultimately contribute to your success as a hearing consultant. Let's say a patient you fit last week is complaining that sounds are "too sharp." This could be a problem related to either loudness or pitch, right? Your job is to solve the problem. Never, fear, you'll be a pro before too long!

Intensity Versus Loudness

The average movie set "blast" on the set of a war movie exceeds 130 dB SPL. All members of the film crew, even the caterers, are required to wear hearing protection during the filming of these scenes.

The intensity of any sound is related to the largest pressure change via the displacement of particles, or the amplitude of the sound wave. Figure 2–8 shows three pure tones of the same frequency with different amplitude. The greater the amplitude or vertical distance between the peaks (maximum compressions) and

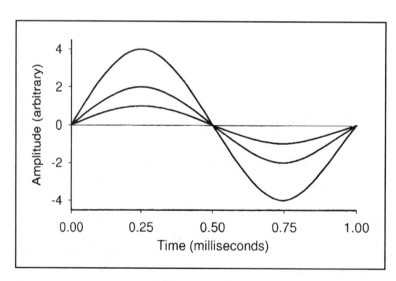

Figure 2–8. Three pure tones of the same frequency with differing amplitude. From *Audiology: Science to Practice* by Steven Kramer. Copyright © 2008, Plural Publishing Inc. All rights reserved. Used with permission, p. 47.

troughs (maximum rarefactions) of the sound wave, the greater the intensity.

The overall amplitude of sound waves is a physical characteristic of the sound and can be easily measured in units of pressure or sound intensity. Loudness, on the other hand, is the psychological interpretation of the physical characteristic intensity and is measured in units called phons. Like mels for frequency judgments, hearing aid fitters don't spend any time thinking about phons (except for maybe on your state licensure exam), so we won't talk much more about them.

Loudness and intensity do not grow at the same rate. This is true for people with normal hearing, but the divergence is even more extreme for people with hearing loss. In fact, you will probably notice during your first week of fitting hearing aids that sounds of the same amplitude or intensity will be judged to have very different loudness levels by two different patients with similar hearing loss.

Humans are equipped with very sensitive ears capable of detecting sound waves of extremely low intensity. The faintest sound that the typical human ear can detect has power intensity equal to 10^{-16} watts/cm^2 and pressure intensity equal to .0002 dynes/cm^2. A sound with an intensity of 10^{-16} watts/cm^2 corresponds to a sound that will displace particles of air by a mere one-billionth of a centimeter. The human ear can detect such a sound! This faintest sound that the human ear can detect is known as the threshold of hearing. The most intense sound that the ear can safely detect without suffering any physical damage is more than one billion times more intense than the threshold of hearing. The sound pressure needed for us to hear a sound also differs significantly across frequencies. We need more pressure (power) in the low and high frequencies, and the least in the 1000 to 2000-Hz range (Figure 2–9).

As the range of intensities that the human ear can detect is so large, the scale that we use is based on multiples of 10. This type of scale is referred to as a logarithmic scale. The scale for measuring intensity is the decibel scale. For the purpose of testing human hearing the threshold of hearing is assigned a sound level of 0 decibels (abbreviated 0 dB); this sound corresponds to an intensity of 10^{-16} watts/cm^2 and a pressure of .0002 dynes/cm^2—which you also will see expressed as 20 micro-Pascals (µPa).

Although the intensity of a sound is an objective quantity that can be measured with appropriate instrumentation, the loudness of a sound is a subjective response that varies given a number of factors. The same sound will not be perceived to have the same loudness to all individuals. One factor that affects the human ear's response to a sound is age. Obviously, hearing for many older people (think of your parents or grandparents) is not what it used to be. The music at a rock concert would not be perceived to have the same quality of loudness to them as it would to you. Furthermore, two sounds with the same intensity but different frequencies will not be perceived to have the same loudness. Because of the human ear's natural tendency to amplify sounds having frequencies in the range from 1000 Hz to 5000 Hz, sounds with these intensities, if delivered with equal SPL, seem louder to the human ear. Table 2–1 summarizes the intensity and pressure ranges of the human ear.

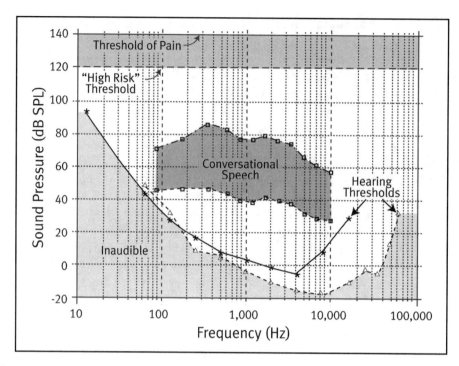

Figure 2–9. The auditory area for listening, expressed in dB SPL, watts/cm² and dynes/cm². Note how hearing sensitivity is best for sounds in the 2000 to 4000 Hz range.

Table 2–1. Intensity and Pressure Ranges from the Least Audible to the Upper Limit Tolerated

	Intensity (w/m²)[a]		Pressure (µPa)[b]	
Upper limit (pain)	100	or 1×10^2	200,000,000	or 20×10^7 (or 2.0×10^8)
Lowest audible (Reference Level)	.000000000001	or 1×10^{-12}	20	or 20×10^0 (or 2.0×10^1)

[a]watts/meter²

[b]microPascals

Source: Audiology: Science to Practice by Steven Kramer. Copyright © 2008, Plural Publishing Inc. All rights reserved. Used with permission, p. 50.

Introducing the Decibel

War is too important to be left to politicians. They have neither the time, the training, nor the inclination for strategic thought.

General Jack D. Ripper, *Dr. Strangelove*

Like the quote from the famous war movie *Dr. Strangelove*, knowledge of the decibel can't be left to others. It's important that you take the time to understand decibels, so that you don't have to rely on others, who don't work directly with patients, to help make important decisions about sound pressure levels. As a hearing care professional you need to know about different measures of sound intensity using the decibel. One measure, expressed as hearing level or hearing threshold level (abbreviated dB HL or dB HTL, respectively) is used primarily in reference to testing hearing levels using the audiometer. The other, expressed as sound pressure level (abbreviated dB SPL), is used in reference to the manufacturing and performance evaluation of hearing instruments, amplification, voice levels, and environmental sounds. You need to understand both scales and how they differ from each other.

Basic Units

The basic unit for measuring sound pressure is the microbar or dyne per square centimeter. The microbar or dyne expresses what we refer to as effective sound pressure or the amount of energy required to move a mass of one gram a distance of one centimeter in one second.

To review, the softest sound that the *best* human ear can detect, in the *best* listening conditions, is an effective sound pressure of .0002 dynes/cm^2 (20 microPascal). Conversely, the loudest sound the normal human ear can tolerate is at an effective sound pressure of about 1000 dynes/cm^2, just below the threshold of pain. At an effective sound pressure of 2000 dynes/cm^2 the human ear will feel pain and may suffer damage if the sound is sustained (see Table 2–1).

Using a dB SPL scale of measurement, the difference between the softest sound that the best human ear can hear and the loudest sound the normal ear can tolerate would be 5 million units. The difference between the softest effective sound pressure and pain would be 10 million units. Because we could not easily test human hearing with such large numerical differences in the range of sound, there needed to be an efficient way to express these values. Enter the decibel.

About the dB

The decibel, (abbreviated dB), which was named after Alexander Graham Bell, literally means 1/10 of a Bel. It is the common term we use to describe intensity or loudness of sound. The decibel is a logarithmic scale that reduces large numbers to the base of 10, giving them the number 10 plus an exponent. For the mathematically challenged, this logarithmic scale basically translates the unworkable range of .0002 to 2000 dynes/cm^2 into a workable range of 0 to 140 dB HL. Table 2–2 summarizes how pressure and intensity measures for human hearing are related to the decibel scale.

The decibel is not a whole number; rather it is a ratio between two pressures and has no fixed absolute value. A specific effective sound pressure is compared to .0002 dynes/cm^2, the standard reference level for effective sound pressure, and expressed as dB sound pressure level (abbreviated dB SPL). Because the decibel is a ratio and has no fixed absolute value, the term dB by itself, offers no information. It must be followed by a reference, for example, dB HL or dB SPL, to identify what measurement scale you are using. But remember, when looking at dB differences, a dB is a dB is a dB! That is, a 2

Table 2–2. Ranges of Human Hearing for Both the Pressure and Intensity Scale in Relation to db SPL

INTENSITY					PRESSURE				
w/m²	ratio (I_{meas}/I_{ref})	Sci Not.	$\log_{10}$	dB IL[a]	µPa	ratio (P_{meas}/P_{ref})	Sci Not.	$\log_{10}$	dB SPL[b]
1×10^{2}	100,000,000,000,000:1	10^{14}	14.0	140	20×10^{7}	100,000,000,000,000:1	10^{14}	7.0	140
1×10^{1}	10,000,000,000,000:1	10^{13}	13.0	130	$20 \times 10^{6.5}$	10,000,000,000,000:1	10^{13}	6.5	130
1×10^{-0}	1,000,000,000,000:1	10^{12}	12.0	120	20×10^{6}	1,000,000,000,000:1	10^{12}	6.0	120
1×10^{-1}	100,000,000,000:1	10^{11}	11.0	110	$20 \times 10^{5.5}$	100,000,000,000:1	10^{11}	5.5	110
1×10^{-2}	10,000,000,000:1	10^{10}	10.0	100	20×10^{5}	10,000,000,000:1	10^{10}	5.0	100
1×10^{-3}	1,000,000,000:1	10^{9}	9.0	90	$20 \times 10^{4.5}$	1,000,000,000:1	10^{9}	4.5	90
1×10^{-4}	100,000,000:1	10^{8}	8.0	80	20×10^{4}	100,000,000:1	10^{8}	4.0	80
1×10^{-5}	10,000,000:1	10^{7}	7.0	70	$20 \times 10^{3.5}$	10,000,000:1	10^{7}	3.5	70
1×10^{-6}	1,000,000:1	10^{6}	6.0	60	20×10^{3}	1,000,000:1	10^{6}	3.0	60
1×10^{-7}	100,000:1	10^{5}	5.0	50	$20 \times 10^{2.5}$	100,000:1	10^{5}	2.5	50
1×10^{-8}	10,000:1	10^{4}	4.0	40	20×10^{2}	10,000:1	10^{4}	2.0	40
1×10^{-9}	1,000:1	10^{3}	3.0	30	$20 \times 10^{1.5}$	1,000:1	10^{3}	1.5	30
1×10^{-10}	100:1	10^{2}	2.0	20	20×10^{1}	100:1	10^{2}	1.0	20
1×10^{-11}	10:1	10^{1}	1.0	10	$20 \times 10^{0.5}$	10:1	10^{1}	0.5	10
1×10^{-12}	1:1	10^{0}	0.0	0	20×10^{0}	1:1	10^{0}	0.0	0

[a]dB IL = 10 log (I_{meas}/I_{ref})
[b]dB SPL = 20 log ($P_{meas}/P_{reference}$)

Source: Audiology: Science to Practice by Steven Kramer. Copyright © 2008, Plural Publishing Inc. All rights reserved. Used with permission, 55.

dB difference in SPL is no bigger than a 2 dB difference in HL even though the reference is not the same. We'll get to that next.

Puzzled by different scales? That's OK. Think temperature. If I tell you that it is 32 degrees outside and we are somewhere in the continental United States, then you will know that it is rather cold and you'd probably put on your coat before you go outside. However, if we were on the European continent and the announced temperature was 32 degrees, it would be hot and you would be very miserable (not to mention looking foolish in that coat).

This disparity is due to the fact that temperature measured in degrees (°) also offers no information unless it is referenced to a specific scale of measurement, in this case, degrees Fahrenheit or degrees Celsius. For example, water freezes at 32°F. It also freezes at 0°C. Same temperature, different scale.

Decibel Sound Pressure Level (dB SPL)

When talking about hearing instruments, voice levels, and environmental sounds, (which cover pretty much everything you encounter in everyday life) dB SPL is used. With the exception of audiometric testing and audiograms you'll be working a lot with dB SPL, so there are a few things you need to know.

When 2 + 2 Isn't 4!

Because the decibel is a calculated ratio, decibels only can be added or sub-tracted exponentially. For example, imagine you were in a laundromat and two adjacent washing machines were operating at an intensity of 70 dB SPL each (perhaps you remember this from your younger days). If you were to add one 70 dB SPL sound to another 70 dB SPL sound as you would add 2 + 2, then the obvious SPL level of the two washing machines would be 140 dB SPL. This is louder than a jet airplane at takeoff, which should tip you off that this is not the correct way to add dB. The actual combined *pressure* level of 70 dB SPL + 70 dB SPL is 76 dB SPL. This is because when identical SPL values are added, there is an increase of 6 dB. When the difference between the two values is not equal, the effect is much smaller and often is very similar to the louder of the two signals. That is, if you were to add 60 dB SPL to 70 dB SPL, the sum would only be a few tenths higher than 70 dB. Too bad it doesn't work that way when adding calories to our dinner.

In terms of loudness, you should know that if the intensity of a sound increases by 10 dB, the perception of loudness of that sound doubles over most of the range of intensities. For example, most people would judge a 1000-Hz tone at 80 dB SPL as two times as loud as 70 dB SPL and one-half as loud as 90 dB SPL.

We mentioned the film *Apocalypse Now* at the beginning of this chapter. Not only do we like the fear and pain analogy as it relates to the study of physics, but there are plenty of good examples of sounds, like the ones listed on the next page. Table 2–3 gives you an idea of the relative intensity level of many "military" sounds.

Table 2–3. A Comparison of dB SPL Levels for Various Military Sounds

Sound Origin	dB SPL
Jet engine at 30 m	150 dB
Rifle being fired at 1 m	140 dB
Threshold of pain	130 dB
Party at Officer's Club	85 dB
Party at NCO Club	95 dB
Hearing damage can occur	85 dB
Shouting sergeant at 1 m	75–80 dB
Normal conversation	50–60 dB
Whisper of Col. Kurtz	35–40 dB
Leaving rustling outside barracks	20 dB
Auditory threshold at 2 kHz	0 dB

TAKE FIVE: Watching TV

Have you ever been watching a nice peaceful movie on a network TV station, and then on comes an obnoxiously loud commercial? At one time or another you probably have said: "Why do they have to make those darn commercials twice as loud as everything else?" The fact is, you were probably listening to the movie at an intensity of about 65 dB SPL and the commercial was only 5 dB or so louder (certainly not 130 dB!), but the *loudness perception* is much different from the relative change in intensity. And hopefully, by the time you read this the new laws will have taken effect, and this will no longer be a problem.

Decibel Hearing Level (dB HL)

When performing a hearing test using an audiometer or referring to an audiogram, you will use dB hearing level (abbreviated dB HL) to express the hearing threshold values.

We do this because the human ear is an incredibly interesting sense organ. As mentioned earlier, it is more sensitive to frequencies in the 1000 to 5000-hertz range. Because of the ear's frequency selectivity, many sounds do not have to be very intense (loud) for the ear to hear them. If then, someone had excellent hearing and heard all the sounds across a wide range of frequencies at the softest levels, their test results would have big numbers for some frequencies and small numbers for others, making the results difficult to interpret for anyone who was not a trained audiometrist. It was discovered early on that these divergent numbers needed to be "equalized."

The American Standards Association (ASA) introduced the dB HL scale in 1951 creating the standard Audiometric Zero reference level. At each frequency, the different sound pressure intensity levels (dB SPL) required for the "best" human ear to hear the tone are "built into" the audiometer, so that the result is 0 dB HL across all the test frequencies. The initial ASA standard was revised by the International Standards Association (ISO) in 1964, and revised again by the American National Standards Institute (ANSI) in 1969. Table 2–4 illustrates dB SPL values for each of the test frequencies.

Table 2–4. dB SPL to dB HL Conversions from ANSI Standard

Frequency (Hz)	dB SPL	dB HL
250	27	0
500	14	0
1000	7.5	0
2000	9	0
4000	12	0
8000	16	0

Although you may find these values important later when you begin to fit hearing instruments, it is not necessary to concern yourself with them while learning how to operate and perform hearing tests with the audiometer. For now you will simply record all hearing threshold values in dB HL (and assume that someone has calibrated your audiometer properly). The differences observed in Table 2–4 show how much variation between dB SPL and dB HL there is across frequencies. Fortunately, the dB SPL to dB HL corrections for each frequency are built into the audiometer. There is no need to do the calculation, but you do need to know the difference between dB HL and dB SPL.

TIPS and TRICKS: When "Zero" Is Something!

When conducting audiograms, it is important to remember that 0 dB HL is the *average* for people with normal hearing. As you know, that means that some people with "normal hearing" have better thresholds than 0 dB, whereas others are worse. You probably will have patients with auditory thresholds *below* zero (assuming you have a test booth with good attenuation). Now, the interesting thing about all this is that when people get out of the test booth and are in a typical room with ambient noise, the real-world thresholds of the people with –10 dB HL thresholds will be no different from those who have 0 dB HL thresholds, or even those with +10 dB HL thresholds. More on that in later chapters.

Sensation Level (dB SL)

Sensation level (abbreviated SL) may be used as a third scale of measurement or reference, but this term only is meaningful after establishing a hearing threshold level or levels in dB HL. By definition, a person's hearing threshold is the softest (lowest intensity) level they are able to hear a pure-tone stimulus and respond 50% of the time. Sensation level refers to any audiometric procedure performed at a dB level above the patient's threshold at any frequency. This is referred to as suprathreshold testing. In other words, dB SL is a scale of measurement that has a baseline determined by the thresholds of the individual that you are testing.

For example, Patient A has a hearing threshold of 10 dB HL at 1000 Hz and Patient B has a threshold of 20 dB HL at 1000 Hz. Each patient is then asked to listen and comment on a 1000-Hz tone presented at 50 dB HL. When recording the results it would be more meaningful if we noted that Patient A was asked to comment on a tone delivered at 40 dB SL, whereas Patient B was asked to respond to a tone delivered at 30 dB SL. Same tone delivered at the same intensity; different results. Why? If Patient A's threshold was 10 dB HL and the presentation level of the comparison tone was 50 dB HL, then we subtract the threshold from the presentation level or 50 − 10 = 40. For Patient B we would calculate 50 − 20 = 30.

Sensation level is often used during speech audiometry because starting intensity levels for some of the tests are determined relative to patient threshold levels. To learn about how the decibel can be applied to daily practice go to Chapter 4 on the measurement of hearing.

The Speech Spectrum

Before we move on, let's focus our attention to something called the speech spectrum. Knowing the relationship between the intensity level of speech and hearing threshold levels is an important concept when it comes to fitting hearing aids. Although the intensity level of speech naturally fluctuates over time, it is common to average the intensity of speech over a given period. When we average the intensity levels of speech over a long period of time we come up with something called long-term average speech spectrum (LTASS). The LTASS is helpful because it can be used to quantify the relationship between speech levels and hearing thresholds. This is particularly important when making predictions about speech intelligibility for hearing aid wearers.

Even though there are published LTASS's which differ somewhat because of the methods in which the samples were collected, for the most part they are all quite similar. The characteristic pattern for average vocal effort reveals a peak around 500 Hz and a spectral slope (drop in level across frequency) of about 9 dB per octave. The differences in the LTASS for three different intensity levels are shown in Figure 2–10. These curves show the average intensity across frequencies—see Figure 2–11 to observe how the different frequencies impact on this average. Notice the effects distance has on the average intensity of speech. For example, the average level of speech produced at 16 feet from a hearing aid should be about 54 dB SPL. For a quiet talker, however, it could be as low as 44 dB SPL, and as much as 70 db SPL for a loud talker. The hearing aid user's own speech at a distance of six inches will be about 84 dB SPL, but might be as high as 94 dB SPL, if he speaks with a loud voice. The bottom line, which is illustrated in Figure 2–10,

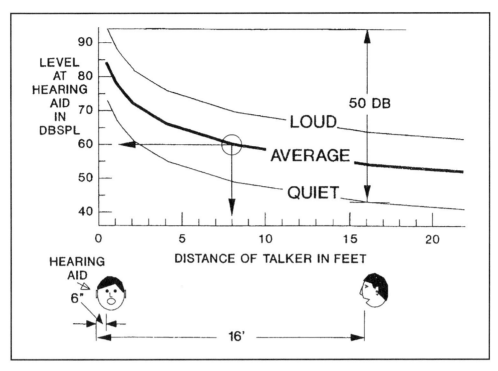

Figure 2–10. The long-term average speech for three intensity levels. Notice that a typical talker, speaking with average effort at a distance of 8 feet, generates an average level of about 60 dB SPL. Reprinted with permission from Unitron, all rights reserved.

is that there is an approximately 50-dB range of speech intensities.

The LTASS has important consequences on hearing aid fitting and use. When a talker varies the volume of their voice not only does the overall intensity of the sound change, but the frequency shape of their voice changes as well. This is illustrated in Figure 2–11. Notice how the energy peak of speech shifts to a higher frequency as the intensity of speech rises from a whisper to a shout. Also, notice how the overall shape of shouted speech differs from a whisper.

Dynamic Range of Speech

Directly related to the LTASS is the dynamic range of speech. The dynamic

range refers to the difference between the lowest level (speech minima) and highest level (speech maxima) parts of speech that are produced in the same frequency range. Like the LTASS, calculating the dynamic range of speech is complex with many variables affecting it. When it comes to fitting hearing aids, however, a dynamic range of 30 dB is used for making predictions of speech recognition. It's important to know that the 30 dB dynamic range is not symmetric around the average of the LTASS; rather it may be best represented as the average LTASS +12 and −18 dB for the speech maxima and minima, respectively. Clinically, it is common to assume a dynamic range of 30 dB which is symmetric around the

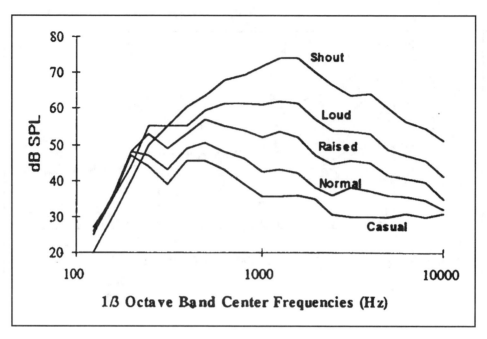

Figure 2–11. Long-term average speech spectrum produced at various vocal levels. Reprinted with the permission of Unitron (Adapted from Pearson, K, et al., EPA Report 60011-77-025, 1977), all rights reserved.

center point of LTASS. To get an idea of how the LTASS compares to the threshold of audibility, take a look back to Figure 2–9.

Filters

Another important concept in acoustics is filtering. Hearing aids rely on filters to allow certain sound to pass through the device. High- pass, low-pass, and band-pass filters are shown in Figure 2–12. The excluded or "filtered" frequencies are determined by the slope of the curve, called the attenuation rate. An octave means a doubling or halving of frequency. A steep filter (D) has a slope of 30 per octave. The point where the frequencies begin to be filtered out is called the cutoff frequency. A high-pass

filter is one that attenuates low-frequency sounds (and allows high-frequency sounds to pass through without being reduced). On the other hand, a low-pass filter attenuates high-frequency sounds and allows low-frequency sounds to pass through without losing energy. For evaluating hearing aids, test equipment sometimes conducts low-pass filtering in order to shape the signal to be more representative of real speech. Finally, one type band-pass filter that reduces sound energy in a very restricted range of frequencies is called a narrowband filter.

In Closing

Now that you've read this chapter, you should have a little more insight into

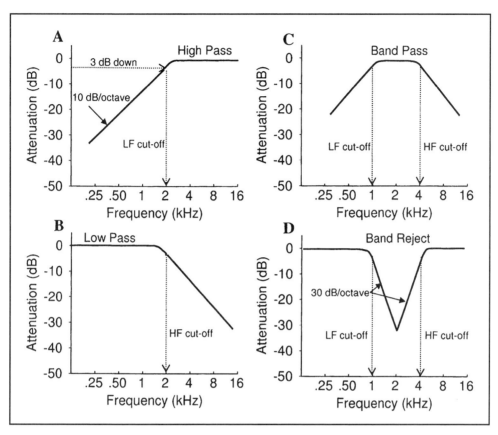

Figure 2–12. Examples of different types of filters. The filter's rate of frequency rejection is indicated by the db/octave. From *Audiology: Science to Practice* by Steven Kramer. Copyright © 2008, Plural Publishing Inc. All rights reserved. Used with permission, p. 62.

some of the basic physics behind dispensing hearing aids. The intention, of course, is to give you enough information to get you started fitting your first hearing aid without it being a harrowing experience. Take a deep breath, you have made it to the end of this chapter. As Robert DeNiro's character in the Oscar-winning Vietnam War movie *The Deer Hunter* said:

"This is this. This ain't something else. From now on, you're on your own."

3

Basic Anatomy and Physiology of the Ear

> *Remember all the old children's songs you used to sing? Before long you'll have the same fondness for ear anatomy and physiology!*

Old MacDonald had a farm
Eee-Eye-Eee-Eye-Oh

Now that you have gotten through one facet of hearing science, we are going to introduce another one. This chapter focuses on the structures of the ear and how the ear gathers and transmits sounds to the speech and language centers of the brain. Like the popular children's song above, while reading this chapter you may experience a couple moo-moos or snort-snorts, but at the end you'll be singing *Eee-Eye Eee-Oh*. You will have some preliminary knowledge of the mechanics of hearing, be able to explain how the different parts of the ear transmit sound to the brain, and know some of the differences between normal and abnormal auditory physiology. It will not be everything you need to know, but certainly enough to give you a general understanding of ear mechanics and transmission systems.

Sometime during health class in elementary school we all learned that the ear is divided into three major parts. Although this certainly is the case, there is considerably more to all this than the *Old MacDonald had a farm Eee-Eye-Eee-Eye-Oh* tune.

In simple terms, the ear (with all its subsequent neural connections) acts as an input mechanism for the language centers located in the auditory cortex of the brain. The brain, in turn, decodes and processes these messages. The final stage of language is the output, which is speech. Think about someone you know or have met who has had a severe hearing loss since early childhood. Notice how this person's speech is affected by the loss. Now compare this person to an older adult with the same amount of hearing loss (the people you mainly will see in your office). Adults who lost their hearing later in life after language development have near-normal sounding speech in most cases.

Of course, there are even more subtle relationships between input and output for people with normal hearing. When people from Wisconsin or North Dakota travel to Nashville, the people in Nashville think that they "talk funny." (We know of course that this isn't true!) The point is, there is a very strong connection between hearing and speech. Hearing processing in the cortex of the brain, and the resulting speech production centers are closely connected.

In this chapter we outline the essentials of ear anatomy. Toward the end of the chapter we provide some answers to the common questions you might have about the functional anatomy and physiology of the human ear. These are designed to help you understand how to better fit hearing aids and answer patient questions. Like the songs we all learned as children, we hope you can commit this information to memory.

Let's start with a grand tour of the ear. Take a few minutes to study Figure 3–1. Notice that the important mechanical and neural processing components of the ear are actually embedded in the temporal bone of the skull. Also notice where these components are located in proximity to the brain.

The Outer Ear

Do your ears hang low?
Do they wobble to and fro?
Can you tie them in a knot?
Can you tie them in a bow?

The part of the outer ear that we see is called the pinna, or auricle and, hopefully, it doesn't hang too low. Besides being a place to hang glasses, earrings, and Bluetooth receivers, the pinna is responsible for gathering

sound, and also assists in localization. In many animal species (and even a few cartoon children's characters, like Dumbo), the pinna performs the important role of gathering and focusing sounds to the ear canal. Both Dumbo and Bambi are two good make-believe examples of animals that have large pinnae that can be moved in the direction of sound to facilitate this process. In the real world many animals really do have large pinnae that move so that they can stay aware of the location of their predators and prey. In fact, some humans have the ability to move their ears, which is probably a vestigial function of our cave dwelling ancestors and their attempt to stay away from saber tooth tigers.

TIPS and TRICKS: Sound Localization

It is tempting to think that the external ear is critical for sound localization, but we do much of our localization (especially side to side) by a right ear versus left ear comparison of intensities. This is not impacted too much by the external ear. This is why our patients wearing BTE hearing aids (with the microphone above the ear) can still do pretty well for lateral localization. Where the pinna does come into play is for front-to-back localization. For this reason, some manufacturers have added "pinna effects" to the gain of the hearing aid when sound originates from behind the user.

In humans, the pinna does not play much of a role in sound localization,

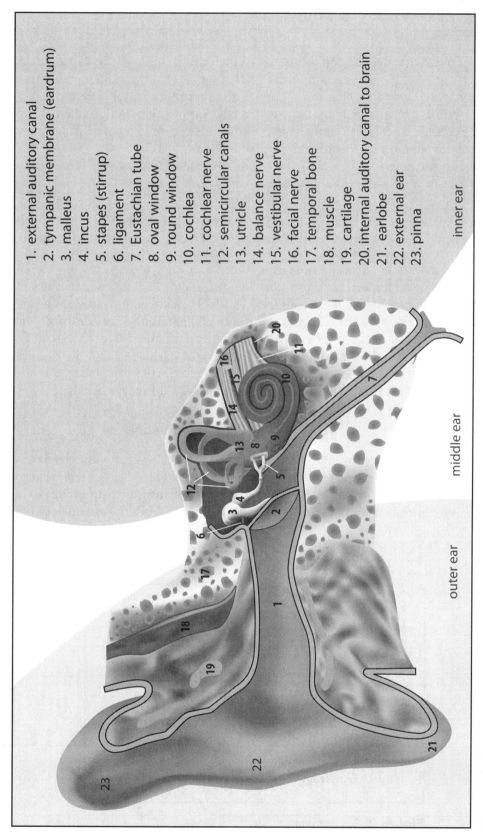

1. external auditory canal
2. tympanic membrane (eardrum)
3. malleus
4. incus
5. stapes (stirrup)
6. ligament
7. Eustachian tube
8. oval window
9. round window
10. cochlea
11. cochlear nerve
12. semicircular canals
13. utricle
14. balance nerve
15. vestibular nerve
16. facial nerve
17. temporal bone
18. muscle
19. cartilage
20. internal auditory canal to brain
21. earlobe
22. external ear
23. pinna

outer ear   middle ear   inner ear

Figure 3–1. A detailed drawing of the anatomic parts of the human ear. Image from Shutterstock®. All rights reserved.

but its somewhat uneven convolutions of cartilage do shape sounds in a distinctive way. Due to the size and shape of the pinna, driven mostly by the area of the concha, it acts as an acoustic resonator for sounds in the higher frequencies (around 3000 to 5000 Hz). This means that the pinna provides a natural boost for sounds in this frequency range. The key landmarks of the human pinna are shown in Figure 3–2. You might find it fascinating that the pinna provides a natural boost for some of the most important sounds for understanding; the very speech sounds that happen to be the softest speech.

The ear canal, also called the external auditory meatus, is the other important outer ear landmark. The ear canal is lined with only a few layers of skin and it is a highly vascularized area, especially the medial one-third or so (the portion nearest the eardrum). This means there is an abundant flow of blood to the ear canal. This is important to know when you are taking an ear impression for earmolds and custom hearing aids, which we'll talk about in detail in Chapter 7. For now, just remember that if the procedure is not performed correctly, it can it be painful to the patient, embarrassing for you, and it just may bleed a lot.

The primary purpose of the external ear canal is to protect the deeper structures of the ear. It does this primarily through the production of cerumen, commonly called earwax, that highly scientific term you probably already were familiar with. The ear canal length is about 2.5 cm, which is about 1 inch. The ear canal dead ends at the tympanic membrane, or eardrum. The first third of the ear canal is made entirely of cartilage, and the second two-thirds partially consist of bone, covered by a thin layer of skin.

Ear Canal Resonance

The ear canal also has an important resonant characteristic which relates directly to hearing aid fittings. Since we know that it is a tube closed on one end,

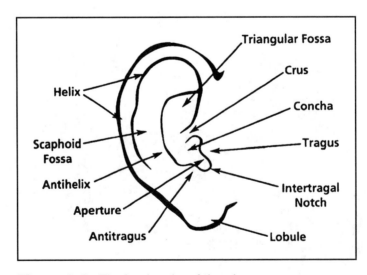

Figure 3–2. The landmarks of the pinna.

with a diameter around 7 mm, and a length around 25 mm, we can calculate the average resonant frequency using some third grade math. We'll save you the trouble, and just tell you that it's around 2700 Hz, creating a boost in this region of about 15 dB. This is a very good region to have a boost, as many soft consonants occur in this frequency range. But what happens when we put an earmold or hearing aid into the ear canal? We change the size of the tube (make it much smaller) and these resonant frequencies move to a much higher frequency (you learned all about this in Chapter 2). Somehow we need to bring this "natural gain" back and we'll tell you how before this book is finished! As you will read in Chapter 10, the average outer ear resonance is easy to measure in your clinic with the right equipment. Figure 3–3 shows what a typical unaided ear canal resonance looks like.

The Middle Ear

Oh those bones, oh those bones, oh mercy,
  how they scare
With the toe bone connected to the foot bone
  and the foot connected to the ankle bone
  and the ankle bone connected to the leg
  bone
Oh mercy, how they scare

Dem Bones (or Skeleton Bones)
James Weldon Johnson (1871–1938)

The famous children's song above might be a good way to learn the interconnectedness of the 206 bones of the human body. Fortunately, there are only three bones, which we address in this section that interconnect in the middle ear. With the correct amount of lighting, if you gently pull up and back on the pinna, and look into the ear canal with an otoscope, you can see the pearly white reflection of the tympanic membrane (TM). The right tympanic

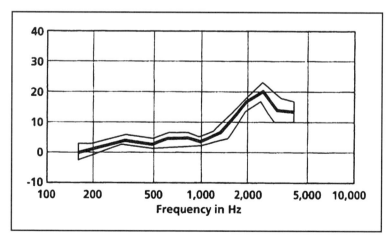

Figure 3–3. The average ear canal resonance of a healthy adult ear. Note the sound level pressure peaks at approximately 2700 Hz. The bold line is the average ear canal resonance and the two thin lines surrounding it designate 1 standard deviation from the average. Reprinted with permission from Unitron, all rights reserved.

membrane, or eardrum, is shown in Figure 3–4, along with the quadrants or sections used to help us describe the location of areas of concern during otoscopy.

The eardrum, or tympanic membrane is the dividing line between the outer and middle ear. This greater part of the drum is called the pars tensa. A small triangular-shaped area at the top edge of the drum is called the pars flaccida. The umbo (head of one of the middle ear bones) usually can be observed in the central most part of the TM. The cone of light, or light reflex, is a landmark of the normal tympanic membrane. It is produced by the reflection of the otoscope light from the concave eardrum. The TM is connected to the bony wall of the ear canal by a tough fibrous ring called the annular ligament.

The Ossicular Chain

Let's now move to the other side of the eardrum and jump into the middle ear (Figure 3–5). The ossicles are the three tiny bones of the middle ear (what you maybe learned as the hammer, anvil, and stirrup in grade school). They are fully developed at birth. They serve as a mechanical link between the tympanic membrane and the inner ear. In order, starting at the eardrum and heading toward the inner ear, the three bones are:

- Malleus. The malleus (Latin word for hammer) is the largest of the three bones and is embedded in the fibrous layer of the eardrum (remember, we mentioned earlier that you often can see the head of this bone shining through the eardrum when looking into the ear canal). It is approximately 9 mm in length.
- Incus. The incus is 7 mm in length and it joins the malleus to the third bone, the stapes. And yes, it does look a little like an anvil.
- Stapes. The stapes is the smallest bone in the human body. The footplate of the stapes, which indeed does look like a stirrup, is fixed in the oval window (membrane) of the inner ear.

Middle Ear Mechanics

The ossicles, or ossicular chain, have one primary function: They serve as a compensation for the impedance mismatch. Impedance is a technical term for resistance to flow. In the case of the ear, sound has to travel from the low-impedance air pressure waves of sound to the high-impedance hydraulic, fluid-filled system of the cochlea. The ossicular chain with its lever and funnel

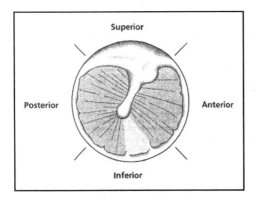

Figure 3–4. A healthy right eardrum. Notice the "cone of light" in the 5 o'clock position.

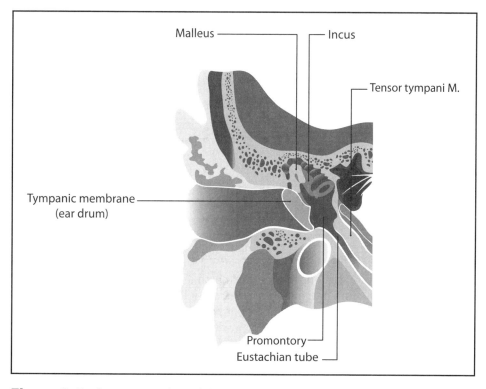

Figure 3–5. A cross-section of the middle ear space showing the major landmarks of the middle ear. Image from Shutterstock®. All rights reserved.

action boost sound as it travels between these two mediums. The advantage of this action is about 30 to 40 dB, although if the chain is disrupted (which does happen, called ossicular disarticulation), there can be an even greater hearing loss (more like 50 to 60 dB), as without the chain, the eardrum acts as a sound attenuator. As we'll discuss later, this would be referred to as a *conductive* hearing loss.

Prior to the occurrence of biomechanical impulses in the inner ear, sounds undergo a vibratory-to-mechanical transformation, which occurs when sound pushes up against the eardrum and the eardrum begins to then push on the ossicles, and, in particular, the stapes

pushes up against the oval window of the cochlea. As mentioned in the previous paragraph, the role of the ossicular chain is to overcome the differences in how sound travels in air compared to fluid. If we tried to transmit the energy of sound traveling in the air directly into a fluid medium, only 1% of the sound energy would be transferred. That means that 99% of the sound would be reflected away from the fluid and lost. This concept is shown in Figure 3–6.

The functional role of the middle ear system is to overcome this impedance mismatch between air and fluid. Without the middle ear system, people would have a substantial 30 to 40 dB HL hearing loss.

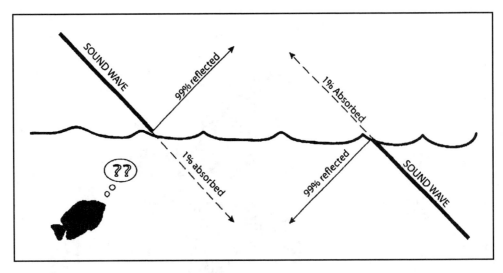

Figure 3–6. Illustrates the impedance mismatch between aid and water. Note that the transfer of energy from one medium to the other is a two-way street, as the same amount of impedance occurs whether energy is moving from a less dense to a denser medium or from a denser medium (water) to less dense air. From *Basics of Audiology: From Vibrations to Sounds*. By Jerry Cranford. Copyright © 2008 Plural Publishing, Inc. All rights reserved. Used with permission, p. 27.

Impedance Mismatch Solved

Build it up with needles and pins
Needles and pins, Needles and pins
Build it up with wood and clay
Wood and clay, Wood and clay
Build it up with iron and steel
Iron and steel, Iron and steel

If you remember all the verses to "London Bridge Is Falling Down," there are many ideas of how to repair it. We have a good thing going in the middle ear to repair the loss of energy caused by the aid to fluid transfer of sound. There are three separate mechanisms used by the middle ear to overcome this impedance mismatch. They are shown in Figure 3–7.

■ Because the area of the tympanic membrane is 14 times greater than the area of the oval window, a funnel action is created (think of the head of a thumb tack versus the point), thus concentrating energy over the narrower area of the oval window. The funneling action provides about a 15 to 20 dB boost to sound as it travels through the middle ear (Figure 3–7A).

■ Because the malleus is significantly longer than the other two middle ear bones, it provides a fulcrum-like action, similar to how a heavier child can be lifted by a lighter child on a seesaw (Figure 3–7B). This fulcrum action magnifies sound another 5 dB or so as it travels through the middle ear.

■ The third mechanism for overcoming impedance mismatch is the buckling effect of the tympanic membrane (Figure 3–7C), which occurs as a result of not being completely attached to the malleus.

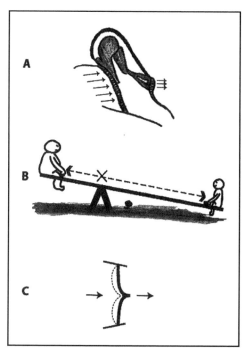

Figure 3–7. Three middle mechanisms that overcome the air-fluid impedance mismatch. From *Basics of Audiology: From Vibrations to Sounds*. By Jerry Cranford. Copyright © 2008 Plural Publishing, Inc. All rights reserved. Used with permission, p. 29.

This action is akin to being stung in the backside by a flicked towel—something we all probably experienced during our childhood. The whiplike action of the loose end of the suddenly stretched towel hitting your skin really hurts. In the middle ear this buckling action boosts sound about 10 dB (with no pain). When you add up the boost in sound provided by these three actions of the middle ear (22, 5, 10 dB) you get amazingly close to the 30 to 40 dB loss that would have been produced by the air-fluid impedance mismatch.

Middle Ear Structures

Let's spend a little more time on the middle ear before we hopscotch to the inner ear. The ossicles, which are suspended by a series of ligaments, work very much like a suspension bridge. Because of the delicate nature of this suspension within the middle ear cavity, they are vulnerable to trauma and disease. (Chapter 5 addresses some of the more common middle ear disorders you are likely to identify when testing patients). The ossicular chain is supported in the middle ear by ligaments and two muscles. The two muscles are called the stapedius and the tensor tympani.

- The *stapedius* muscle attaches to the stapes and draws the stapes in a posterior direction when it contracts.
- The *tensor tympani* attaches to the malleus. When the tensor tympani contracts it pulls in opposition to the stapedius muscle thereby tightening the tympanic membrane.

The stiffening actions of these two muscles together (although the stapedius has the greatest effect) create the acoustic reflex. The acoustic reflex then changes the ear's overall impedance, which provides some protection to the ear from loud sounds (the reflex only occurs for signals around 85 dB or louder). However, because it takes 60 to 120 milliseconds to activate, and then tires or fades over time, the acoustic reflex does not completely protect the ear from either sudden impact sounds (e.g., gunfire, explosives, etc.) or sustained loud sounds (e.g., sirens, machinery noise, etc.). The acoustic reflex is easily measured with a machine referred to as an immittance meter, and is an integral part of a routine audiologic evaluation in most hearing centers.

TAKE FIVE:
Guided Tour of the Ear

It may not be as fun as an old-fashioned hayride, but you sure can learn a lot by going on this guided tour.

To view a narrated overview of how the ear works, go to your favorite search engine and type in the key words "Sinauer + Associates + sound + transduction". Choose from one of several animations demonstrating how various parts of the ear work.

Eustachian Tube

The eustachian tube is the middle ear's air pressure equalizing system. The middle ear is encased in bone and unless some unwanted pathology is present, does not communicate with the outside atmosphere except through the eustachian tube. The eustachian tube is 35 to 40 mm long in adults; the first 10 mm of bone and then 25 to 30 mm of cartilage. In adults the eustachian tube is at a 30 to 40-degree downward angle from the horizontal. In children, it is closer to the horizontal plane, and is shorter and wider. The eustachian tube is *normally closed*, but its ability to open periodically ventilates the middle ear space. If it does not open regularly, a negative pressure develops in the middle ear. If this continues, fluid will be pulled from the mucous lining and collect in the middle ear space. This is referred to as middle ear effusion, a common pathology among children. The fluid can become infectious, but often it is not. Eustachian tube dysfunction, as it is commonly called, is a fairly normal consequence of an immature eustachian tube, with part of the problem being that the downward angle has not yet developed. Most children outgrow this when their eustachian tube has completely developed around the age of six or so.

TIPS and TRICKS:
Blow Your Nose

For most adults, we usually only think about our eustachian tubes when we are descending in an airplane. Often the cabin pressure is not well controlled and we develop a negative middle ear pressure (much like someone would with eustachian tube dysfunction). It's usually a little uncomfortable and you probably also notice a slight hearing loss. To fix this you need to open your eustachian tube. Sometimes chewing or a good large mouth opening works. The easiest technique, however, is what is called the Valsalva procedure (you guessed it, named after Antonio Maria Valsalva, the 17th century physician and anatomist from Bologna, probably a distant cousin of Bartolomeo Eustachius, the noted Italian anatomist of the 1500s) The procedure is simple: You hold your nostrils closed with your finger and thumb, keep your mouth closed, and then try to blow air out of your nose. With a little practice you'll feel (and hear) your ear "pop," which means you've forced open your eustachian tubes. Although you might look a little goofy at the time, the induced comfort is well worth the stares from the other passengers.

The Inner Ear

The inner ear (Figure 3–8) is a series of channels and chambers embedded within the temporal bone. It is also called the *bony labyrinth*. This term alone should tell you how convoluted the inner ear is. The inner ear, specifically the cochlea, is the part of the ear that you'll need to spend the most study time with. Nearly all the people you'll fit with hearing instruments will have a deficit that can be pinpointed to the cochlea. Knowing many details about how the cochlea works will be critical to your professional success. The better you understand how a normal cochlea functions compared to a damaged one, the more effective you will be in identifying hearing loss and fitting hearing instruments. Let's tackle some of the fundamental details of cochlear physiology.

The Role of the Cochlea

Oh my darling, oh my darling
Oh my darling, Clementine
Thou art lost and gone forever
Dreadful sorry, Clementine
    "Oh My Darling, Clementine"
    Percy Montrose 1844

Like the song of a young lost love ("Clementine"), once the tiny microstructures within the cochlea have been lost, they are gone forever. Unlike the ear canal or middle ear, which are both air filled, the cochlea is completely filled with fluid. This fluid is similar to seawater in its consistency.

Deftly Engineered

The cochlea changes mechanical sound energy into a sequence of electrical discharges that is the language of the auditory nervous system. This deftly

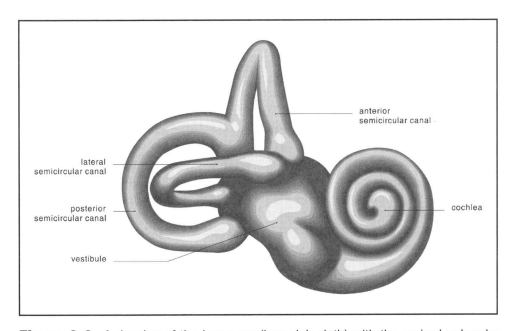

Figure 3–8. A drawing of the inner ear (bony labyrinth) with the major landmarks labeled. Image from Shutterstock®. All rights reserved.

engineered sense organ completes the transduction in several stages. Let's first return to the middle ear ossicles. The mechanical vibrations of the eardrum-to-maleus-to-incus-to-stapes are delivered to the cochlea at the oval window, where a hydromechanical disturbance or wave is created. This wave, traveling through the membranous structures of the inner ear, acts to displace two highly specialized types of sensory cells, called inner and outer hair cells.

These hair cells convert mechanical energy into electromechanical energy. Outer hair cells act as a sort of a biological amplifier, boosting the electromechanical traveling wave. This process, in turn, produces synaptic transmission between the hair cells and the neurons of the auditory portion of the eighth nerve. Finally, the electrical energy created from this outer hair cell activity is directly transmitted from the inner hair cells to the eighth nerve. The electrical impulses then travel along the length of the eighth nerve to the central nervous system. All of this is performed over and over again in a few milliseconds by an organ considerably less than 1 mL in volume. The intricacy of the cochlear mechanism is one of the most fascinating tales in sensory biology. In fact, many of its workings were not fully understood until rather recently.

The Intricate Design

The cochlea is an elongated, fluid-filled cavity housed in the petrous portion of the temporal bone. This cavity is coiled into a tight spiral that resembles the shell of a snail. The broad end of the spiral, which lies close to the middle ear, is called the base. The narrow end is known as the apex. The cochlea is divided lengthwise into three channels by the basilar membrane and Reissner's membrane (Figure 3–9).

- Scala vestibule. The channel formed by the upper bony wall of the cochlea is known as the scala vestibule.
- Scala tympani. The channel between the basilar membrane and the lower bony wall is called the scala tympani.
- Cochlear duct. The third channel, which lies between the two membranes, is called the cochlear duct.

> ### TAKE FIVE: Another (Virtual) Three-Hour Tour
>
> If you want to learn more about the interconnectedness of the inner, middle, and outer ear, take a virtual tour by going to your favorite search engine and entering "guided tour of the ear". There are several interesting Web sites to choose from. One that we like is hosted by Perry Hanavan of Augustana College in Sioux Falls, SD. You can access it at: http://www.augie.edu/perry/ear/ear.html

The Channels

One of the most important characteristics of the cochlear duct is its elasticity. Because it is bound on two sides by tissue membranes, it responds to pressure from either side by moving in the appropriate direction.

The cochlear duct throughout the length of the cochlea separates the scala vestibuli and scala tympani, except at the apical end, farthest from the middle

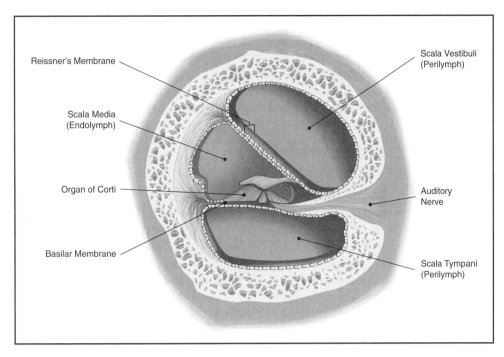

Figure 3–9. A cross-section of the cochlear partition with major landmarks labeled. From *INTRO: A Guide to Communication Sciences and Disorders.* By Michael P. Robb. Copyright © 2010 Plural Publishing, Inc. All rights reserved. Used with permission, p. 76.

ear. Here the cochlear duct abruptly ends, and the two canals communicate through an opening called the helicotrema.

Two Important Fluids

- Perilymph. The outer chambers, scalae vestibuli and tympani, are filled with a high-sodium low-potassium fluid called perilymph.
- Endolymph. The cochlear duct contains a second fluid known as endolymph, perilymph's opposite, having low sodium and high potassium content.

The Windows

The fluid-filled spaces of the cochlea are separated from the air spaces of the middle ear by the bony wall and two openings or windows. One opening, the oval window, leads from the middle ear directly into the scala vestibuli. As already mentioned, the smallest bone of the middle ear, the stapes, fits loosely into the oval window via the stapes footplate. The footplate is held in place by the flexible annular ligament that seals in the perilymph while allowing the stapes to move in and out of the oval window creating the wavelike movements in the fluid-filled inner ear.

The second opening is known as the round window. This opening, covered by a thin, flexible membrane leads directly into the scala tympani, on the side of the cochlear duct opposite the oval window. When pressure is applied to the cochlear fluids via the oval window, the round window acts as a pressure release structure, compensating by bulging outward or inward in response to the movement of the fluid.

The basilar membrane, which separates the cochlear duct from scala tympani, supports the structures that are directly responsible for the hearing sensory function in the cochlea. These include the organ of Corti and the tectorial membrane. Together, along with the basilar membrane, these structures make up what is called the cochlear partition. Because the cochlear partition plays a very important part in the hearing mechanism we discuss its anatomic features in some detail.

Cochlear Partition

The cochlear partition changes as it progresses from the base of the cochlea to its apex in three ways that are especially important to its function.

- The width of the partition increases, from base to apex, by approximately tenfold.
- The mass increases with the width.
- The flexibility of the partition changes from being quite stiff at the base to becoming progressively more elastic toward the apex.

This change in elasticity is more than one hundredfold from base to apex. The consequences of these physical characteristics are discussed when we review traveling wave theory.

Figure 3–9 is a cross-section of the cochlear partition. The organ of Corti rests directly on the basilar membrane. The organ of Corti consists of sensory cells embedded in an array of supporting cells. As the basilar membrane moves, the sensory cells follow its motion closely. These sensory cells occur in rows that run along the organ from end to end of the cochlea. The top of each sensory cell forms part of the upper surface of the organ of Corti with a group of stiff cilia. For this reason, these sensory cells are known as hair cells. Atop each sensory hair cell, tiny sensory "hairs" occur in several rows of increasing length, so that the bundles rise in staircase fashion above the surface of the organ of Corti.

As we stated previously, there are two types of hair cells typically found in the cochlea.

IHCs. The inner hair cells (IHCs) lie in a single row close to the inside of the cochlear spiral. They are flask-shaped, and very rigid. Only the IHCs move when sound is transmitted.

OHCs. The outer hair cells (OHCs) form three rows that lie on the outer edge of the cochlea. Outer hair cells change shape when sound is transmitted. The movement of the IHCs allows the OHCs to change shape. Most of the cylinder-shaped OHC is suspended in the fluid spaces just inside the organ of Corti. These spaces are filled with a fluid called cortilymph.

Outer hair cell damage is the most common site of problems you will see in your practice. Most of your patients with sensorineural hearing loss will have extensive damage to the outer hair cells due to noise exposure and/or age. That is, their damage is more "sensory" than "neural." Today's digital hearing in-

---

TIPS and TRICKS: Outer Hair Cell Damage

Outer hair cell damage is the most common site of problems you will see in your practice. Most of your patients with sensorineural hearing loss have extensive damage to the outer hair cells due to noise exposure and/or age. That is, their damage is more "sensory" than "neural." Today's digital hearing instrument technology, using a type of processing known as wide dynamic range compression is designed primarily to compensate (in amplitude adjustment) for this outer hair cell damage.

---

strument technology, using a type of processing known as wide dynamic range compression, is designed primarily to compensate (in amplitude adjustment) for this outer hair cell damage.

Lying directly above the organ of Corti, but separated from it by narrow space, is the tectorial membrane. It's pretty easy to spot on Figure 3–9. This gelatinous structure is attached at its inner edge to the lining of the bony cochlear wall. The tallest hairs of the outer hair cells are in firm contact with the underside of the tectorial membrane. The fluid underneath the tectorial membrane is endolymph.

Energy Supply to the Inner Ear

Being tiny does not stop the inner ear from consuming a great deal of energy. The inner ear possesses its own extensive network of blood vessels to supply oxygen and nutrients. The cochlear artery enters the inner ear alongside the eighth nerve and then divides into two major pathways. One artery branches into an extensive network of capillaries that occupy the outer wall of the cochlear duct supplying the stria vascularis, and spiral ligament. These structures con-

sume large quantities of energy. The outer wall structures and especially the stria vascularis are thought to be responsible for generation of the endocochlear potential (a resting potential critical to the function of the inner ear). The second source of arterial blood is the spiral vessels that run along side the spiral ganglion and spiral limbus, and just beneath the basilar membrane. It is this second arterial vessel that supplies oxygen to the organ of Corti.

Eighth Cranial Nerve and Central Auditory Pathways

Ring around the rosie.
Pocket full of posies.

There are few of us who haven't sung the song, "Ring Around the Rosie." But what exactly is a "rosie"? And for that matter, what are "posies"? When you're a child, you can get by, with using words that you don't really know what they mean, but when it comes to explaining the transmission of sound to a patient, it sure helps if you know what you're talking about. Listen up. The fibers of the eighth (auditory) nerve enter the cochlea through the center of the cochlear spiral.

Most (95%) of these afferent fibers (e.g., going from the cochlea to brain) approach the closest inner hair cells to form a one-to-one connection (about 20 fibers per hair cell). The remaining 5% of these fibers travel across the organ of Corti turning down the cochlea toward the base to connect with groups of outer hair cells. There, each fiber may be connected to approximately 20 to 50 OHCs, and each outer hair cell may receive processes from approximately 20 afferent fibers. Obviously, given the disparity in the pattern of innervation for these two types of hair cells, their behavior could be quite different. It would appear that most of the sensory information going to the brain would originate from the inner hair cells and very little from the outer hair cells.

A small number of the fibers in the eighth nerve are efferent (e.g., sending impulses from the brain to the cochlea). These fibers arise from neurons whose cell bodies are located in the brainstem, mostly on the side opposite from the ear to which they travel. For now, however, we focus our attention on the 95% of fibers connecting the IHCs to the eighth cranial nerve.

The neural transduction process occurs at the synapse lying between the IHC and dendrites of the auditory neurons. Thus, biochemical activity is changed to neural activity at this connection. There are two phases of activity at this connection point. One is excitatory, which means that there is an increase in the release of neurotransmitter substance at the synapse. The other is inhibitory, which means there is a reduction in the neurotransmitter substance at the synapse. The dendritic connection is sensitive to the amount of neurotransmitter substance and the nerve fiber "fires" when there is enough there is enough of the neurotransmitter substance present at the synapse. Once the fiber "fires" there is a chain reaction along the axon through the auditory pathway from the eighth cranial nerve all the way to the cochlear nucleus of the brainstem. The brain codes these "spikes" in neural activity patterns as changes in intensity and frequency of sound. This is shown in Figure 3–10.

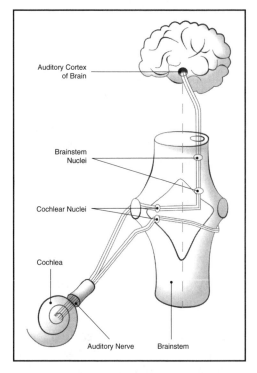

Figure 3–10. A schematic of the various subcoritcal and cortical neural centers that comprise the auditory pathway from the cochlea to the temporal lobe. From *INTRO: A Guide to Communication Sciences and Disorders.* By Michael P. Robb. Copyright © 2010 Plural Publishing, Inc. All rights reserved. Used with permission, p. 78.

Balance Function

Baa baa black sheep
Have you any wool
Yes sir, yes sir
Three bags full

None of us are too sure why the black sheep had three (not two or four) bags of wool, but it makes good sense why we have three semicircular canals.

Not just an organ of hearing, the inner ear is also responsible for maintaining your balance. The three semicircular canals and vestibule are responsible for this function. Collectively, this series of canals keep you aware of your position (lateral, vertical, or horizontal) in space as you move in different directions. The vestibule and semicircular canals share the same perilymph and endolymph found in the cochlea, which we discussed earlier.

Because of this close relationship between the cochlea and the semi circular canals it should be of no surprise to you that disorders of hearing and disorders of balance sometimes go hand in hand, as many hearing disorders are accompanied by balance-related problems. Therefore, questions related to vertigo and dizziness are always part of a good audiologic case history. In fact, some audiologists who specialize in this area see patients more patients with balance problems than they do with hearing problems.

A common type of dizziness that originates in the vestibular organs of the inner ear is called vertigo. Vertigo is usually described by patients as a sensation of the "room spinning." The balance system is quite complex and even a cursory review of it is beyond the scope of this text. For now, it's good to remember that the balance system is comprised of the peripheral vestibular organs of the inner ear, the visual system as well as the proprioceptive system. These systems are integrated with the brainstem, cerebellum, and cerebral cortex to maintain a person's balance.

Frequently Asked Questions About "How the Ear Works"

The final section of this chapter will help you integrate your burgeoning knowledge of the cochlea into the daily practice of fitting hearing aids. It will at least get you started by reviewing some of the important concepts that you will encounter often. Just like your favorite children's song you can memorize these basic principles next time you are playing (studying) with friends.

How Does the Cochlea Analyze Sound?

Let's go back to the traveling wave theory. If you haven't yet read the chapter on acoustics (Chapter 2) you may be asking, "What wave are you talking about, and why does it travel?" Don't worry. These concepts are pretty straightforward. It's important to address this topic here for one important reason: It is the damaged cochlea's inability to precisely amplify sound that gives you the primary reason to fit hearing aids on most of the patients you will see.

Remember that the basilar membrane of the cochlea is finely tuned to different frequencies. Tonotopic means that specific parts of the cochlea are more sensitive to specific frequencies or pitches of sound.

Recall that the base of the cochlea, which is narrow and stiff, is tuned to high-frequency sounds. The apex of the cochlea, which is wide and heavier, is tuned to low-frequency sounds. In other words, high-frequency sound waves primarily stimulate the base of the cochlea whereas low-frequency sound waves primarily stimulate the apex of the cochlea. This tuning is shown in Figure 3–11. Georg von Békésy

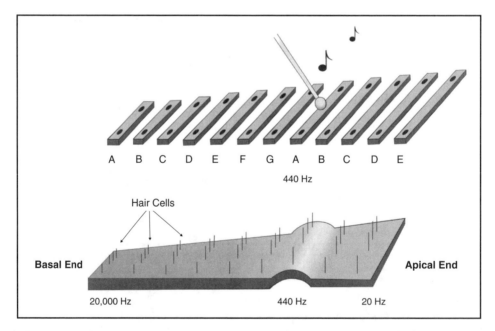

Figure 3–11. A drawing of the cochlea showing its tonotopic arrangement. Note that the base is tuned to high-frequency sounds and the apex is tuned to low-frequency sounds. From *INTRO: A Guide to Communication Sciences and Disorders.* By Michael P. Robb. Copyright © 2010 Plural Publishing, Inc. All rights reserved. Used with permission, p. 77.

first theorized the concept of the traveling wave in the 1950s through his work with cadavers. (Gruesome yes, but keep in mind, the cochlea was, at that time, completely inaccessible in the living.) Besides, he was nobody's ghoul; in 1961 von Békésy was awarded the Nobel Prize for his research on the traveling wave.

From his observations, von Békésy believed that the cochlea was passive, rather than sharply tuned (remember, he was working with *cadavers*). In other words, he believed that the acuity of human hearing ability did not occur in the cochlea; rather, he attributed all fine-tuning to central nervous pathways located higher-up in the system. The cochlea was thought to function as a simple sound transmitter, sending auditory information along to wherever it would be "amplified" by the auditory nervous system. Although von Békésy was a brilliant scientist, in this case he was mostly wrong.

OHCs at Work

Twenty-five years ago we recognized the cochlea as being a sharply tuned cochlear amplifier and more recently that the OHCs are primarily responsible for this sharp tuning. As each point along the basilar membrane is precisely tuned to a specific sound frequency, the OHCs located at that point are equally sensitive to that same specific sound. Through the active mechanics of the OHCs, the cochlea actually adds energy to the sound before it travels up to the brain via the auditory nerve. OHCs are an active biological amplifier, not a passive mechanical filter.

TAKE FIVE: Buff and Fluff

It is now well accepted that both the traveling wave theory and the activity of the OHCs are primarily responsible for our keen ability to detect the smallest differences in intensity and frequency. And it is this acuity that allows those of us with normal hearing ability to readily differentiate between similar speech sounds found in words like "buff" and "fluff" and pick out one voice we want to hear out of a roomful of people talking.

What Happens When Someone Has a Hearing Loss?

So far we have learned a lot about the cochlea's complexity. We've seen that it not only transmits sound to the brain's cortex via the auditory nerve, but that it also provides selective amplification to these sounds. We also know that to accomplish these incredibly intricate feats, the cochlea needs a steady blood supply while generating a stunningly awesome amount of biochemical activity. Most of us know the old adage, "the more complex something is, the more that can go wrong with it." This is also true of the human cochlea; noise exposure, infection, diet, medication, the aging process, disease, and other harmful agents can damage an otherwise healthy inner ear.

Because OHCs are the primary site of all that biomechanical activity (they move faster than any muscle in the

human body) they are the most susceptible to damage. When OHCs are damaged two important things happen:

■ There is a mild-to-moderate loss of
hearing. (which can be as great 50
to 60 dB from OHC damage)
■ The cochlea loses its ability for
sharp tuning.

When these two things occur at the
same time, people not only will notice
an inability to hear softer sounds (e.g.,
birds singing, a baby crying from
another room, the sound of their car's
turn signal, etc.) but will also complain
that they frequently miss (or misunder-
stand) words during normal conversation, even when they hear the word.
Two of the most common types of damage to the cochlea are the result of aging
(presbycusis) and exposure to high levels of sound (noise-induced hearing
loss). Both of these generally affect
OHC function, and often in similar frequency regions (typically greatest effect
in the 3000 to 8000 range, and little
effect in the 250 to 1000-Hz range).

Outnumbered by OHCs (4 to 1),
inner hair cells or IHCs are tougher and

TAKE FIVE: A Quick Guide to Essential Cochlear Anatomy and Physiology

You may pat yourself on the back if
you have just read this entire this
chapter on the anatomy and physiology of the cochlea. This is some
heavy stuff! You should now appreciate that, when you are sitting in
front of a patient trying to solve their
communication problems, you won't
need to know or regurgitate all the
details. Just take a look at the
following Quick Guide and familiarize
yourself with the key differences
between outer and inner hair cells.
Any information you retain will help to
emphasize these differences when
helping patients in the selection of
hearing instruments (Figure 3–12).

Outer Hair Cells (OHCs)

1. Shaped like a cylinder.
2. End of OHC is embedded in the
   tectorial membrane.
3. Efferent: they receive information
   from the auditory nerves of the
   lower brainstem

4. OHCs mechanically boost soft
   incoming sounds. OHCs are
   sometimes called cochlear
   amplifiers.
5. OHCs sharpen the peaking of
   the traveling wave.
6. OHC damage results in up to
   60 dB hearing loss.

Inner Hair Cells (IHCs)

1. Shaped like a flask.
2. Do not touch the tectorial
   membrane.
3. Afferent: they send information
   to the brain via the auditory
   nerves of the lower brainstem.
4. IHC damage results in severe
   hearing loss (greater than 60 dB)
   and/or very poor word understanding ability. This is because
   sound is not only reduced in
   amplitude, but even when amplitude is increased, distortions
   are present.

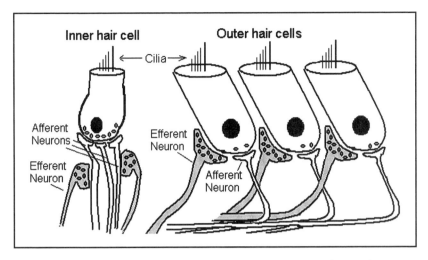

Figure 3–12. The structure of the inner hair cell (*left*) and the outer hair cells (*right*). From *The Hearing Sciences*. By Teri A. Hamill and Lloyd L. Price. Copyright © 2008 Plural Publishing, Inc. All rights reserved. Used with permission, p. 201.

more difficult to damage. However, because IHCs are directly connected to the auditory nerve, the subsequent hearing loss and distortion effects are more severe when they are damaged.

In the beginning you won't have to be too concerned whether or not the impaired hearing of your patients is the result of IHC or OHC damage. For now when the hearing loss is both sensorineural and mild-to-moderate (<50 dB HL), you can assume there is primarily OHC involvement, whereas more severe impairments (>60 dB HL) typically will involve both OHC and IHC damage.

What Are You Actually Doing When You Fit Hearing Aids?

Okay, let's stop for a moment and see how all this fits together. It is easy to get overwhelmed by all the terminology and jargon associated with cochlear mechan-

ics; you can leave most of that up to your hearing scientist friends to sort out the details. It may help if we relate cochlear mechanics to the day-to-day fitting of hearing instruments.

The cochlea is buried deep in the temporal bone of the skull right behind the pinna. Whenever someone (like you!) pushes an amplifier encased in a hard plastic shell into a patients tight, humid, waxy ear canal you apply more force (SPL) to the eardrum and ossicles (one hopes not more SPL than they were designed to absorb).

When this amplified sound eventually reaches the damaged cochlea, the boosted sound energy excites any remaining undamaged outer hair cells. The primary purpose of all hearing aids is to restore the missing sounds of soft to average speech. When more sound energy is delivered to the brain through the damaged cochlea, there is a good chance that much of the desired sounds of speech will be perceived, especially if you do your job correctly by matching the right hearing aid programming to the hearing loss. Unfortunately, normal cochlear function cannot be completely restored with amplification. Hearing aids do a great job of restoring inaudible sounds, but at this point they cannot bring back the cochlea's ability to sharpen the peaks of the traveling wave.

Why Do People with Hearing Loss Complain About Hearing in Noise?

For anyone who has spent more than a few days visiting with patients in a hearing aid office, one thing is obvious: The most frequent complaint or comment for someone with a mild-to-moderate hearing loss is an inability to understand speech in background noise. Why?

First, it is important to realize that it is hard for anyone, normal hearing or otherwise, to hear in noise. The din of a crowded restaurant often has more intensity that the typical volume of the average talker. Although talkers do raise their voice somewhat in background noise, they only stay ahead of the noise up to about 70 to 75 dB SPL (its common that background noise at parties is >80 dB SPL). Once the signal-to-noise ratio approaches 0 dB (noise = speech) even people with normal hearing have trouble understanding.

A second reason, as discussed in Chapter 2, is that speech is a very dynamic sound. It has unique distribution of intensity that is always moving and changing. There is a large range between soft speech and loud speech, low frequency energy and high frequency energy.

A third reason is that people with mild hearing loss frequently miss the softest consonant sounds of speech in noisy environments. When this occurs, speech may sound like it is loud enough, but it is not really clear or distinct. These folks can hear the hubbub of the ongoing noise, but because the damaged cochlea has lost some of its sharp tuning, it becomes difficult to accurately cue in on all the quick changes in intensity of speech, especially when it is masked or buried in a sea of noise.

Finally, many people with hearing loss are older, and the noise causes a processing confusion in the higher auditory levels of the brain. They may also have additional cognitive problems that can contribute to poor speech communication.

Are you now feeling as confused as the person trying to understand speech in background noise? For a visual analogy, think of the Where's Waldo puzzle pictures that were so popular a few years back. The task was to find the tiny Waldo figure (distinguishable mostly by his red and white striped cap) in a visual sea of bodies and activities. With normal vision it was difficult enough, but with eyes crossed or mildly blurred vision it would have been impossible. Remember that damage to the OHCs in the cochlea have eliminated the fine tuning of hearing, incoming sounds may be *louder* in noise, but they may be no more distinguishable than the red and green dots to a colorblind person.

Hearing instruments, even the high-end modern digital ones with directional technology and noise reduction, cannot correct for this problem completely enough for a hearing-impaired-patient to function as good as normal in all listening situations. Modern hearing aids with noise reduction features help soften the hubbub of background noise, keeping the sound environment more comfortable, but they still do not make one speech sound more distinct than another. They just can't sharpen those peaks. In fact, sad to say, in many well-controlled research studies, where speech-in-noise has been presented at relatively high levels, hearing-impaired participants understand no better with hearing aids than without.

Before you get too discouraged, remember, hearing aids really do help people hear better in *most* listening situations. It's just that there are no substitutions for a normally functioning healthy cochlea. That being said, you will learn in later chapters about highly specialized hearing aids on the market that take advantage of directional microphones and do a better job of helping people to hear and understand in background noise. Stay tuned, the best is yet to come.

Is Fitting the Ears with Hearing Instruments Different from Fitting the Eyes with Glasses?

This is a question your patients are bound to ask you, so we thought we'd give you the answer. The human retina, like the cochlea, is a complex sensing organ; however, *most people with vision problems have normal retinas*. Most vision problems are conductive; for example, they result when the eyeball shortens or lengthens and incoming light falls short of or overshoots the retina. Either way,

shortfall or the overshoot, near-sighted or far-sighted, may be corrected by simply refocusing the light on the retina. Once the optician is able to refocus the light through a prescriptive lens, normal vision is restored.

The job of correcting a sensorineural hearing loss never is as simple as fitting a pair of glasses. This is because, although some of our patients will have what we call a "conductive" loss of hearing (loss resulting from damage to the outer and/or middle ear), *most of the patients with hearing loss you will see will have damage to the cochlea*. For the latter, hearing instruments will not restore normal cochlear function. And it is this damage to the cochlea that makes fitting hearing aids (unlike fitting glasses) extremely challenging. Given time, you will learn that it is your knowledgeable application of what we call "compression" in a hearing instrument that will compensate for some of this irreversible damage to the cochlea.

The ants go marching one by one, hurrah, hurrah.
The ants go marching one by one, hurrah, hurrah.

Those are some pretty easy lyrics to remember!

Table 3–1 summarizes all the transduction processes that occur in the peripheral auditory system. And yes, it's a little more complicated than remembering the words to your favorite children's song. For those who want more details we encourage you to pick up a copy of Kramer's text, *Audiology: Science to Practice* published by Plural in 2008. It is filled with details on the subject of auditory physiology and it is highly readable.

Table 3–1. Summary of the Auditory Transduction Processes and Their Related Locations, Mechanisms, and Functions

Process	Part of Ear	Structures	Mechanism	Function
Acoustic	Outer	Auricle; ear canal	Resonance	Amplify mid to high frequencies to overcome impedance mismatch
Mechanic	Middle	Tympanic membrane; ossicles; oval window	Area, lever, and curved membrane advantages; route vibrations to oval window	Amplify low to mid frequencies to overcome impedance mismatch
Hydro-mechanic	Cochlea	Oval and round windows; scalae	Reciprocal in and out movements of oval and round windows	Instantaneous pressure variations in fluid-filled cochlea
		Basilar membrane	**Passive Process:** Traveling wave dependent on width and stiffness gradients of basilar membrane	Tonotopic place principle; Highs at base and lows at apex; produces broad tuning curves.
		Tectorial and basilar membranes; Stereocilia	Bends stereocilia back and forth due to different pivot points of the two membranes; controls K+ flow into OHCs and IHCs.	Activates hair cells; towards modiolus = excitation; away from modiolus = inhibition
Chemical-motoric	Cochlea	OHCs	**Active Process:** OHC motility, from fluctuation in K+ flow, adds displacement to traveling wave to allow direct bending of IHC stereocilia.	Increases sensitivity and sharpens tuning; responsible for sharp tip region of tuning curves
Chemical-neural	Cochlea	IHCs	Increase and decrease of intracellular potential resulting from fluctuation in K+ flow.	Controls release of neurotransmitter substance
Neural	8th Nerve	Auditory nerve fibers	Uptake of neurotransmitter substance; if adequate, cells initiates all or none discharges down 8th nerve axons to cells in cochlear nucleus.	Neural discharge patterns provide intensity and frequency information to central nervous system.

Source: Audiology: Science to Practice by Steven Kramer, copyright © 2008. Plural Publishing Inc. All rights reserved. Used with permission, p. 95.

In Closing

This chapter provides a minimal overview of ear anatomy and physiology. We recommend that you dig deeper into the topic by adding a couple of other books to your professional library. Affectionately known as the "Zemlin book" and the "Pickles book," *Speech and Hearing Science* by Zemlin and *An Introduction to the Physiology of Hearing* by Pickles are two classics. Another Plural book that has an excellent review chapter on applied ear physiology is, *Basics of Audiology: From Vibrations to Sounds* by Jerry Cranford.

Now that you've become more familiar with the properties of sound and the basic function of the auditory system, it's time to switch our focus to clinical audiology and hearing disorders in the next couple of chapters. Before you turn the page, however, we hope you have a better appreciation of how all landmarks in the auditory system are interconnected. It may not be as simple to learn as that classic children's song about anatomy, but you should now have a clearer picture of how each part of the ear works in harmony to transduce sound.

If you're happy and you know it clap your hands
If you're happy and you know it clap your hands
If you're happy and you know it, your face will surely show it
If you're happy and you know it clap your hands

Measurement of Hearing

> *Nothing really goes better with the measurement of hearing than a few good movie quotes!*

May the Force be with you.
> Harrison Ford, *Star Wars Episode IV*

We're not certain if Irish scientist Robert Boyle had the "Force," or if he ever was in a movie, but he also had a memorable quote:

If you want to improve something, you first have to measure it.

Boyle is the scientist who discovered the inverse relationship between the pressure and volume of a gas, which explains the relationship between ear canal volume and sound pressure level. During Sir Robert's laboratory experiments he also discovered that to better understand something you first have to measure it. This concept certainly holds true for hearing care professionals because when we take the time to accurately measure hearing, we better understand how a hearing loss affects communication.

The aim of this chapter is to familiarize you with the basic procedures of the hearing test battery, help you understand why each test needs to be completed, and how to do each test in an accurate and efficient manner. Our focus is on testing that is conducted during the initial prefitting evaluation before we have determined if the patient is a hearing aid candidate. This basic test battery is designed to identify the type and degree of hearing loss. There are other more advanced tests that we also will mention; however, these tests typically are conducted by a clinical audiologists as part of a complete diagnostic exam.

Before tackling the basic test battery, we'll first introduce you to the all important audiogram, and its cousin, the audiometer. You have probably had a chance to at least press the "power on" switch for the audiometer, so now is the time for a test drive and to start learning about the essential skills you need to actually use it. This chapter focuses on how to conduct a complete and accurate hearing test. It's designed to supplement any hands-on experience you receive during a clinical practicum or apprenticeship program. But, before getting started, let's review two important lessons.

Lesson #1:
You Must Master Five
Core Clinical Skills

1. Otoscopy
2. Pure-Tone Air Conduction Audiometry
3. Pure-Tone Bone Conduction Audiometry
4. Speech Audiometry
5. Effective Masking

The main point is that knowing just a couple of these is not enough. All five of these core skills are interconnected and sometimes serve as a cross-check of another. *Primum non nocere* is a Latin phrase that means "First, do no harm." Since at least 1860, it has been one of the principal precepts all medical students are taught in medical school. We mention it here, as conducting this testing incorrectly easily could lead to erroneous results, which easily could lead to an inappropriate hearing aid fitting. More importantly, glaring mistakes in the test results could lead to life-altering, or even life-threatening consequences for the patient.

Once you have mastered all five skills you will be able to effectively test any cooperative adult arriving at your office. This will take time, and hands-on practice, but you must put in the time to learn. That leads to the second essential preliminary lesson.

Lesson #2:
Technique Counts.
Never Compromise It

The absolute importance of using a standardized technique for these five core skills cannot be emphasized enough. This is because you will conduct these tests on virtually every patient you see in your office. In fact, you cannot complete the job of fitting hearing aids unless you do these tests efficiently. The application of a consistent technique is important for a number of reasons. Most importantly, using a consistent test technique allows you to be efficient and accurate. The test techniques we'll discuss below are all field-tested and accepted by all licensed hearing instrument specialists and audiologists worldwide. In short, you must know these techniques. Last, there is no substitute for direct hands-on learning of these core skills.

Because these skills cannot be learned completely simply by reading a book, they are presented here in a cookbook manner. You can think of the audiometer and otoscope as your kitchen appliances. That makes you the chef, and it's going to be more difficult than boiling water. Like any gourmet chef there is some minimal training required before you can make a complicated dish. In the case of conducting a hearing test, there are a few prerequisite skills you need to master before you start, and unless you're Emeril, you need a good recipe. We've put together some good recipes for you; so let's get started making our first dish.

Otoscopy

Before you grab an otoscope and peek into someone's ear, it is important to be familiar with the basic anatomy of the outer and middle ear. We discussed that in Chapter 3, so if you need a review, now is the time to go back and look things over again. Remember, that the external ear canal is a sensitive area; therefore you need to be gentle in your approach.

Equipment

The otoscope, as shown in Figure 4–1, is like a magnifying flashlight. Otoscopes consist of a handle and a head. The head contains an electric light source and a low power magnifying lens. The front end of the otoscope has an attachment for disposable plastic ear speculums. Specula come in several different sizes. The size that you use should correspond to the size of the patient's ear canal. If the patient is a child, a small-diameter speculum should be used; for large adult ear canals a larger size is necessary. You don't have to worry too much about this, as the standard size will work for most adults.

Many models have a detachable sliding rear window which allows the examiner to insert instruments through the otoscope into the ear canal, such as tools for removing earwax.

Otoscopes come in a large variety of styles and sizes. They, of course, also vary significantly in cost, ranging from a disposable otoscope for under $10 to the common Welch-Allyn clinical models in the $100 to $200 range. Some are wall mounted (which makes them easier to find in a busy office), whereas others are portable. Wall-mounted otoscopes are attached by a flexible power cord to a base, which serves to hold the otoscope when it's not in use and also serves as a source of electric power, being plugged into an electric outlet. Portable models are powered by batteries in the handle; these batteries usually are rechargeable and can be recharged from a base unit.

In addition to or instead of traditional otoscopy, it's possible to use video otoscopy, an otoscope attached to a video monitor to that the observations can be easily observed and stored. Recent surveys have shown that about 50% of dispensing offices use this equipment. One of the pioneers of the use of this equipment is Roy Sullivan, Ph.D. and a wealth of information regarding its use is available at his Web site: http://www.rcsullivan.com

Advantage of Video Otoscopy

There are several advantages to using this equipment. First, it is much easier to visualize minor abnormalities on the large video screen than when using the traditional hand-held otoscope. Secondly, the patient is able to see what you see. If there is something abnormal (e.g., an ear canal plugged with cerumen), this assists greatly in counseling. Sometimes, after using hearing aids, new users develop pressure sores in the ear canal, these also may be visible. A second advantage is that the "view" of the patient's ear canal and eardrum can be printed for part of their permanent record. This is useful for follow-up visits, or if you refer the patient for medical care, they

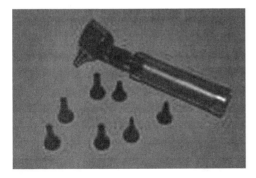

Figure 4–1. A typical otoscope along with several different sizes of speculums.

can take a photo of their ear along to their primary physician or otolaryngologist. There are several video otoscopes on the market. A good place to investigate your options is http://www.med rx-usa.com and http://www.welchal lyn.com

General Purpose

Otoscopy is the process of visually observing the ear canal and eardrum with the otoscope. Unlike physicians who use otoscopy to diagnose many ear disorders, we primarily rely on otoscopy to ensure that the ear canal is not obstructed prior to completing the hearing test.

The complete otoscopic examination, however, is more than simply looking into the ear canal. Before even picking up the otoscope from the table, it is important to carefully look at the outer ear (pinna) and the mastoid process behind the ear (Figure 4–2). Signs of previous ear surgery and other malformations should be noted.

Before placing the speculum into the ear canal, it's important to inform the patient of what you're going to do. The instruction would go something like this:

I'm going to use this special magnifying light to look into your ear. It might feel just a little uncomfortable, but it shouldn't hurt. Please hold real still while I take a peak. I just need to see what the inside of your ear canal and eardrum looks like.

After you complete this procedure briefly explain what you saw to the patient. For example, "You ear canal is clear, it looks normal." Show them on

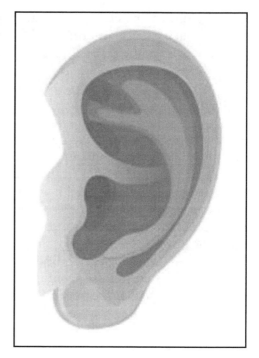

Figure 4–2. The normal adult pinna.

the video otoscope what it looks like, or use a picture of a normal eardrum as a reference.

Examination Process: Step-by-Step

After you have visually observed the outer ear and mastoid process, and noted its appearance, pick up the otoscope (Figure 4–3).

1. Turn it on and set it to maximum brightness.
2. Place the largest size speculum (ear tip) appropriate for the patient's ear gently into the opening of the ear canal.
3. Hold the otoscope like a pencil with the lighted end about where the tip of the pencil would be.

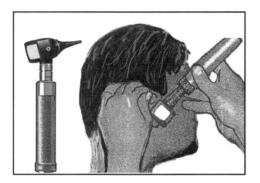

Figure 4–3. The proper way to hold an otoscope when conducting an otoscopic examination. From *Basics of Audiology* by Jerry Cranford, © 2008 Plural Publishing Inc. Used with permission. All rights reserved, p. 58.

Face the light toward the patient's ear canal opening.

4. Place both hands (one still has the otoscope) up to the patient's ear along the patients' face. It is important to use both hands. This technique, called bracing, will prevent the speculum from scraping the ear canal, if the patient moves suddenly. It is important that you are on the same plane as the patient. If the patient is seated, you should be seated right next to him.

5. The posterior (back) portion of the pinna should be gently pulled up and back in order to straighten the ear canal. While you are pulling back on the pinna with one hand, place the tip of the otoscope into the open ear canal. Look into the ear.

6. The first thing that should be noted is the condition of the external ear canal. Are there excessive amounts of cerumen?

The normal ear canal should be smooth and pinkish in appearance. Scratches, blood, redness, and excessive wetness are all signs of an abnormality.

7. As you continue looking into the ear canal (which might require turning the speculum at a slightly different angle), at the end of the canal you will see the tympanic membrane, commonly called the eardrum. Don't worry, both terms are acceptable. The eardrum should be a light gray color and very shiny. The cone of light, your most important visual landmark, should be clearly visible on the bottom half. Also, note the other landmarks present such as the malleus and the annular ligament. The condition of the eardrum should always be noted on your history form. Some of the most obvious examples of abnormal TMs can be viewed at the Web site we cite below.

TIPS and TRICKS:
Learn from the Photos

Okay we know you're having fun reading all this, but to fully understand how the eardrum looks, what is normal and what isn't, you need to look at some good color photos. Go to the Web site of Roy Sullivan that we mentioned earlier: http://www.rcsullivan.com. Scroll to the portion of the opening page where Dr. Sullivan has provided examples of the normal earcanal and eardrum, and many different kinds of abnormalities. Take some time to view these excellent photos.

The Hearing Test Battery

Well, it's not really a battery like you would find in your car or cell phone, and we certainly hope it's not the kind of *battery* that means injury to someone! When we do a group of tests we call it a battery, probably derived from the days when different artillery pieces were aligned in a battery. Let's hope your "battles" with this section will be minimal.

When you test someone's hearing in order to obtain a complete picture of the way their ear works, you must do a series of tests. This series of tests complement each other. In a short while, you will be able to look at the results of a hearing test battery and explain the amount and the type of hearing loss. Right now, let's learn how to do the hearing test battery, step by step.

The Audiometer and the Pure-Tone Audiogram

Toto, I've got a feeling we're not in Kansas anymore.

Judy Garland, *The Wizard of Oz*

When you first sit down behind an audiometer, you might get the sense,

like Dorothy, that you're not in Kansas anymore. But we're here to help.

Before learning how to complete a basic hearing test, it's time to get formally introduced to the pure-tone audiometer. Without a doubt the audiometer is your most essential tool. It is the instrument you will use to measure a patient's ability to hear. The audiometer is a sound generator producing pure tones (and other signals we'll talk about later) that you will present at various frequencies and intensity levels to establish hearing thresholds.

The typical audiometer used in a dispensing practice will have an output for air conduction, bone conduction and speech, the ability to have either pulsed or warble pure tones, and a variety of different masking noises (e.g., narrowband, white noise, and speech noise). Figure 4–4 shows an example of a commonly used clinical audiometer. There is a frequency selection dial and a hearing level dial (often referred to as an attenuator) for selecting the intensity level. Some audiometers are PC-based, and actually may not have a "dial" for some of these functions. There also is a talk-forward/talk-back feature that allows you to talk to the patient through the earphones, and also hear what the patient is saying using a

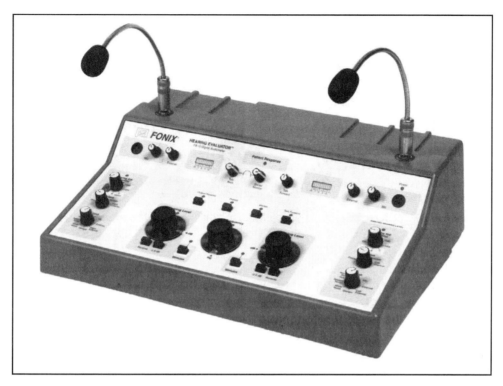

Figure 4–4. A standard clinical audiometer. Photo reprinted with the permission of Frye Electronics, Inc., Tigard, OR.

monitor microphone. It is best to have a "two channel" audiometer, which means that different input signals and intensities can be delivered independently (e.g., speech from one channel, noise from the other, both delivered to the same ear).

TAKE FIVE:
Many Shapes and Sizes

Audiometers come in all shapes and sizes (see Figure 4–4). Some are stand-alone, quite large, and cover a desktop. Others are computer-based audiometers that allow you to use your laptop to test someone's hearing. There are even hand-held audiometers. One can be viewed at http://www.otovation.com

---

About Earphones

An essential component to conducting air-conduction testing is the earphones (Figure 4–5). The selection of earphones is critical, as these earphones are part of the calibration of your audiometer. And, yes, earphones are color coded: red for right and blue for left. Historically, the most commonly used earphones have been the Telephonics supra-aural TDH-series (e.g., Model 39, Model 49P, etc.). These earphones are attached to a rubber cushion and are calibrated in a 6-cc coupler. The earphones are held in place using headband designed with a specific tension. Care must be taken to ensure that these earphones are placed correctly on the ear, or invalid thresholds can be obtained (e.g., typically worse than the correct

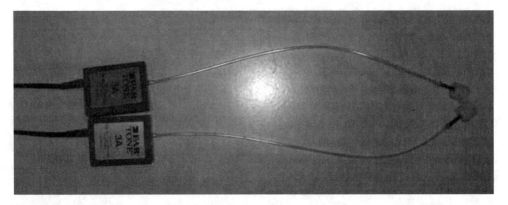

Figure 4–5. A pair of Etymotic Research 3A earphones with standard adult foam eartips.

thresholds for the higher frequencies). Also, if the tension is not correct, thresholds also may be elevated, and sounds are more prone to leak around the head.

An additional limitation of this traditional earphone style is that the pressure of the earphone placement can cause the ear canal to push together or "collapse," which will act as an earplug and elevate hearing thresholds (particularly in the higher frequencies).

For the reasons just discussed, the preferred earphones for audiometric testing are called "insert earphones," most commonly used are those from Etymotic Research (e.g., ER-3A; go to http://www.etymotic.com for an example). Figure 4–5 shows ER-3A earphones. With this type of earphone, the signal

---

TIPS and TRICKS: Calibration Is Key

It is critical that audiometers are calibrated, and that they meet the ANSI 3.66 standards. This service usually is conducted annually by regional equipment specialists. This calibration and supporting documentation is important to ensure accurate test results, and of course is examined very closely when medical-legal actions regarding hearing loss are involved. Don't try to save a few bucks and put off this important maintenance. Biologic calibration also is important. The operation of your audiometer should be checked daily before it is used for any audiometric testing with patients. This is most easily accomplished by conducting air-conduction testing for someone with known stable hearing. Any deviation of more than 5 dB from known thresholds would be cause for concern. If you work in a small office, where there are not many others to test, you can have your own hearing tested. Then, even if no one else is available for assistance, you can use yourself as a reference to ensure that the output of the earphones is correct. During this testing, also listen carefully to ensure that no distortions or unwanted noises from the earphones are present.

is taken from the receiver box (clipped on to the patient clothes) via a tube, which then terminates in a foam plug (similar to what you have used for hearing protection). This foam plug is "rolled down," and then inserted into the ear canal. These earphones are calibrated in a 2-cc coupler, just like hearing aids, which helps a little when conversion between the two is needed.

Advantage of Inserts

There are several advantages of insert earphones compared to the older TDH styles:

- Improved interaural attenuation (less sound leaking to other ear around the head).
- Improved patient comfort (the tight fitting headband of the TDH earphones is very uncomfortable for some patients)
- Improved infection control (the foam tips are designed for one-time use and are discarded following testing)
- Better attenuation of ambient room noise
- Elimination of collapsed canal
- Increased reliability due to better placement

TAKE FIVE: Simulations

Thanks to the wonders of the Internet, you can now download a virtual audiometer simulator. If you do not have a real audiometer to practice with, this one is an excellent substitute. You can use this simulation to gain some much needed hands-on experience prior to testing your first patient. Currently, we know of at least two audiometer simulators available on the Web for purchase. Go to http://www.audsim.com or http://www.innoforce.com to learn more about them.

Air Conduction Testing

As discussed in Chapter 3, we perceive sounds in two different ways. Sound either can be transmitted via sound waves in the air through the outer ear (ear canal to the eardrum), through the middle ear and to the inner ear (cochlea), or directly to the cochlea via bone conduction. When testing a patient's hearing using the air conductive pathway of sound from the outer to the inner ear we use earphones and perform what is termed "air conduction audiometry." The pure tone or speech stimulus that you introduce via the earphones travels through the outer ear and middle ears, to the inner ear, then along the eighth nerve, the brainstem and finally to the auditory cortex of the brain where it is perceived. Sounds arriving at the auditory cortex via the *entire* auditory system can be classified as air conduction stimuli. Almost all sounds we hear start their journey through the ear as an air conducted sound (Figure 4–6).

Bone Conduction Testing

When we deliver pure tones or speech signals by placing a bone conduction

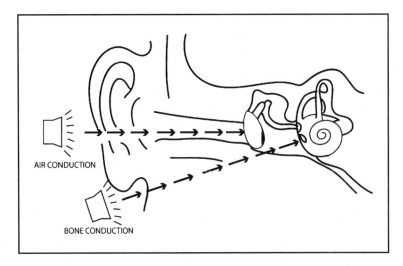

AIR CONDUCTION

BONE CONDUCTION

Figure 4–6. The pathway sounds takes to ear via air conduction and bone conduction. Note how the bone conduction pathway bypasses the structures of the middle ear and directly vibrates the entire skull, which is then transferred to the fluid contents of the cochlea. From *Basics of Audiology* by Jerry Cranford, © 2008 Plural Publishing Inc. Used with permission. All rights reserved, p. 68.

oscillator directly on the mastoid bone behind the ear (or on the forehead) we are bypassing the outer and middle ear structures. A properly placed oscillator literally vibrates the bones of the skull stimulating neural activity in the cochlea, then on to the auditory cortex via the eighth or auditory nerve and the brainstem auditory centers. These vibrations directly move the structures of the inner ear and allow us to eventually perceive sound in the exactly the same way we perceived the air conducted signal.

During a routine hearing test, we usually conduct different procedures in which either air conducted or bone conducted sounds are presented to the ears. Comparing air and bone conduction thresholds helps us to determine the site of lesion of the hearing loss. Site of lesion testing tells us very important information about where the problem contributing to the hearing loss lies: the outer, middle, or inner ear. For example, if person has a significant loss by air conduction, but excellent hearing by bone conduction, we know that the problem must lie in either the outer or middle ear. On the other hand, if the results indicate that air conduction and bone conduction thresholds are exactly the same, we can assume that the problem is at the cochlea, or a more medial location.

Physicians and the medical community are particularly interested in hearing loss resulting from problems in the outer or middle ear. These usually are treatable, either by prescription drugs or by surgery. As hearing health care providers, we primarily are involved with hearing loss resulting from damage to the inner ear or cochlea, as this type of hearing loss does not usually respond to prescriptions or surgery, and the use of hearing aids often is the only treatment.

The Audiogram

There are very few things in life as common as the audiogram (if you spend your time in a hearing dispensing office!). Despite the fact that it's upside down to most people, it is the graph nearly every professional around the globe uses to plot the type and degree of hearing loss—we briefly introduced you to this chart in Chapter 2. The audiogram tells us the threshold of hearing for a series of frequencies we present to the patient during a routine hearing test. Threshold is a measure of sensitivity and corresponds to the softest sound a person hears half the time it is presented. Yes, believe it or not there actually is a scientific way to find out when a person is hearing something 50% of the time; you will learn all about this shortly.

Getting to Know the Symbols

The audiogram and its symbols have been around for decades. Instead of spending time on their origins, let's just say that most symbols on the audiogram are internationally recognized to stand for *something*. An audiogram should have a key on it describing what each symbol represents. Over the years several different types of forms and symbols have been used. For example, we happen to prefer to put the right and left ear results on different audiograms displayed side by side, as we find this easier to interpret and less messy. Others simply write the thresholds in rows, no graphing, symbols, or audiogram per se at all.

But, like most things, it's usually best to go along with some type of consensus. We have that for audiometric symbols, and they are shown in Figure 4–7.

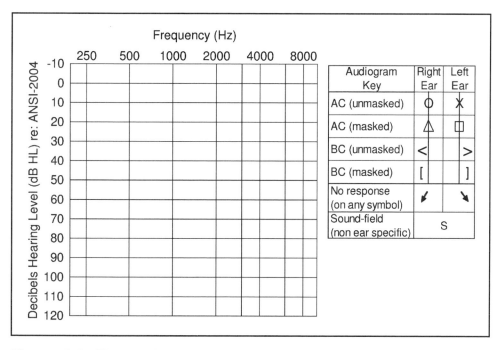

Figure 4–7. The standard audiogram and symbols for air and bone conduction testing. From *Audiology: Science to Practice* by Steven Kramer. © 2008 Plural Publishing, Inc. All rights reserved. Used with permission, p. 138.

This chart of standard symbols is from the American Speech-Language-Hearing Association (ASHA). If you'd like to read more about the history, you can find the original document posted at http://www.asha.org/docs/html/GL2005-00014.html#r6 . We recognize that this lengthy address is probably more typing than you may care to do; a quick Google search on "audiometric symbols" should do the job. It's a good article to print and keep in your files for reference.

The "Normal" Audiogram

Let's get started with a normal audiogram, shown in Figure 4–8. You will notice on this audiogram that the "O" denotes the right ear and the "X" represents the left ear. We have handwritten the symbols on the audiogram to add an element of realism, even though we know many clinicians now record perfect X's and O's with the aid of their computerized audiometer. As Robert Boyle didn't have a computer when he

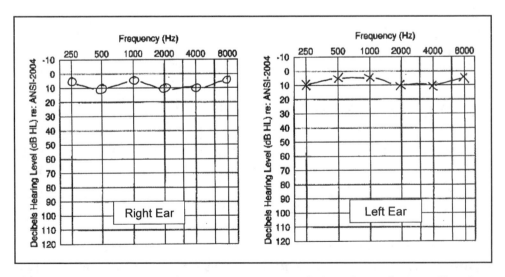

Figure 4–8. An example of normal hearing recorded on the audiogram. Note how all the thresholds are between 0 and 20 db HL in this example.

made his contributions to science, we figured we didn't need to rely on one either! As mentioned earlier, historically the right ear is displayed in red, and the left ear is displayed in blue, although if a person cannot tell the difference between a black "O" and "X," we might question if they really are qualified to interpret an audiogram in the first place (see our "Take Five" on this topic). These two symbols, regardless of color, are what we use for plotting air conducted sounds. The other thing you should notice is that in this case, all the symbols are at the top of the audiogram, between 0 and 20 dB HL. If the symbols representing the left and right ear are between 0 and 20 dB the hearing thresholds are considered normal.

Also notice that there are six X's and O's plotted on the audiogram. Each of these six symbols represent a discrete frequency is which sound is presented. Recall from prior chapters that the ear is tonotopically arranged. The audiogram represents the sensitivity of a relatively wide range of the cochlea by displaying sounds at six discrete octaves. For simplicity in this example, we have only used six key frequencies. In most cases, however, you will also want to do testing at other frequencies. For example, thresholds at both 1500 and 3000 Hz often are helpful in the programming of hearing aids.

TIPS and TRICKS: When to Test Extra Frequencies

There is no hard-fast rule when to test 1500 and 3000 Hz. Some might say "always," others may say "never," and most will say, "whenever the thresholds of the octave frequencies differ by X dB or more." What is X? Because these frequencies are important for fitting hearing aids, we say, "whenever the difference is greater than 10 dB."

The next set of essential symbols you need to know represent the threshold for bone conducted sounds. As we will learn later, people with hearing loss confined to the middle or outer ear have normal inner ear thresholds. In the example in Figure 4–9, the patient has

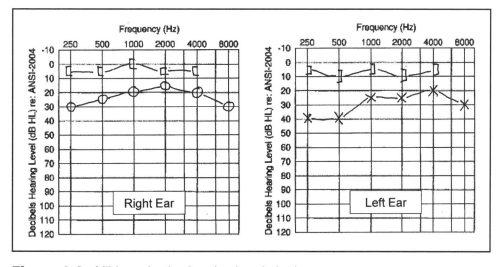

Figure 4–9. Mild conductive hearing loss in both ears.

a conductive hearing loss in the right ear. Notice now how the air-conduction symbols are around 30 to 40 dB, but the bone-conduction symbols are around 5 to 10 dB, causing a "gap" between the two symbols. This is referred to as the air-bone gap, a telltale sign of a conductive hearing loss, typically involving the middle ear.

Notice how intensity is plotted. Although, as we mentioned earlier, it might seem a little counterintuitive, the more intense sounds are found at the bottom of the audiogram. As you raise the intensity of sounds you are presenting to the patient, and lower the plotting on the audiogram, you are identifying a hearing loss of greater degree. Once you get a little practice with audiogram symbols and shapes we encourage you to visit this Web site where you can complete some interactive audiogram exercises (http://www.audstudent.com). This Web site has a wealth of information on understanding audiograms.

Audiogram Shapes

Mama always said life was like a box of chocolates. You never know what you're gonna get.

Tom Hanks, *Forrest Gump*

Like a box of chocolates, audiograms have quite the variety. Just like the shape of someone's body might tell you a little about their lifestyle, or at least their eating habits, the shape of someone's audiogram can tell you a lot about the status of their ears (and maybe a little about their lifestyle, too). There are two broad classifications of audiogram shapes: flat and sloping.

A sloping audiogram means the degree of hearing loss is much greater in one frequency region than another, highs versus lows. Typically, the hearing loss is greater in the high frequencies compared to the lows. Figure 4–10 is an example of downward sloping (high frequency) hearing loss. Notice that as the frequency becomes higher, more sound pressure (intensity) is

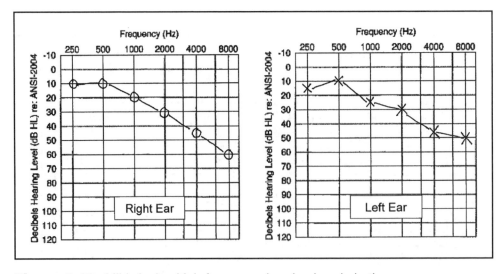

Figure 4–10. Mild sloping high-frequency hearing loss in both ears.

needed to reach threshold. On the other hand, a flat hearing loss means that all the thresholds fall right around the same intensity level. As you'll learn in Chapter 5, sloping and flat losses can sometimes help determine the origin of hearing disorders.

Now that we are on the subject of shapes, it's a good time to introduce to you some other important shapes and terms you will need to know.

- Symmetric Hearing Loss: Hearing loss is similar in both ears (usually 10 to 15 dB at all frequencies).
- Asymmetric Hearing Loss: One ear is significantly different than another (usually 20 dB or more) for a range of frequencies. Pay attention to these, as most "routine" patients will have a symmetrical loss.
- Flat: Relatively equal hearing loss (within 20 dB or so) across frequencies 500 to 4000 Hz.
- Gradually Sloping: Hearing loss becomes progressively, but gradually worse as the frequencies become higher.
- Presbycusic: General pattern of a gradually downward-sloping hearing loss, observed in older individuals
- Precipitously Sloping (ski slope): Hearing loss becomes rapidly worse as frequencies become higher (e.g., change of 20 dB per octave).
- Reverse Slope: Significant hearing loss in lower frequencies with hearing loss becoming better (or normal) in higher frequencies.
- Noise Notch: Normal or relatively normal hearing in the low and mid range, with a hearing loss in the 3000 to 6000 range, and then improved thresholds for 8000 Hz.

- Cookie-Bite: Normal or near-normal hearing in the low frequencies, a significant loss in the 1000 to 4000-Hz range, then returning to normal or near-normal in the high frequencies (when plotted, gives appearance that a "bite" has been taken out of normal hearing).
- Corner Audiogram: Hearing loss in the very low frequencies, with no measurable hearing in the higher frequencies (the entire audiogram is plotted in the "lower-left corner" of the audiogram.

Pure-Tone Air Conduction Audiometry

Now that you have gained some familiarity with how sound is conducted through the human ear, and how it's recorded on the audiogram, let's begin to learn more specifically how to measure it with pure-tone audiometry. The accepted procedure for determining threshold is called the Hughson-Westlake procedure. It's been used for more than 50 years, and is casually known as the "Up 5, Down 10" procedure. It is outlined step-by-step on the next page.

Purpose

Virtually every patient you see will need a hearing test, and the basic test is air conduction threshold testing using pure tones. The preciseness of these measures is critical. In addition to assuring that no medical attention is needed, these thresholds will be used later to program the hearing instruments. Invalid thresholds leads to invalid programming, and ultimately, an unhappy hearing aid user (or maybe a *nonuser!*)

Equipment

A calibrated audiometer with the appropriate earphones is needed.

Equipment Preparation:
1. Turn the audiometer on.
2. Be sure that you can identify and operate all the important components of the audiometer needed for air conduction testing:
   a. Power switch
   b. Output selection: Right or left ear
   c. Input: Pure tone
   d. Frequency selector: 250 to 8000 Hz
   e. Hearing level (HL) dial: −10 to 120 dB HL
   f. Tone presentation bar
   g. Talk-over system: Allows the tester to talk to the patient through the earphones
   h. Talk-back system: Allows the tester to hear the patient
3. Set Channel 1 to tone and to the desired ear. Start with the right ear, unless you know that the patient's hearing is significantly better in the left ear.
4. Set the frequency selector to 1000 Hz and the tone presentation (hearing level dial) to 40 dB.
5. Make sure that both the talk-over and talk-back are set at the appropriate loudness.

Instructions to the Patient

After I place these phones in your ears, please listen for the soft beeping sounds and press the button (raise hand) each time you think you hear the tones. Listen carefully for the quiet sounds way off in the distance. It's okay to press the button (raise your hand) even if you are not sure. I will begin the test in your right ear. Do you have any questions?

Standard Procedure

1. The patient should be seated so he is not looking directly at you, or the dials of the audiometer.
2. The response mode depends on the individual being tested and the personal preference of the tester. Either ask the patient to raise his hand when he hears the tone, or push a button when he hears the tone. You may also ask the patient to say "yes" when he hears the tone.
3. Place the earphones on the patient. Hair should be pushed away from the ear canals. If using the older supra-aural earphones glasses, hearing aids, and earrings must be removed before placing the headphones on. The red earphone is placed on the right ear and the blue ear phone is placed on the left ear. (If you are using traditional headphones, make sure the diaphragm of each phone is placed so that it is centered directly over the ear canal of both ears. The headband should be tightened to ensure that the earphones do not move.)
4. Begin the test in the right ear (if you know what ear hears better, start in that ear) at 1000 Hz and 40 dB unless there is a reason to start at a louder level. This starting place is used because it is important that the first tone can be heard at a comfortable level.
5. Present the first series of beeping tones. The duration of each tone should be no more than a second.

If your audiometer has a pulsing tone presentation mode, this is preferred (200 m/sec on/off works well).

6. It is extremely important to use different time intervals between each series of tone presentations to prevent a presentation pattern that might cue the patient to respond.

7. If there is no response at the starting level of 40 dB raise the intensity 10 dB until the patient responds to the presentation of the tone.

8. As soon as a response is elicited, either at 40 dB or at the raised level, the intensity of the tone is decreased (made softer) in 10 dB steps, until no response is given. At this point, it is assumed that the level of the tone is below the patient's threshold, and threshold determination begins.

9. The intensity of the tone is raised (made louder) in 5 dB steps, until a response is again observed.

10. As soon as a response is obtained, the intensity is lowered (made softer) by 10 dB.

11. If a response is not obtained, the intensity is increased in 5 dB steps until you see a response.

12. This procedure is repeated ("down 10, up 5"). The lowest intensity level at which at least three out of six presentations produce responses is considered to be the patient's threshold.

13. The threshold is recorded on the audiogram with an "X" for the left ear and an "O" for the right ear. Record the patient's responses as neatly on the blank audiogram (Figure 4–11) as possible.

14. After obtained the threshold on one ear at 1000 Hz, stay in the

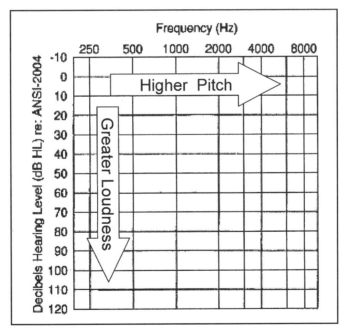

Figure 4–11. A standard blank audiogram. A visual reminder that "right" takes you to the higher frequencies and "down" represents higher intensities.

same ear and test is ascending order (2000 Hz, 4000 Hz, 8000 Hz).

15. After testing at 8000 Hz, go back and recheck the threshold at 1000 Hz. This second threshold should be at ±5 dB of the first one. If this is not the case, the reliability of the test is in question and the patient must be re-instructed and all previously measured thresholds must be re-measured.

16. After rechecking 1000 Hz, 500 Hz is tested, followed by 250 Hz.

17. The other ear is now tested using the identical procedure Since the patient is now familiar with the test, it works best to simply start testing the other ear at 250 Hz (that's the last thing he heard, and saves you a little time switiching). Then just continue ascending to 8000 Hz. A purist might say to go back and start at 1000 Hz, but why?

Recording Results

As stated previously, record the responses on the audiogram using an "X" for the left ear and an "O" for the right ear. Refer to the key shown in Figure 4–7.

Interpretation

The air-conduction pure-tone thresholds tell you how *much* hearing loss a person has. In simple terms, the amount of hearing loss is the difference (in dB) between 0 dB HL (average hearing level for people with excellent hearing) and the patient's threshold at each frequency. In order to communicate the amount of hearing loss to other professionals and to the patient, there are gen-

Table 4–1. The Degree of Hearing Loss

−10 to 20 dB = Normal hearing
21 to 40 dB = Mild hearing loss
41 to 55 dB = Moderate hearing loss
56 to 70 dB = Moderate-to-severe hearing loss
71 to 90 dB = Severe hearing loss
>90 dB = Profound hearing loss

eral categories that are used to describe the amount of hearing loss. The categories are shown in Table 4–1.

The average air conduction hearing loss for the speech frequencies usually is calculated using the **three-frequency pure-tone average (PTA)**. You can calculate the PTA by adding the thresholds obtained at 500, 1000, and 2000 then divide the sum by 3. This is the PTA for each ear. Use the PTA and the degree of hearing loss chart to summarize the amount of hearing loss for each ear. The audiogram interpretation section will elaborate on this.

Pure-Tone Bone Conduction Audiometry

Go ahead, make my day.

Clint Eastwood, *Sudden Impact*

Recall that there are two different and unique paths sounds can take before they are perceived. When a hearing loss is present, you need to locate the origin, and indeed your handy bone conduction results just might "make your day." As we mentioned earlier, bone conducted sounds essentially bypass the outer and middle ear and directly vibrate the cochlea. Bone conduction audiometry can be as part of test battery to determine the site of lesion within the auditory system. Figure 4–12 shows a standard bone oscillator used for bone conduction tests.

Purpose

When a hearing loss is observed, bone conduction (BC) audiometry is completed after air conduction audiometry. BC audiometry will determine if the patient has either a conductive, sensorineural or mixed hearing loss.

Equipment Preparation

1. Turn the audiometer on
2. Set channel 1 to "tone" and "bone conduction"
3. Select 1000 Hz
4. Set the hearing level dial to the appropriate intensity (e.g., 30 dB HL, or the patient's AC threshold)
5. BC testing is done for all frequencies between 250 to 4000 Hz and for intensities between –10 to 70 dB HL.

Instructions to the Patient

You are going to hear more beeping tones. This time they will be presented

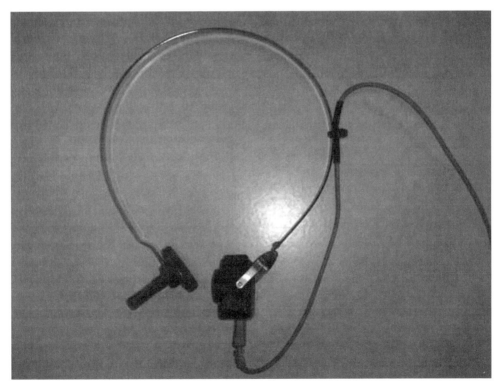

Figure 4–12. A standard bone conduction oscillator connected to a headband used for bone conduction testing.

from the device I have placed behind your ear. Press the button when you hear the tone. Listen for the softest sounds. You might hear them in your right ear or your left ear, it doesn't matter—push the button regardless. Do you have any questions?

Procedure

1. The patient is seated with his back to the audiometer—just like for AC testing.
2. The bone oscillator is placed, concave side down, on the patient's head. In most cases the oscillator is placed on the mastoid bone behind the outer ear. The oscillator's concave surface should rest flat on the mastoid bone (or forehead, if this placement is used).
3. Begin the test at 1000 Hz, 30 dB HL
4. Use pulsed tones as you did for AC testing.
5. If there is no response at 30 dB HL raise the intensity to 50 dB HL. Keep raising the intensity in 10 dB steps until the patient responds.
6. As soon as the patient responses reduce the intensity in 10 dB steps. The process of obtaining threshold has begun.
7. The intensity of the tone is raised in 5 dB steps until another response is observed. As soon as a response is obtained, the intensity is lowered by 10 dB.
8. If a response is not seen, the intensity is increased in 5 dB steps until a response is seen. The procedure starts again ("down 10, up 5")
9. The lowest level where three responses are seen in six stimulations is considered to be the patient's threshold.

10. Record the threshold on the audiogram in the appropriate place. Use the key on the audiometer to determine the appropriate symbol to use.
11. Thresholds are then obtained at other frequencies: 2 kHz, 4kHz, 500 Hz, and 250 Hz (we do not test above 4 kHz for BC).
12. Move the oscillator to the opposite ear, and complete the same threshold procedure.
13. Determine the need to use effective masking. (see the next section for details)

Interpretation

1. The difference between 0 dB HL and the BC threshold is the amount of sensorineural hearing loss at each frequency.
2. The difference between the AC threshold and the BC threshold is called the Air-Bone Gap. This is the amount of conductive hearing loss at each frequency. An air-bone gap is not considered significant unless it is 10 dB or more, as there are test-retest variances for both the air conduction and bone conduction measures.
3. Because the same cochlea is involved for the perception of both the air conduction and bone conducted signals, it is not theoretically possible for bone conduction thresholds to be *worse* than air conduction. Because of test-retest issues, it is possible, however, that a small difference could be observed. If a 10 dB or more difference is noted (i.e., bone thresholds 10 dB *worse* than air), you should question if you have

the oscillator positioned correctly. If this difference is observed on several different patients, the calibration of your equipment should be checked.

TIPS and TRICKS: More on Bone Conduction Testing

It is important to understand that when any sound stimulus is presented to the head via bone conduction, both cochleae (given that both are functioning equally) will respond as the entire skull vibrates at essentially the same time. So, when you place the bone oscillator behind the right ear and present a stimulus and obtain a threshold response, you may mark the results using the appropriate symbol for right bone conduction thresholds on the audiogram, but without further testing you cannot be sure exactly which cochlea heard the signal. You can only say that the best cochlea heard the signal and that a response was obtained with the bone conductor on the right side of the head. Many clinics use a special symbol for "Best Ear Bone Conduction" which simply means the patient heard it, but you don't know which ear. For example, if the patient has an air conduction threshold of 40 dB in each ear, and their "Best Ear Bone" threshold was also 40 dB, you really don't care whether they heard it in the right ear or the left ear, as you know they do not have an air/bone difference in either ear. How about that—a little knowledge about ear anatomy and physiology might actually save you some time.

Effective Masking

We're gonna need a bigger boat.
Roy Scheider, *Jaws*

It's not quite as bad as a giant shark attack, but masking can be a very perplexing subject. It is easy to get bogged down in its complexity. To get started, let's briefly discuss what masking is and why you need to do it. For our purposes, masking is defined as the condition in which one sound (noise) is introduced into one ear while measuring the threshold of the other ear. When conducting a hearing test, it is important to test each ear independently. When sound reaches a certain intensity level (which can be as soft as 0 dB in the case of bone conducted sound for someone with normal hearing) you don't know which ear is actually hearing it. Therefore, masking is needed to keep the non-test ear busy, while you accurately determine the threshold of the test ear. Knowing when to mask and how much masking noise to use takes some time to learn. Perhaps, the best way to really "get" the concept of masking is to actually do it. We start with the following exercise that will demonstrate how a masking noise can shift the threshold level.

Effective masking (EM) is defined as the masker level (dB HL) required to produce a threshold shift for a given stimulus. For example, 20 dB EM just masks a 20 dB signal presented to the *same* ear. This exercise allows for the opportunity to determine the EM correction factors for each audiometer. Only persons with normal hearing should be used for this exercise.

1. Set the audiometer so that the signal and masking noise (narrow

band noise—NBN) are routed to the same ear.

2. Set the attenuator dial for the pure tone to 30 dB HL.
3. Set the noise channel to 0 dB HL.

Instructions

You are going to hear a tone and some noise in the same ear. Raise your hand (push the button) when you hear the tone, not the noise, and just try to ignore the noise.

Procedure

1. Set the frequency of the tone channel to 1000 Hz
2. Introduce the tone to the test ear at 30 dB HL. The subject will respond.
3. Set the intensity of the noise in the masking channel to 0 dB HL.
4. Set the masking noise so it is on continuously.
5. Increase the level of the noise in 5 dB steps and present a tone at 30 dB HL at each 5 dB noise increment until the subject does not respond to the tone.
6. The procedure should be repeated to check for accuracy.
7. Record the noise level on a sheet of paper. In order to determine the amount of masking that is effective, and calculate correction factors, subtract 30 dB from the level of the noise. For example if it required 35 dB of noise, to mask a 30 dB tone, your correction factor for effective masking would be +5 dB.

8. Repeat steps 2 to 7 for each frequency.

Occlusion Effect

The occlusion effect (OE) is the enhancement in loudness of bone-conducted sound when the ear canal is plugged or occluded. During BC testing you may need to occlude the non-test ear with the earphone. This will create an enhancement of BC hearing in the NTE for the lower frequencies; therefore, you need to compensate for this by adding more noise. When doing bone conduction testing, you need to correct for the OE by adding 10 to 15 dB more masking noise than you would normally use to the non-test ear (NTE). Correcting for the OE only is done for low frequency tones (250 and 500 Hz).

To familiarize yourself with how the occlusion effect can alter the bone-conducted signal, try the following exercise with someone with relatively normal hearing. This demonstration will work best if your "subject" has thresholds of 15 dB or worse in the lower frequencies. Otherwise, the lower limits of the audiometer and/or ambient room noise might prevent observation of the shift (i.e., to see the shift, you'd have to measure a threshold of −5 dB or better). Here are the steps to use:

1. Determine the unmasked BC threshold for one ear at 500 Hz.
2. Cover the NTE with an earphone (or foam plug from insert). Do not present any noise to the NTE. Re-establish the threshold for the test ear.

3. Subtract the difference between the two thresholds obtained for at 500Hz. Was there a difference?
4. Repeat the same procedure for 250 and 1000 Hz.

Interaural Attenuation

An important concept of masking is interaural attenuation. To simplify this concept, imagine two people trying to hear one another on either side of a wall (perhaps you have experienced something similar to this in a cheap hotel room). How loud does one person have to talk to pass through the "attenuation" of the wall? Well, the head also can be thought of as an attenuation device. How loud does a sound have to be presented to one ear (through an earphone or bone conduction device) before it crosses over to the other ear? The point of crossover is called interaural attenuation.

Interaural attenuation varies considerably depending on what device is used to deliver the signal. Interaural attenuation is the biggest for insert earphones; because they are seated tightly in the ear canal, it is difficult for sound to leak out and pass around the head. At some point, however, there is a stimulation of the cochlea of the opposite ear. That is, the air conducted signal is loud enough to cause skull vibrations and a bone conducted signal has occurred.

With supra-aural earphones, interaural attenuation is not as large, as it is easier for the sound to leak out from under the earphone cushion. Interaural attenuation for air conducted sounds also varies as a function of frequency, smaller for low frequencies (because of their longer wavelengths it's easier for them to go around the head).

In general, taking into consideration the variables that we have just discussed, the attenuation effect is about 50 to 70 dB. However, we want to be conservative when we apply masking. Heed the following:

> **It's much better to mask when masking isn't needed than to not mask when masking is needed.**

The rule for applying masking for air conduction, therefore, is the conservative value of 40 dB. That is, whenever the presentation level to one ear is 40 dB (or more) greater than the bone conduction threshold of the non-test ear, masking is applied to the non-test ear.

Masking for Bone Conduction

Tell 'em to go out there with all they got and win just one for "the Gipper."
    Pat O'Brien, *Knute Rockne, All American*

Yes, there are times that in order to get the masking right for bone conduction, you'll have to go out there with all you've got! That's because the rules for masking for bone conduction are much different. Recall as we stated earlier, that whenever we deliver a bone conducted sound to the skull, we must assume it is going to both cochleas. It is tempting to think that because the oscillator is sitting behind the right ear we are primarily stimulating the right cochlea. That line of thinking, however, can get you into trouble. It is best to assume that there is no inter-aural attenuation for bone conduction.

As just stated, because the interaural attenuation (IA) for bone conduction is considered to be 0 dB, this means that a response from the nontest ear is always possible during BC testing. Masking, therefore is nearly always needed to remove the nontest ear from participation in the test.

When to mask: Any time there is an A/B gap of greater than 10 dB masking must be introduced into the nontest ear.

Equipment Preparation

1. Set the test ear channel to "tone" and "bone conduction"
2. Select the desired frequency
3. Adjust the hearing level dial to the previously determined unmasked threshold
4. Set the masking channel to NBN.
5. Direct the NBN masking to the nontest ear
6. Adjust the hearing level dial of the masking channel to the minimum effective masking level. The EM level is equal to the threshold of the non-test ear, plus the occlusion effect at that test frequency.

Instructions to the Patient

You are going to hear some beeping tones. Every time you hear the tone press the button (raise your hand) even if you barely hear the tone. You will hear a rushing sound in the other ear through the headphone. Just ignore it and only raise your hand when you hear the tone, not the noise. Do you have any questions?

Procedure

1. Position the bone oscillator on either the mastoid or the forehead.

2. If you are using headphones, place the other earphone on the side of the head above the ear. Tighten the headband so it doesn't slip. The placement of the BC oscillator should not be disrupted by the headphone placement. The oscillator cannot touch the pinna of the test ear.
3. Set the masking channel so that the noise is on continuously. Start at 0 dB HL.
4. The intensity of the noise is slowly increased to the EM level. The EM is the AC threshold of the ear being masked plus 10 dB for the occlusion effect in the low frequencies (250 and 500 Hz).
5. Present a tone to the test ear through the oscillator. If the patient responds, the masking procedure is complete.
6. Record the threshold and amount of EM on the audiogram.
7. If the patient does not respond, increase the intensity of the tone 5 dB and present it again. If the patient now responds the masking procedure is finished and you can record the results on the audiogram.
8. If the patient does not respond, you must plateau to ensure the actual threshold.

The Plateau Method

Although knowing and using effective masking levels usually will ensure correct thresholds, some people prefer to use a "plateau" method when they apply masking. This provides some additional "safety" in knowing that masking is correct. Here's how to use the plateau method when applying masking:

1. Set the noise in the non-test ear to EM. Again, this is the AC threshold in this ear plus 10 to 15 dB for the occlusion effect in the low frequencies.
2. Raise the level of the tone in 5 dB steps in the test ear until the patient responds
3. Once the person responds, the level of the noise in the nontest ear is raised three times in 5 dB steps.
4. If the patient responds to the tone with each increase in the intensity of the noise, a plateau has been reached, and you can assume that the threshold obtained in that ear is accurate.
5. Record the threshold with the appropriate symbol and EM level in each ear.
6. If the patient does not respond to the tone three consecutive times with the 5 dB increases in the noise level, increase the level of the tone in the test ear by 5 dB or until a response is obtain and repeat the procedure. Continue until a plateau has been established or until you have reached the limits of the audiometer.

TAKE FIVE: More on Masking

All students and trainees need some hands on time to really understand masking. We've learned that this procedure is the leading reason why individuals fail the practical portion of their state hearing aid licensing exams. If you're having trouble understanding these concepts, we recommend obtaining a copy of Linda Donaldson's book, *Masking: Practical Applications.* You can purchase a copy at the International Hearing Society Web site, which is http://www.ihsinfo.org

---

Masking for Air Conduction

Purpose

As discussed earlier, even with an air conducted signal, there is a point when the tone can cross to the nontest ear via bone conduction. When this is expected, it is necessary to eliminate this ear from participation using masking.

When to Mask

You need to mask during AC testing whenever the AC threshold of the non-test ear, minus interaural attenuation (IA) is more than the BC threshold of the non-test ear. IA can be estimated. The IA can be as low as 40 dB when using supra-aural headphones, and is more like 60 to 70 dB when using insert receivers. We want to be conservative, so if the difference is greater than 40 dB different between the two ears, then masking must be used.

Equipment Preparation

1. The earphones are placed in both ears.
2. The tone is presented to one ear and the masking noise presented

to the other ear using the other channel

3. The masking level used should be 5 dB above the AC threshold of the nontest ear.

Procedure

Follow the same procedure outlined for BC masking using the plateau technique as needed.

Speech Audiometry

Speech audiometry has a long and complicated history within the test booths of the typical hearing aid practice. Several decades ago, speech audiometry was developed as a diagnostic tool (e.g., middle ear versus cochlea versus 8th nerve). Today, that is still the primary purpose for conducting speech audiometry; however, it is also now part of the prefitting hearing aid assessment. Although there are dozens of speech tests to choose from that can be conducted in quiet or in noisy conditions;

our focus here will be on the two most basic speech audiometry procedures: Speech Recognition Threshold and Word Recognition Testing.

Speech Recognition Threshold (SRT)

The main purpose of the speech recognition threshold (SRT), sometimes called the speech reception threshold, procedure is to check the reliability of the pure-tone thresholds. The SRT should be within ± 10 dB of the average of the pure-tone thresholds at 500, 1000, and 2000 Hz for each ear, or for a precipitous downward sloping hearing loss, within ± 10 dB of the 500 and 1000 Hz average. After this exercise, you should be able to determine an SRT and make judgments as to the reliability of pure-tone results. The stimuli used for SRT testing are spondees, which are two-syllable words that have equal stress on both syllables. Both syllables should peak at 0 on the VU meter of the audiometer. A list of spondees is shown in Table 4–2. Spondees differ in difficulty

Table 4–2. One List of Spondee Words from CID W-1 Word List

airplane	eardrum	iceberg	railroad
armchair	farewell	inkwell	schoolboy
baseball	grandson	mousetrap	sidewalk
birthday	greyhound	mushroom	stairway
cowboy	hardware	northwest	sunset
daybreak	headlight	oatmeal	toothbrush
doormat	horseshoe	padlock	whitewash
drawbridge	hotdog	pancake	workshop
duckpond	hothouse	playground	woodwork

(e.g., intensity at which they are understood) so it is important to use the words from the list, not simply repeat words from memory (after conducting several tests, most clinicians will remember several spondees. Unfortunately, they tend to remember all the easy ones, as those were the ones that patients responded to correctly).

The SRT is often the first test of the audiologic battery. When it is completed first, there is no bias in the testing, which can occur if pure-tone thresholds are already known, and it can be used as a reliability check, as described earlier. Speech can be delivered using recorded material, or by monitored live voice (MLV). MLV is the process of reading the words using a microphone with careful visual attention paid to the volume units (VU) meter of the audiometer. Recorded speech is the preferred method.

Equipment Preparation

1. Before testing the patient the level of the preamplifier for the VU meter on the audiometer must be set.
   a. If MLV is to be used the audiometer's input is set to "microphone." The microphone level knob is adjusted while presenting the spondees, until both syllables peak at 0 on the VU meter.
   b. A calibration tone is provided on pre-recorded (CD or tape) materials that can be played while the VU meter is adjusted to 0 dB.
2. Set the test channel to the "microphone" position for MLV, or "disk" or "tape" for prerecorded materials.

3. Set the output to the appropriate earphone. The non-test channel should be set to "speech noise" or to "white noise" if speech noise is not available.
4. The patient should not be allowed to see your face.

Instructions to the Patient

The patient must be seated so that lip movements of the examiner are not visible, especially if monitored live voice is used. Speechreading the stimulus words often can produce test results that will suggest that the patient's speech understanding is better than it truly is.

You are going to hear some words. Repeat every word you hear. The words will get softer and softer, so soft, in fact that they will be very difficult for you to hear. It is very important that you try to repeat the words, even if you have to guess. Do you have any questions?

Procedure

1. An important part of the SRT test is the initial patient familiarization with the test words. It is important to remember that this is a test of recognition, not speech understanding. It is "okay" for the patient to know the list of words that will be presented. One way to familiarize the patient is to use live voice. The spondees are presented through the microphone/speech channel or through the talk-over channel on the audiometer at a comfortable loudness level (60 dB HL or louder).

This method allows you to verify that the patient understands all the spondees. If the patient cannot repeat a given spondee at a comfortable loudness level, then that spondee should not be used to determine the SRT. Please note the Spondee Word list in Table 4–2.

2. The starting level is 30 dB HL.
3. One spondee is presented.
4. If the patient repeats the word correctly, the hearing level is decreased in 10 dB steps while presenting one word at each level. This procedure is continued until a spondee is missed.
5. If the patient does not respond at the initial 30 dB HL, raise the hearing level to 50 db HL, and then in 10 dB steps, while presenting a spondee at each level, until the patient correctly repeats a word.
6. When a word is repeated correctly, start the descending procedure in 10 dB steps.
7. As soon as a patient misses the first spondee, the threshold determination procedure begins. At this point, the level is raised in 5 dB steps, presenting one spondee at each level, until the patient is able to repeat the spondee.
8. The procedure is the same "down 10, up 5" one used for pure-tone threshold determination. Each time the patient gets a word correct, the hearing level is decreased 10 dB, and another spondee is presented. Every time the patient does not respond correctly at a given level, the level of the word is increased by 5 dB and another spondee is presented.

9. When a level is reached where at least 3 out of 6 of the spondees are repeated correctly, the procedure is terminated, and the SRT is recorded.
10. Each ear is tested independently under earphones.

TIPS and TRICKS: SRT Measurement

There is little reason to conduct a "bilateral" SRT, as the findings essentially will be the same as the best ear. Likewise, there is little reason for conducting a soundfield SRT, unless for some reason earphones cannot be used. Again, when soundfield testing is conducted, the response obtained will only represent the best ear (unless some type of masking from an earphone is used).

Results

1. There is a place on the audiometric worksheet for the SRT to be recorded in dB HL for each ear.
2. If the SRT does not agree with the pure-tone average, the overall results are considered unreliable, and pure-tone thresholds should be retested.

Interpretation

1. The SRT should be within 10 dB of the pure-tone average, unless there is some unusual shape of the

audiogram (e.g., sharply falling or sharply rising configurations).

2. The difference (in decibels) between 0 dB HL and the patient's SRT is the amount of hearing loss for speech.

3. The SRT should *not* be used as a determination for the use of amplification. Many individuals with significant high-frequency hearing loss will have SRTs within normal limits.

Word Recognition Testing

Purpose

Word recognition (WR) testing is the first suprathreshold test in the audiometric evaluation. Suprathreshold means the test is conducted at an intensity level above threshold. It typically is performed at a presentation level that is somewhat louder than "comfortable" (or slightly loud but okay) to the patient —it's important to maximize audibility, which usually doesn't happen at the patient's MCL. Of all the tests in the basic test battery, word recognition (WR) is the most misunderstood and incorrectly conducted. For our purposes we outline basic WR procedures that are best for determining if a pathology requiring medical attention is present, and for assessing candidacy for amplification. WR testing is conducted in each ear separately.

The purpose of the WR testing is to evaluate an individual's ability to recognize single-syllable words from a phonetically balanced (PB) word list. The testing is sometimes casually re-ferred to as "PB," "discrimination," or "discrim" testing (even though the test itself is a recognition, *not* a discrimination measure). It is critical that WR testing be conducted at a level in which the words are both comfortable, yet loud enough to be audible. If possible, audible in the higher frequencies (e.g., 2000 to 3000 Hz), as many of the words contain high-frequency consonants.

The primary purpose of WR test is to determine the patient's maximum score for single syllable, phonetically balanced words (PBmax). That is, if we make the words loud so that audibility is not a major limiting factor, what is the maximum performance a patient can attain. In order to find the PBmax, it often is necessary to conduct WR testing at more than one presentation level (e.g., testing might be conducted at both 60 dB and 75 dB HL for someone with a mild-to-moderate hearing loss). Because of the inconsistencies surrounding word recognitions procedures, we will discuss each important aspect point by point below.

Word Lists

There are several different monosyllabic words lists, often named after the laboratory where they were developed. The lists are similar, but slightly different WR scores will result. We recommend using the Northwestern University List #6 (NU-6), which is the most common list used in the U.S. Many word lists, including the NU-6 lists are available from Auditec located in St. Louis (http://www.auditec.com).

Number of Words Presented

I feel the need—the need for speed.
                    Tom Cruise, *Top Gun*

While we certainly encourage you to develop an efficient test battery, don't let "the need for speed" compromise your test protocol. This is especially true when conducting WR testing.

The standard word lists are 50 words in length, and all Best Practice Guidelines state that 50 words are presented to each ear for each patient (with a valve 25 words are presented (with a value of 2% per correct word). Unfortunately, sometimes examiners "feel the need for speed" and only use 25 words). The latter is referred to as using a "half-list." Although using a half-list does save a little time, accuracy is sacrificed. The words differ in difficulty, and because the lists were not intended to be halved, the most difficult words may not be equally distributed between the first and second half. We, therefore, recommend always using the full 50-word lists.

TIPS and TRICKS:
The 10 Best Words

A modification of the traditional word lists have been made in recent years, which can be used for WR screening. A special recording is available that has the most difficult 10 words of each list presented first. If the patient correctly recognizes all or nine of these 10 words, it can be assumed that their true speech understanding for the entire list is within normal limits. This recording also is available from Auditec and is listed as: "NU-6 Ordered by Difficulty."

Presentation Level

As already mentioned, WR testing needs to be conducted at a "loud MCL." The most comfortable level (MCL) is in range between the SRT and LDL. We recommend starting at 70 dB HL or higher. Exactly what level yields PBmax for individuals with hearing loss has generated considerable discussion, but very little conclusive research over the years. A common practice among experienced clinicians is to routinely conduct WR testing at 30 to 40 dB above the SRT (30 to 40 db SL). We do know that this is *not* a good idea for routine practice.

Recent research from Lesli Guthrie and Carol Mackersie has shown that if you are going to select a single presentation level for finding PB-Max, two procedures yielded the best results for mild, moderate gradual sloping, and steeply sloping hearing losses:

1. Set the WR presentation level 5 dB below speech UCL,
2. Set the WR presentation level above the 2 kHz threshold using the following guidelines:
   - If 2 kHZ threshold <50 dB HL, add 25 dB SL
   - If 2 kHz threshold = 60 to 65 dB HL, add 15 dB SL
   - If 2 kHz threshold = 70 to 75 dB HL, add 10 dB SL

We suggest that you take a note card and copy the 2000 Hz SL values shown above, and then keep the note card handy when you do your speech testing. This will give you a good chance of obtaining PBmax for a single level, although we still recommend speech testing at multiple levels if time permits.

Presentation Mode

Word recognition testing must be conducted using speech material from a standardized CD or wave file. The given talker for the words can make a large difference in the resulting score, which is why conducting this test using monitored live voice (MLV) is poor practice. This is much like creating your own new test, a test with *no norms!* Even when CD/wave file recordings are used, the talker matters. We recommend using the NU-6 recordings on CD from Auditec of St. Louis (http://www.auditec.com).

Equipment Preparation

1. The audiometer input is set to "tape" or "CD." The output is set to the test ear (start with the ear with the best thresholds).
2. All pre-recorded tests of PB word lists contain a calibration tone. While the tone is playing, the level control for the tape or CD is adjusted to the point where the needle on the VU meter reads "0." This should be completed before the test begins. The recording should be advanced so that the introduction to the test is not heard by the patient.

Test Procedure

1. Select a presentation level (see guidelines on previous page). Determine if masking is needed. A full 50-word list per ear needs to be used (hopefully you'll never have to record this).

2. Instruct the patient, using the following instructions below:

The patient should not be allowed to watch the examiner, especially if monitored live voice testing is used. A written response may be substituted for a verbal one, if desired.

You are going to hear some sentences. Please repeat the last word in each sentence. For example, if you hear "Say the word BOY," just repeat "BOY." If you are unsure of a word, say whatever you think you heard. Don't be afraid to guess. Do you have any questions?

3. Present the recorded word list.
4. Keep track of the number of correct and incorrect words.
5. Begin the test in the opposite ear using another word list
6. Once you have completed the test in each ear at the initial intensity level, raise the intensity level and repeat the test in each ear using another word list. The second presentation level needs to be 5 to 10 dB below the patients LDL or approximately 20 dB higher than the first presentation level.
7. If the WR score at the higher intensity level is the same or better than the score at the lower level, stop the test and record this score.
8. If the WR score obtained at the lower intensity level is better by more than 8%, additional testing is required in order to determine PBmax and to determine if there may be significant rollover. (See section on PI-PB rollover.) Testing should continue in 20 dB increments until PBmax is obtained.

Scoring

1. The type of word list used, and the sensation level at which the list was presented are always recorded on the audiometric worksheet. Also a notation should be made if a half-list was used.
2. The WRS is calculated as follows: the number of words missed is counted, multiplied by 2% (50 words), and this value is subtracted from 100%. This number is recorded in the appropriate box on the audiometric worksheet
3. PBmax: In many cases, to determine PBmax, you will have to present words lists at more than one intensity level. PBmax is the term used to describe the best score in each ear for word recognition testing.

TAKE FIVE: What Is PBmax?

The primary purpose of WR testing is to assess the auditory system using speech. There are several auditory disorders we will cover in Chapter 5 that can be identified from low WR scores. Because a low WR score can be a "red flag" for a medical pathology involving the auditory system, it is important that we don't falsely identify a medical condition that doesn't really exist. Conducting WR testing at multiple levels and finding the PBmax will help reduce the number of unnecessary referrals.

In order to determine the PBmax, you need to conduct WR testing at multiple intensity levels. This is called a performance intensity function for phonetically balanced words or simply, a PI-PB function. Figure 4–13 shows PI-PB functions for normal hearing and a cochlear hearing loss. Notice that as the presentation level increases, the WR score increases. At a certain point, increasing the intensity does not improve the WR score. The point is which the best WR score is obtained is called the PB Max. For certain types of retrocochlear disorders, the scores actually become significantly worse at high intensity level. On a PI-PB function, this would show a drop off at higher intensity levels. This phenomenon is known as "rollover." If the rollover ratio is greater than .25, it is a red flag for a retrocochlear pathology, and the patient should be referred for further testing. The rollover ratio can be calculated using this formula:

$$\text{Rollover Ratio} = \frac{\text{PBmax} - \text{PBmin}}{\text{PBmax}}$$

Interpreting WR Test Scores

We typically report the WR score on the audiogram as a percent correct as well as giving a brief description of the degree of impairment. When talking to the patient or other professionals, it sometimes is helpful to use general terms to describe a percentage range. Table 4–3 gives some common cate-

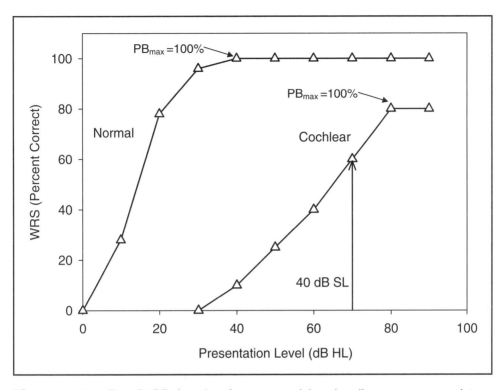

Figure 4–13. The PI-PB function for a normal hearing listener compared to a patient with cochlear hearing loss. PBmax is the point where the score plateaus. From *Audiology: Science to Practice* by Steven Kramer. © 2008 Plural Publishing, Inc. All Rights Reserved. Used with permission, p. 195.

Table 4–3. Categories Commonly Used to Describe WR Test Results

WR score	Degree of Impairment	Word Recognition Ability
92–100%	None	Excellent or Normal
84–91%	Slight	Good
70–83%	Moderate	Fair
56–69%	Poor	Poor
<56%	Very Poor	Very Poor

gories used to describe the degree of impairment for a given percent score. These are only general guidelines—you may see somewhat different ranges published elsewhere, as there is no standard for these classifications.

Significant Differences or Changes in WR Scores

One of the common questions associated with WR testing is, "When is a difference really a difference?" In other words, when your patient has a score of 72% in the right ear and 56% in the left ear is this difference something you need to pay attention to or does it simply reflect normal variability between scores. We have the answer—something called the binomial distribution is a statistically derived table of probabilities that is used to determine a real difference from normal variability.

The variability in WR testing decreases as the number of words increases. Therefore, a 50-word list has less variability than a 25-word list. In practical terms, this simply means that a greater difference between scores is needed when you use a 25-word list compared to a 50-word list. For example, if you are using a 25-word list and the difference between the right ear and left ear score is 16%, this difference is not significant because it likely reflects the expected amount of variability as a result of using a shorter list of words.

There is quite a bit of statistical analysis behind the calculation of the binomial distribution, but for now, there is no reason to get bogged down in the details (we can leave that up to our Ph.D. audiologist friends). Using Table 4–4 you can take the scores you have obtained from the right and left ears, or compare the scores today from those of the last test you did two years ago to see if there is a critical difference.

Using Table 4–4 to see if a difference is really a difference is easy. Just take the lower of the two scores you are comparing and find it on the chart. (Hint: it's a number between 0 and 100). Next look under one of the four columns (10, 25, 50, or 63) which designate the number of words or phonemes you are scoring. It's unlikely you will ever use the 63 column unless you are one of the very few clinicians who do testing on the phoneme level.

For example, if you are using a 50-word list and the lowest of the two scores is 52%, the other score has to be

---

TIPS and TRICKS: A Practice Case

Let's do one more case study using Table 4–4. You tested a patient a year ago and his PBmax was 84% in his left ear. He is now telling you that he can't understand as well in his left ear. Is it the hearing aid you sold him? Is it not working correctly? Or did his speech understanding change significantly over the past year? You repeat the testing using the same procedures.

This time your score is 62%. Is this significantly worse than 84%? Let's find out. Go to Table 4–4 and locate 62% (it was the lowest of the two scores). Now move over three columns to the right, to the "50" column (that's the number of words you used). Notice that the number is 80%. Was your score from a year ago larger than 80%? Yes it was! This means that the two scores are indeed significantly different. Pretty easy, huh?

Table 4–4. Critical Difference Values for PB Words Based on the Bimodial Distribution

95% Confidence		Number of items (phoneme scoring = 2.5 number of words)									
		10	25	50	63			10	25	50	63
The lower of the two scores being compared (in %)	0	33	15	8	6	The lower of the two scores being compared (in %)	50	91	77	70	68
	1	36	17	10	9		51	91	78	71	68
	2	38	20	12	11		52	92	79	71	69
	3	40	22	14	13		53	93	80	72	70
	4	41	23	16	14		54	93	81	73	71
	5	43	25	18	16		55	94	81	74	72
	6	45	27	19	17		56	95	82	75	73
	7	47	29	21	19		57	95	83	76	74
	8	48	30	22	20		58	96	84	77	75
	9	50	32	24	22		59	96	84	78	76
	10	51	33	25	23		60	97	85	78	77
	11	53	35	27	25		61	97	86	79	77
	12	54	36	28	26		62	98	87	80	78
	13	55	38	29	27		63	98	87	81	79
	14	57	39	31	29		64	99	88	82	80
	15	58	40	32	30		65	99	89	83	81
	16	59	42	33	31		66	100	90	83	82
	17	61	43	34	32		67	100	90	84	82
	18	62	44	36	34		68	100	91	85	83
	19	63	45	37	35		69	100	92	86	84
	20	64	47	38	36		70	100	92	87	85
	21	65	48	39	37		71	100	93	87	86
	22	66	49	41	38		72	100	93	88	86
	23	68	50	42	40		73	100	94	89	87
	24	69	51	43	41		74	100	95	89	88
	25	70	53	44	42		75	100	95	90	89
	26	71	54	45	43		76	100	96	91	89
	27	72	55	46	44		77	100	96	92	90
	28	73	56	47	45		78	100	97	92	91
	29	74	57	48	46		79	100	97	93	92
	30	75	58	50	47		80	100	98	94	92
	31	76	59	51	48		81	100	98	94	93
	32	77	60	52	50		82	100	99	95	94
	33	77	61	53	51		83	100	99	95	94
	34	78	62	54	52		84	100	100	96	95
	35	79	63	55	53		85	100	100	97	96
	36	80	64	56	54		86	100	100	97	96
	37	81	65	57	55		87	100	100	98	97
	38	82	66	58	56		88	100	100	98	97
	39	83	67	59	57		89	100	100	99	98
	40	83	68	60	58		90	100	100	99	98
	41	84	69	61	59		91	100	100	100	99
	42	85	70	62	60		92	100	100	100	99
	43	86	71	63	61		93	100	100	100	100
	44	87	72	64	62		94	100	100	100	100
	45	87	73	65	63		95	100	100	100	100
	46	88	74	66	64		96	100	100	100	100
	47	89	75	67	65		97	100	100	100	100
	48	89	75	68	66		98	100	100	100	100
	49	90	76	69	67		99	100	100	100	100

Find where lower score (row) intersects number of items scored (column).

Source: Audiology: Science to Practice by Steven Kramer. © 2008 Plural Publishing, Inc. All Rights Reserved. Used with permission, p. 199.

greater than 71% for the difference, to be significant. When scores exceed the critical difference, and it's not explained by the audiogram (e.g., the thresholds of one ear are significantly worse than the other) it's a "red flag" for a possible medical problem causing the low score, and a medical referral is probably warranted.

Most Comfortable and Uncomfortable Loudness Levels

We leave you with one more important consideration to close out this chapter. As you will see in later chapters about hearing aid selection and fitting, there are several other prefitting tests you can do that quantify the amount of

hearing loss. Most clinicians conduct some type of testing that identifies the dynamic range for speech. These tests are called most comfortable loudness level (MCL), and uncomfortable loudness level (UCL). For now we want to introduce the concept of dynamic range for speech. As you can see in Figure 4–14, there is a significant difference between dynamic ranges depending on the type of hearing loss. As the vast majority of people you will fit with hearing aids have a cochlear (SNHL) loss, notice in Figure 4–14 how much narrower the dynamic range for speech is compared to a conductive loss and normal hearing. Because a patient with a cochlear loss has a relatively narrow dynamic range between MCL and UCL we have to be careful about how we conduct speech testing. Testing at too low of an intensity causes erroneous

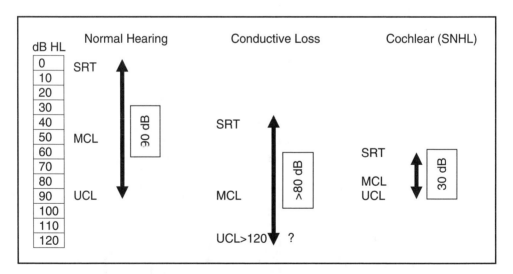

Figure 4–14. An illustration of the dynamic range for speech for normal hearing, a conductive hearing loss and a cochlear hearing loss. The difference between the SRT and the UCL is the dynamic range for speech. Note the narrow dynamic range for cochlear hearing loss and the elevated, yet broad dynamic range for conductive hearing loss. From *Audiology: Science to Practice* by Steven Kramer. © 2008 Plural Publishing, Inc. All Rights Reserved. Used with permission, p. 192.

results and testing at too high of a level can cause discomfort and even pain. Also, notice in Figure 4–14 that the UCL scores for normal and cochlear losses are about the same; just because someone has elevated SRTs and thresholds doesn't mean their UCLs are elevated too! More on that in future chapters.

In Closing

Now that you've read Chapter 4, you should have a better understanding of the basic test procedures needed to quantify a patient's hearing loss. All of the tests reviewed in this chapter are essential to the prefitting process. In other words, you need to know how to conduct these tests before you can fit someone with hearing aids. Next, we turn our attention to many of the common hearing disorders you will identify when properly conducting the basic test battery. Even though conducting a basic hearing test is different from discovering Boyle's law of gases, taking the time to measure hearing is the first step in improving a patient's communication ability with hearing aids.

And it all goes a little better with a few quotes from movies—with a little work you might be saying, "I'm king of the world." Here's a quote to end on:

Elementary, my dear Watson.

Basil Rathbone
The Adventures of Sherlock Holmes

5

Hearing Disorders and Audiogram Interpretation

> *There are many great unsolved mysteries of the world. Maybe we can solve some of them in this chapter!*

As someone new to conducting hearing tests, you might find the process of uncovering various types of hearing disorders somewhat mysterious. You might even think that interpreting your first audiograms is like trying to uncover one of the great unsolved mysteries of the world. Although some of the hearing disorders we review might seem a little mysterious to you right now, we seriously doubt that you'll get lost in the Bermuda Triangle or get carried off by Bigfoot.

We've already solved a couple of the world's mysteries—after the previous chapter you have a good working knowledge of the normal auditory system and how to measure its function. Let's turn our attention to various disorders than can affect it. The primary purpose of this chapter is to provide you with a basic understanding of hearing disorders, characteristics of the hearing loss, and, most importantly, the audiometric configuration that is most

closely associated to the disorder. The goal is not for you to memorize every possible disorder, along with the audiometric pattern, but when you are finished reading this chapter you should have a better understanding of how the results of the hearing test relate to the diagnosis of some common hearing disorders.

The first thing you need to know about hearing disorders is that it is critical to have a good understanding of when to refer a patient to a physician for a medical evaluation. In fact, before you even begin to discuss hearing aids with a patient it is imperative that you have ruled out a treatable medical problem involving the auditory system. This means that you have to recognize what a hearing disorder looks like on an audiogram. Before reviewing the various types of hearing disorders, let's discuss the difference between a symptom and an etiology.

Symptoms Versus Etiology

Understanding the difference between a symptom and an etiology is important. When someone walks through your door for a hearing test, they may be experiencing several symptoms related to any number of possible hearing disorders.

- A symptom is a description by the patient of what they are feeling, or an observation you make (e.g., dizziness, pain, etc.).
- An etiology is the underlying cause for the disorder. It is only through an accurate hearing test, which may lead to a diagnosis by a physician, that you may know the cause or etiology.

In some cases the etiology is never known. It is common to conduct medical tests to "rule out" pathologies that require further medical attention. A person with an unexplained unilateral loss, for example, may have an MRI to rule out a space occupying lesion. Once the MRI shows there is no obvious pathology, the patient is cleared for the fitting of a hearing aid, although the true cause for the hearing loss still remains unknown.

With accurate audiometry you often will be able to quantify the extent of the ear problem. In most cases, regardless of the etiology, once a treatable medical problem involving the ear has been ruled out, you will fit the patient with hearing aids.

Typically, the hearing disorders you will encounter will involve the inner ear. Not only are they much more common, but disorders of the cochlea usu-

ally require the use of hearing aids as part of the treatment process, and for the most part, hearing aids are the *only* treatment.

Case History

Before completing any diagnostic audiometry, it is important to carefully complete a case history. The case history should always be completed face-to-face with the patient, rather than having the patient complete a case history checklist or questionnaire in the waiting room. During the taking of the case history, your job is to find out if the patient has recently experienced any of the common symptoms listed below. Given that these symptoms occasionally are an indication of a more threatening medical problem, they are important to know and understand.

Common Symptoms

The symptoms listed below are ones you will frequently encounter, and are used by physicians and audiologists on a regular basis.

Tinnitus

This is the perceived sensation of ear noise, often described as a ringing or buzzing in the ear. It is not a disorder, just the sensation to hear sounds generated by the auditory system. Tinnitus, however, is often associated with hearing loss and hearing disorders. For example, most people with noise-induced hearing loss have tinnitus. In this case, there is no medical treatment. On the other hand, someone with an acoustic nerve neuroma also may have tinnitus and, in this case, a medical workup is critical. Tinnitus can be an occasional occurrence, or it can be constant. Tinnitus is actually more common than hearing loss, as it believed that over 50 million Americans experience tinnitus to some degree. In case you're wondering, tinnitus can be pronounced either as ti-NIGHT-us or TIN-i-tus; the latter is preferred by most professionals.

Vertigo and Dizziness

True vertigo is a severe spinning sensation usually of short duration. It can be spontaneous, or associated with head movement. The patient can have the sensation the patient of spinning themselves or that the room is spinning around them. There are almost as many causes of dizziness as there are ways in which patients describe it. Recall from Chapter 3, that the balance and auditory system are located in the inner ear. Therefore, it is fairly common to encounter patients with hearing loss (especially if it is of relatively sudden onset) who are also experiencing vertigo.

Otalgia

Simply put, this is ear pain, sometimes called an "earache." Otalgia is not always associated with hearing disorders, as it can be caused by conditions such as impacted teeth, sinus disease, and inflamed tonsils. If directly related to the ear, it may be due to middle or outer ear pathology. It's common for

there to be a generalization of pain. That is, the external ear could be painful resulting from an ear canal problem.

**TAKE FIVE:
Medical Terminology**

This chapter introduces you to many of the common terms used to describe hearing disorders and their symptoms. If you receive referrals from physicians and other medical professionals you are likely to encounter terms you don't know. One way to find out about them quickly is to use an on-line medical dictionary. One example is http://www.medterms.com.

Aural Fullness

The perceived sensation of a plugged ear that often accompanies vertigo and sudden hearing loss. Aural fullness can also be a symptom of a problem involving the middle ear, often related to poor eustachian tube function.

Hyperacusis

An abnormal sensitivity to sound. Hyperacusis is an internal overamplification of environmental sounds by the auditory system. Environmental sounds of ordinary intensity that do not bother most people, really bother those suffering from hyperacusis—e.g., a sound of 65 dB SPL might be perceived like a 100 dB SPL input. This is different from people who simply are "bothered" by loud noise.

TIPS and TRICKS: More on Tinnitus

Tinnitus is a condition that still is not completely understood. In fact, experts are still not in complete agreement regarding the underlying causes of tinnitus. To complicate matters, there is a wide range of treatment options that go well beyond the scope of this book. To learn more about the etiology of tinnitus, along with some of the treatment options supported by research evidence, here are a couple of useful Web sites:

http://www.tinnitus.org—A British Web site devoted to a specific type of tinnitus therapy called Tinnitus Retraining Therapy (TRT)

http://www.ata.org—Sponsored by the American Tinnitus Association, it contains plenty of information for professionals and consumers.

TIPS and TRICKS:
Cochlear Hearing Loss, Loudness, and Recruitment

As mentioned a number of times already, the majority of your patients will be individuals with cochlear hearing loss. This population is unique regarding their loudness growth pattern; because of their hearing loss they need a loudness boost for soft sounds, but because of the way the cochlea works (see Chapter 3) they do not need a loudness boost for loud sounds. Their loudness perceptions for loud sounds are very similar to someone with normal hearing. In other words, their floor has been raised, but the ceiling has remained in the same. As a result, there is a rapid growth of loudness between the point of audibility and the point of discomfort. This abnormal growth of loudness often has been referred to as *recruitment*. Recruitment is perhaps the most common, and most commonly talked about, yet most misunderstood, symptom of cochlear hearing loss. It is a *normal* nonpathological phenomenon associated with a damaged cochlea.

Sample Case: Your Monday morning patient has a 60 dB hearing loss, but when you did LDL testing, you found that he found things uncomfortably loud at 100 dB, the same point as many people with normal hearing, a dynamic range of only 40 dB. Does he have recruitment? Yes. Does he have "a lot of recruitment"? Well, if there were such a thing, maybe yes. Is this something to be concerned about? No. It is the *expected* finding. What *is* something to be concerned about is the patient with a 60 dB hearing loss who *doesn't* have recruitment. That would mean that the hearing loss is probably caused by a middle ear, eighth nerve, or brainstem pathology, and the patient should be referred for medical evaluation.

Common Hearing Disorders

A close encounter is an event in which a person witnesses an unidentified flying object or makes contact with an alien. According to ufologist (yes, that's a real word) J. Allen Hynek, there are four types of close encounters. Close encounters of the first and second kind are sightings of unidentified flying objects, whereas close encounters of the third and fourth type involve contact and even abduction by an alien. In a clinic the only type of encounter you are likely to find is one is which you could uncover a hearing disorder.

The following is a summary of some of the most common hearing disorders you will "encounter" in your daily practice—and some probably will be a mystery. This is not an exhaustive list. It is simply a summary of some of the most common conditions, their causes, and audiometric patterns. To make things fairly straightforward, we have organized the disorders as they relate to parts of the ear. Thanks to the World Wide Web, you can find many more examples of hearing disorders that we did not cover here. Among the Web sites devoted to hearing disorders are http://www.merck.com.mmpe and http://emedicine.medscape.com/ otolaryngology

Hearing Disorders of the Outer Ear

Most disorders of the outer ear are easy to observe, respond to treatment, and usually do not cause significant hearing loss. We review five of the most common in this section.

Collapsing Ear Canal

Recall that we discussed the advantages of using insert earphones in Chapter 4; let's talk about an important reason for using them in a little more detail. Some people, especially the elderly, have ear canals that are collapsing. This means that the tissues lining the ear canal have become very soft. This is a normal condition and does not cause hearing loss in the vast majority of cases, because sound only needs a small opening to pass through. But for patients with this problem, this could change when you do a hearing test. When you place supra-aural headphones on someone with collapsing ear canals, it's possible that the pressure will totally collapse the ear canal, and you are actually causing a hearing loss. It is as though the patient is wearing an earplug. This condition results in an audiogram that has the appearance of a conductive hearing loss (usually greatest loss in the higher frequencies, as they are the easiest to attenuate). This easily can be prevented, however, by using insert earphones. Figure 5–1 gives an example of an audiogram of a patient with collapsing ear canals. The audiogram on the right is after the use of insert phones. Note how the loss returns to near normal levels (e.g., "correct" values) when the appropriate earphones are used.

Failure to recognize collapsing canals, and the resulting erroneous assumption that there is a conductive hearing loss present, is a good way to lose credibility with the physicians that you refer to, as their physical examination clearly will be normal. Of course, if your scope of practice includes the use of immittance audiometry, these results will quickly alert you that the measured air-bone gap is erroneous.

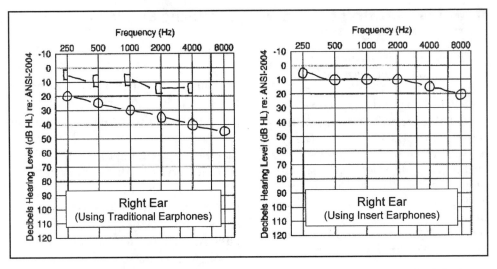

Figure 5–1. The effects of a collapsing ear canal. The audiogram on the left shows a mild conductive loss when traditional earphones are used. The audiogram on the right shows how air conduction thresholds return to normal levels for the same ear when an insert earphone is used. High frequency conductive losses are rare, so always consider collapsed canals when this pattern is present; the routine use of insert earphones of course will mostly eliminate the problem from the onset.

Impacted Cerumen

Cerumen (or ear wax) is a normal byproduct of a healthy ear. It lubricates the ear canal and protects the canal and tympanic membrane. As cerumen is produced by the subcutaneous glands of the ear canal, it migrates out of the ear canal by way of the tiny hairs lining the outer layer of the external ear canal.

Some people produce more cerumen than others, especially the elderly. Additionally, other people may disturb the natural cerumen excretion process by inserting Q-tips and other foreign objects into their ear canal, attempting to remove the cerumen. These objects often irritate the canal, which then results in increased cerumen production, which then results in more probing by the individual, not a good thing. Addi-

tionally, using foreign objects to attempt to remove cerumen can result in an impaction, a total blockage of an area of the ear canal.

For individuals who produce excessive cerumen, impaction sometimes also occurs because of hearing aid use. That is, the hearing aid (in the case of a custom instrument) or the earmold at the time of each insertion continues to push the cerumen to a given point (usually about 10 to 15 mm from the ear canal opening) and, eventually, a total (or near total) blockage will occur.

Impacted cerumen results in a temporary conductive hearing loss of varying degree (in severe cases, an air-bone gap as large as 30 to 40 dB will be present). Once the cerumen is removed by a qualified professional, hearing returns to pre-impact levels. A good otoscopic examination will reveal if impacted cerumen exists. If you observe this, you may want to have the cerumen removed before conducting the hearing test, as there is little reason to conduct a test when you know a priori that the results do not represent the patient's "true" hearing.

TIPS and TRICKS: Cerumen Management

Some audiologists and a few hearing instrument specialists have specialized training in the removal of cerumen from the ear canal. Known as cerumen management, your ability to conduct this service should only happen after you have checked with your state licensing board to see if you can offer it, and had additional training on it.

To find locations where cerumen management courses are offered check with the International Hearing Society or your state licensing board.

External Otitis

Otitis externa is an inflammation of the outer ear and ear canal. Along with otitis media, which we address shortly, external otitis is one of two conditions commonly referred to as an "earache." One common name for this condition is "swimmer's ear" because it frequently develops in people who have been swimming and have had water trapped in their ears.

External otitis is an extremely painful condition requiring treatment from a physician. Hearing tests often cannot be conducted on patients with external otitis because the ear is too painful to allow for the placement of earphones.

Acute external otitis often occurs suddenly, rapidly worsens, and becomes extremely painful. Because the tissues lining the external ear canal are extremely thin they are easily torn or abraded by minimal force. Inflammation of the ear canal can begin when someone tries to self-clean their ear canal with a cotton swab or other small implement. Another cause of external otitis is prolonged exposure to water or extreme humidity. Regardless of the cause, external otitis occurs when active bacteria or fungus begin to infect the skin of the ear canal.

TIPS and TRICKS: External Otitis and Hearing Loss

In general, we would not expect external otitis to cause a hearing loss. If the swelling was such that there was complete closure of the ear canal, then a mild conductive loss would be expected (probably greatest in the higher frequencies). In general, however, expect normal hearing with this pathology.

Some hearing care professionals have been specially trained to remove cerumen from the ear canal. Due to the thinness of the tissues of ear canals it is easy to abrade them, thus causing inflammation and possibly external otitis in some patients.

Pain that worsens on touching of the outer ear is the predominant complaint associated with external otitis. Patients may also experience discharge from the ear canal and itchiness. Swelling of the ear canal is another symptom and when the swelling is severe enough a conductive hearing loss may occur. In advanced cases of external otitis, pain may radiate to the jaw and neck.

Because the ear is a self-cleaning system, milder cases of this condition can be addressed by simply refraining from swimming or not using implements to try and clear wax from the ear canal. Topical solutions or suspensions in the form of ear drops typically are used to treat mild and moderate cases of otitis externa. In more advanced cases a physician may have to use a binocular microscope to clean the ear canal and insert what is called an ear wick to deliver medication to the infected area. Because external otitis is so common and can be caused by the actions of even the most experienced hearing care professional during cerumen removal procedures, it's important to know the common symptoms and to immediately refer your patient to a physician for an evaluation if you suspect it.

Tumors of the External Ear Canal

Both malignant and benign tumors have been found in the external ear canal. Bony tumors, called osteomas, are sometimes seen in the ears of people who have done a lot of swimming in cold water. You may not observe a tumor per se, but rather just a narrowing of the canal. Unless the bony growth or tumor closes off the entire external ear canal, they do not cause hearing loss. A detailed otoscopic exam should reveal this, and, unless this is a long-standing condition reported by the patient, a physician referral is appropriate.

Perforated Tympanic Membrane

There are several ways the tympanic membrane (TM) can become perforated. A perforated eardrum is a rupture or perforation (hole) of the eardrum that can occur as a result of infection, trauma (e.g., by trying to clean the ear with sharp instruments, or even a Q-Tip), explosion, barotrauma, or surgery (accidental creation of a rupture).

Because traumatic perforations often alter otherwise normal tissue, they often heal spontaneously. One common cause of TM perforations is related to the buildup of excessive pressure in the middle ear as a result of a middle ear disorder (e.g., eustachian tube dysfunction, infection, effusion, etc.). In these cases, the excess pressure causes the TM to rupture. Because of the underlying middle ear disorder, TM perforations caused from this excessive pressure need to be managed medically.

Surgical repair of a perforated TM is called myringoplasty or tympanoplasty. In some cases, the "surgical patching" procedures are not successful, and the patient more or less will have a "permanent" perforation. Those with more severe and long-standing ruptures may need to wear an earplug to avoid water (or other liquids) making contact with the eardrum, and entering the middle ear cavity.

Perforation of the eardrum usually leads to conductive hearing loss. The amount of hearing loss caused by a perforated TM varies by both the size of the perforation and the location of the opening. Some perforations can be so small that they cannot be detected during routine otoscopy. With large perforations, it's common to see a conductive hearing loss of 30 to 40 dB. Once the perforation heals, hearing is usually recovered fully (maybe with a slight 5- to 10-dB drop due to scarring), but chronic infection over a long period may lead to permanent hearing loss, as the structure of the TM is altered.

Disorders of the Middle Ear

The Bermuda Triangle is a region in the western part of the North Atlantic Ocean where a number of aircraft and surface vessels allegedly disappeared mysteriously. Popular culture has attributed these disappearances to the paranormal or activity by extraterrestrial beings. Documented evidence indicates that a significant percentage of the incidents were inaccurately reported or embellished by later authors, and numerous official agencies have stated that the number and nature of disappearances in the region is similar to that in any other area of ocean. You can think of middle ear disorders like reports of lost vessels in the Bermuda Triangle. On the surface the disorder might be unexplainable, but on further testing using tympanometry and acoustic reflexes, the disorder is no longer mysterious.

Recall that the purpose of the middle ear is to transmit the airborne sound from the eardrum to the cochlea. This is accomplished quite effectively through the aerial ratio of the TM compared to the oval window, the through the lever action of the ossicular chain. As you would expect, anything that disrupts this flow will cause a middle ear (conductive) hearing loss. We'll describe some of the most common.

Otosclerosis

Otosclerosis is caused by two main sites of involvement of the sclerotic (or scarlike) lesions. The best understood mechanism is fixation of the stapes footplate to the oval window of the cochlea. This greatly impairs movement of the stapes and therefore transmission of sound into the inner ear ("ossicular coupling").

Additionally, the cochlea's round window can also become sclerotic, and in a similar way impair movement of sound pressure waves through the inner ear ("acoustic coupling"). There is some documentation of sclerotic lesions that also are within the cochlea, sometimes referred to as "cochlear otosclerosis."

Treatment of otosclerosis often involves a surgical procedure called a stapedectomy. A stapedectomy consists of removing a portion of the sclerotic stapes footplate and replacing it with an implant that is secured to the incus. This procedure restores continuity of ossicular movement and allows transmission of sound waves from the eardrum to the inner ear. A modern variant of this surgery called a stapedotomy, is performed by drilling a small hole in the stapes footplate with a microdrill or a laser, and the insertion of a pistonlike prosthesis.

Otosclerosis can be hereditary, and at least in the early stages, results in a conductive hearing loss of mild to moderate-severe degree, usually with the greatest loss in the lower frequencies. In the later stages, a mixed hearing loss may be present. Figure 5–2 gives an example of otosclerosis you might see in your office or on an audiogram. While this patient certainly is a heraring aid candidate, and probably would be a successful user of hearing aids, most opt for surgical treatment. Typically, following surgery there is a significant improvement in air conduction thresholds.

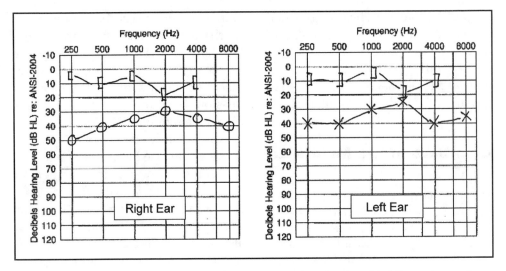

Figure 5–2. A bilateral conductive hearing loss consistent with bilateral otosclerosis. Notice the 2000 Hz or "Carhart" notch in the bone conduction scores in both ears.

TIPS and TRICKS: Carhart's Notch

An audiometric characteristic of otosclerosis is something called "Carhart's notch." This is an apparent bone conduction loss at 2000 Hz, named after the person who first described it, audiologist Raymond Carhart, Ph.D. This finding is not a true sensorineural loss, and usually disappears following surgery.

Negative Middle Ear Pressure and Middle Ear Effusion

As mentioned in Chapter 3, the eustachian tube equalizes the pressure between the air filled middle ear and outside air pressure. This tube is normally closed, but when healthy, opens frequently when we talk, chew, yawn, and so forth. When the eustachian tube becomes blocked or swollen from an allergy or common cold, the air pressure outside the middle ear is greater than the air pressure within the middle ear space. Children are more prone to negative middle ear pressure and effusion, because the eustachian tube has not had the opportunity to grow to the proper angle (~45 degrees) and is much more horizontal.

Eustachian tube dysfunction causes the air trapped inside the middle ear to become absorbed by the tissues lining the middle ear space, resulting in a drop in pressure within the middle ear space. The greater pressure from the outside air causes the tympanic membrane to become retracted or pushed into the middle ear space. This condition can be observed with otoscopy, although sometimes it is quite subtle.

A specific audiologic test battery called immittance audiometry is used to measure the function of the entire middle ear system. Tympanometry, which is part of this battery, easily will reveal a retracted TM, or a middle ear system that is not moving effectively.

If negative middle ear pressure continues to develop, and is present for an extended time, the fluids normally secreted by the mucous membranes are collected in the middle ear cavity, resulting in a condition called serous effusion or middle ear effusion. When fluid partially fills the middle ear space a mild to moderate conductive hearing loss can occur. Often, when a young child has fluid in their middle ears, it is referred to by the lay person (e.g., parents) as an "ear infection." Middle ear effusion, however, is not necessarily infectious.

The audiogram for this patient is directly related to the amount of retraction and/or the amount of fluid in the middle ear. If the patient only has a retracted TM, there probably will be little effect on hearing thresholds. If fluid begins to collect, expect thresholds, especially in the low frequencies, to drop accordingly.

Otitis Media

If middle ear effusion is allowed to continue unabated, otitis media can develop. Otitis media is any infection of the mucous-membrane lining of the middle ear space. Although otitis media is thought of as a disease of childhood, it can occur at any age, and can be quite painful. When these tissues become infected they become swollen, interfering with its pressure equalization function. During this process, the tympanic membrane becomes very vascular, resulting in the TM's red appearance.

There are two types of otitis media, called chronic and acute. As you might imagine, acute otitis media has a very rapid onset time, whereas chronic conditions of otitis media are long-standing. In some cases the fluid in the middle ear becomes thick and sticky and, hence, the nonmedical term "glue ear" sometimes has been used to describe the condition. Like many pathologies of the middle ear, the audiogram will vary with the severity of the problem. It's reasonable to expect a conductive hearing loss of 20 to 30 dB or worse. The configuration might be similar to that shown in Figure 5–2. In severe cases, air-borne gaps of 30 dB or greater are common.

Antibiotics are used in the treatment of otitis media. If otitis media persists, however, pressure equalization (PE) tubes are inserted into the TM by an otolaryngologist. This procedure is called myringotomy with PE tubes. These tubes are also referred to as grommets or tympanostomy tubes. If the tubes are open during audiometric testing (they sometimes become plugged), you would expect to see relatively normal hearing If you conduct immittance testing, volume measures will quickly indicate if the tube is open or closed.

TIPS and TRICKS: Ear Impressions and PE Tubes

It's common for children with PE tubes to obtain ear impressions so that they can obtain custom-fitting earplugs for swimming, showering, and so forth. Although we of course suggest that you always be *very* careful when taking ear impressions, this becomes even more critical when the patient has PE tubes. If impression material goes around the ear canal block, it easily can attach to the tube, and the tube then could be pulled out of the TM when the ear impression is removed. This is not good! It's not common that adult patient have PE tubes, but you will encounter this occasionally.

Cholesteatoma

In general, cholesteatomas are the result of a long-standing middle ear condition. Cholesteatomas form a sac with concentric rings consisting of a protein called keratin; there is some evidence to classify them as low-grade tumors. In patients with TM perforations, the tissue may enter the middle ear through the perforation, producing a cholesteatoma. Cholesteatomas may also be caused by chronic episodes of otitis media. Cholesteatomas are dangerous because they eventually can erode the bones of the middle ear. They potentially also could damage the facial nerve, and will even invade the nose and brain cavity in rare instances. In most cases cholesteatoma are removed with surgery. As with other middle ear pathologies, the patient will have a conductive hearing loss, although the patient with a cholesteatoma will typically have a more severe loss than most other middle ear conditions, due to the extent of the disease. It's common to observe air-bone gaps of 30 to 40 dB. A sample case study is shown in Figure 5–3.

Tympanosclerosis

Tympanosclerosis is characterized by white plaques on the surface of the tympanic membrane and deposits on the ossicles. It often is the result of chronic otitis media, which when untreated leaves this white residue. Tympanosclerosis can have a stiffening effect on the TM, which may result in a conductive hearing loss in the low frequencies. As mentioned earlier, PE tubes are a common treatment for otitis media. It's common for these patients (~30 to 40%) to have resulting tympanosclerosis after the tubes have fallen out, or been removed.

Ossicular Disarticulation

This is also referred to as "dislocation" or "discontinuity." As the name indicates, this condition results in one of the two joints between the three ossicles being pulled apart or disarticulated (the incudostapedial juncture is the most common). It can produce a wide

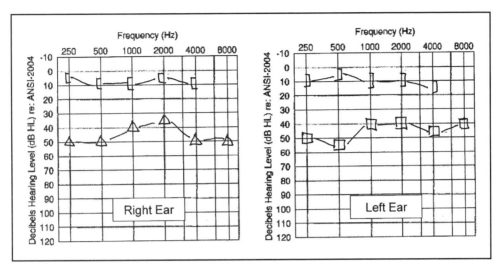

Figure 5–3. A bilateral conductive hearing loss associated with a cholesteatoma in the right ear, and otitis media in the left.

variety of conductive hearing losses depending on the location and extent of the disarticulation. The most common causes of ossicular disarticulation are degenerative diseases and trauma to the head. In severe head trauma a TM perforation also might be observed. Interestingly, the largest hearing loss (conductive) is present when the TM is intact, not perforated. In these cases, it is possible for an ossicular disarticulation to cause up to a 50 to 60 dB conductive hearing loss. This sometimes has been referred to as "maximum" conductive loss, as the cochlea is stimulated via bone conduction for higher levels (see Figure 5–3).

Patulous Eustachian Tube

In some cases the eustachian tube, which is ordinarily closed, is chronically open (patent). These persons often complain that their own voices sound hollow or that they hear their own breathing inside their head. Many of these patients have an overly patent or patulous eustachian tube. One of the more common reasons for having a patulous eustachian tube is a loss of a significant amount of weight. Although a patulous eustachian tube is not a pathologic condition, it can be quite annoying. Immitance audiometry which we briefly mentioned in Chapter 4 can be used to identify patulous eustachian tubes. There is little or no accompanying hearing loss.

Disorders of the Cochlea

The scientific community regards the Loch Ness Monster as a modern-day myth, and explains sightings as a mix of hoaxes and wishful thinking. Despite this, it remains one of the most famous examples of cryptozoology, which is the study of animals long thought extinct. When searching for disorders of the cochlea, in most cases you don't have to search long or hard to encounter a relatively common cochlear problem causing a significant hearing loss.

A significant number of people around the world have sensorineural hearing loss as a consequence of damage to the cochlea. For adults, sensorineural hearing loss resulting from cochlear pathology is by far the most common type of hearing impairment. In this section we spend some time reviewing the most common types of sensorineural hearing loss resulting from cochlear pathology. Because there is very limited medical or surgical treatment of cochlear hearing loss, these are the people that you will likely see for hearing aid fittings.

Presbycusis

Don Juan Ponce de Leon completed Spain's claim on America in 1509, and soon after was made governor of Puerto Rico. Six years later, following Indian rumors, he traveled north to the island of Bimini in search of the Fountain of Youth. Bimini turned out to be the penisula of Florida. If you've ever been to an early-bird dinner in southern Florida, you know that thousands of people are still arriving in search of that elusive fountain.

If your patient is beyond the age of 60 years old, it's possible that the hearing sensitivity has progressively worsened over the years, and this will now be reflected in the audiogram, especially in the higher frequencies. This gradual deterioration of hearing is often a result of prebycusis (sometimes written "presbyacusis"). Simply stated, presbycusis is hearing loss caused by the cumulative effects of the aging process. This progression is somewhat more rapid for men than for women, although this partially could be due to the fact that men experience more noise exposure than women, which is difficult to separate from the aging effects on the inner ear structures.

**TIPS and TRICKS:
Aging or Noise?**

An intriguing question that often comes up regarding presbycusis, is whether this is indeed the result of "aging," per se, or the result of aging in a noise and stress-filled society. Is presbycusis just a different type of noise-induced hearing loss? An often cited study related to this topic dates back to 1962, conducted with the Mabaan tribe in Sudan. Because of their isolation, there was very little noise in their lives. And guess what— there was little or no hearing loss for even the older members of the tribe (~75 years old). Interpretation of this is a little tricky, as there were also other differences (e.g., general health, diet, etc.), but it certainly is something to think about.

Presbycusis affects all parts of the ear, including neural transmissions to the brain, but the primary site of lesion is the cochlea. The outer hair cells within the cochlea are particularly sensitive to the wear and tear associated with the aging process. As a general rule, the higher the frequency, the greater effect of presbycusis (even people in their 20s and 30s experience loss of sensitivity in the >16,000-Hz range).

The classic presbycusis audiogram will show a gradually sloping downward pattern; nearly always, as the frequency becomes higher the hearing loss becomes worse (Figure 5–4). Because this is a generalized aging process, we would also expect the loss to be quite symmetric. In fact, if the loss is downward sloping, but *not* symmetric, other etiologies should be considered.

TAKE FIVE: Taking Advantage of Presbycusis

Given the known effects of presbycusis on high-frequency hearing, a cell phone ring has been developed with a center frequency around 16,000 Hz. The notion is that school children can use it to call each other during class, and their teachers won't hear it! Another technology application related to presbycusis has been to use a very loud high-pitched signal in stores where teenagers loiter. The sound is very annoying and drives them out, but the older adult customers can't hear it! Sometimes presbycusis can be a good thing.

Noise-Induced Hearing Loss (NIHL)

Exposure to loud sounds can result in temporary or permanent hearing loss. This condition is called noise-induced hearing loss (NIHL).

Around 30 million adults in the United States are exposed to hazardous sound levels in the workplace. Among these 30 million people, it's estimated that one in four will acquire a permanent hearing loss as a result of their occupation.

The degree of hearing loss caused by NIHL depends on the intensity of the sound, duration of the exposure, frequency spectrum of the sound, individual susceptibility, along with other variables. Usually, this type of hearing loss is due to continued exposure to

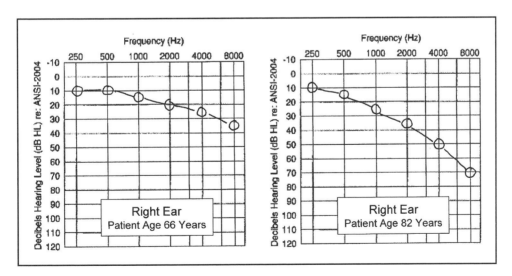

Figure 5–4. The progressive nature of presbycusis for an individual's right ear. The audiogram on the left is from a 66-year-old male. The audiogram on the right is for the same male patient at the age of 82. We only show the right ear thresholds, but typically a symmetrical pattern is observed.

work or recreational noise exposure that has occurred over several years. It is possible, however, for NIHL to occur for only a very short duration of exposure, or even a single blast (referred to as "acoustic trauma"). Because of the shape of the cochlea and the resonant effects of the outer ear, most cases of NIHL show a high-frequency hearing loss, with maximum loss in the 3000 to 6000-Hz range, and usually with some recovery at the highest frequencies. This pattern on the audiogram is called a "noise notch" (see Figure 5–5). NIHL can affect people of all ages.

As NIHL is a fairly common condition it is worth spending a little bit of time discussing the reason for the precipitous slope and noise notch. There are a couple of reasons why the area around 4000 Hz is most susceptible to damage. Although the noise causing

NIHL may be broadband, with roughly equal amplitude at all frequencies, the outer ear and ear canal resonances have amplified the noise in the 2000 to 4000 Hz region by the time the sound reaches the cochlea. This region, therefore, shows the greatest amount of damage from noise exposure. Another reason for NIHL causing more loss in the high frequencies compared to the lows is related to cochlear mechanics and cochlear blood flow; the positioning of the 3000 to 4000-Hz hair cell receptors along the basal turn of the cochlea. It is possible, but quite uncommon, for a noise notch to occur at lower frequencies (e.g., 500 to 1500 Hz; this is most commonly observed when the person was continuously exposed to a unique noise of a narrow bandwidth).

No matter the underlying reason, NIHL is a common etiology of cochlear

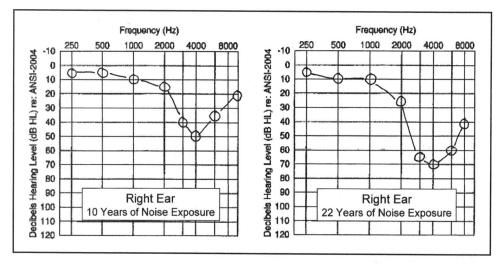

Figure 5–5. The effects of NIHL over time for one individual's left ear. Thresholds were measured 12 years apart for a male patient working in a condition of intense noise (daily carpentry with skill saw). The audiogram on the right shows the progressive nature of the hearing loss consistent with the patient's history of noise exposure. Notice how the dip at 4000 Hz deepens, and other frequencies become more involved. The left ear had the same pattern but was not as severe; perhaps there was some attenuation of the noise from head shadow for this ear.

pathology. Given its prevalence, patients that are exposed to both workplace and recreational noise need to be using properly fitted hearing protection. Counseling regarding the need for hearing protection is part of all audiologic exams.

NIHL in its most common form is of gradual onset. The two audiograms shown in Figure 5–5 are from the same worker taken 12 years apart. Notice that the loss has become worse over this 12-year period. People with significant NIHL routinely are fitted with hearing aids, however, because many with NIHL have normal hearing for low-frequency sounds they sometimes are challenging to fit. Many people with the hearing loss in the audiogram in Figure 5–5 say they can *hear*, but they just can't *understand* completely. This is due to the normal low-frequency hearing, which provides them "loudness," but the missing high frequencies reduces the audibility of critical speech cues for understanding.

Permissible Levels

Our review of noise-induced hearing loss would not be complete without a discussion of permissible levels of noise exposure. There is a direct relationship between the intensity of noise, the duration of the exposure, and the degree of potential NIHL. When counseling patients about noise exposure, it's good to have a general idea of what is "safe," and when hearing protection is needed. The Occupational Health and Safety Agency (OSHA) is an arm of the federal government responsible for ensuring that workers are safely protected from dangerous amounts of noise. Table 5–1 indicates when the intensity and duration of exposure becomes dangerous for individuals. If a worker is exposed to levels of sound greater than 90 dB for 8 hours per day, they are required to wear hearing protection. Notice that as the intensity increases the exposure time needed to cause damage is reduced.

TAKE FIVE:
Personal Stereo Systems

In the past few years there has been a lot of discussion regarding young people obtaining noise-induced hearing loss from listening to iPods and other personal stereo systems. It probably isn't as bad as suggested by some of the articles, but there is a real problem in that many of these devices can be turned up quite loud and many people use them for several hours without giving their ears a "rest." The rest period each hour is critical (and less loud, of course, is good too).

Table 5–1. Maximum Permissible Noise Levels

90 dB	8.0 hours
92 dB	6.0 hours
95 dB	4.0 hours
97 dB	3.0 hours
100 dB	2.0 hours
102 dB	1.5 hours
105 dB	1.0 hours
110 dB	30 minutes
115 dB	15 minutes

Source: Downloaded from http://www.quiet solution.com/Noise_Levels.pdf

It may be obvious to some, but workplaces are not the only conditions causing NIHL. There are plenty of recreational activities, like hunting, drag racing, and going to the disco that can cause NIHL. Even though OSHA's Permissible Noise Exposure chart wasn't created with them in mind, if you have a sound level meter, you can determine if your nightclub activities are causing some permanent hearing loss.

Ototoxicity

There are several drugs used for therapeutic treatment of diseases that have the potential side effect of causing damage to the inner ear. Because the cochlea is such a delicate organ it is susceptible to damage from medications and chemical agents. Such drugs and agents are considered to be ototoxic or poisonous to the ears.

Ototoxic drugs have one thing in common: they cause a sensorineural hearing loss. The amount of ototoxic hearing loss depends on the exact dosage and duration of use. When you encounter a patient who has used or been exposed to an ototoxic medication or agent you should consult a physician or pharmacist. A ototoxic hearing loss can present itself in different ways, but, typically, the high frequencies are the first affected, and the hearing loss is usually downward sloping. Some facilities conduct high-frequency audiometry (10,000 to 18,000 Hz) to monitor early changes in hearing.

There are hundreds of otoxic medications and agents. The most common ones along with their therapeutic uses are listed in Table 5–2. Also listed is whether the drug causes a permanent or reversible hearing loss. The majority of drugs cause a permanent hearing loss, but some cause reversible hearing loss.

Table 5–2. A Summary of Common Drug Types and Their Effects on Hearing

Type of Drug	Type of Hearing Loss	Reversible? (Y/N)
1. **Aminoglycoside Antibiotics** • streptomycin • gentamycin • kanamycin • vancomycin	Sensorineural	No
2. **Cancer Chemotherapeutics** • cisplatin • carboplatin	Sensorineural	No
3. **Loop Diuretics (Furosemide)** • lasix • bumax	Sensorineural	Yes
4. **Salicylates** • aspirin	Sensorineural	Yes
5. **Quinine**	Sensorineural	Yes

This list is by no means exhaustive; rather, it is designed to represent a sample of the most common ototoxic agents you will encounter. Because new medications are always being introduced into the market it is best to consult with your local physician or pharmacist for the most current information.

Ototoxic hearing loss is relatively common in patients receiving platinum-based chemotherapy drugs. According to several studies, between 23 and 61% develop sensorineural hearing loss as a result of receiving these chemotherapy drugs. In many cases these hearing losses develop 100 to 135 days following the onset of the chemotherapy regiment. Some of the more common platinum-based agents include cisplatin, carboplatin, eloxtin, and vincristine.

Figure 5–6 shows two audiograms from a patient who had been receiving large doses of cisplatin for lung cancer. The first audiogram is 1 month after the first treatment and the second audiogram is 60 days later. Note the difference in the thresholds due to the treatment duration. As a dispensing professional you probably will not be directly involved in collecting these types of serial audiograms; however, it's important to note how and when various treatments may affect someone's hearing and associated hearing aid use.

> ## TAKE FIVE:
> ## Important Resource
>
> In addition to causing hearing loss, prescriptive medications can cause tinnitus, hyperacusis, dizziness, and otalgia. Dr. Robert DeSogra, an audiologist in New Jersey, has created a Web site devoted to audiologic reactions to medications. By going to http://www.earserv.com and looking up a medication you quickly can find the side effects.

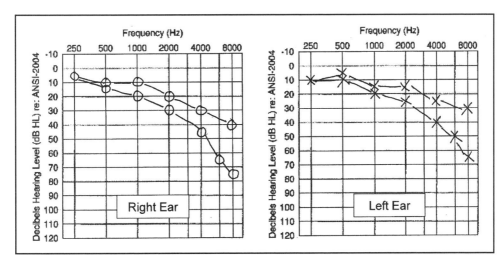

Figure 5–6. Audiograms for a patient taking larges doses of cisplatin. The upper (better) is 30 days after the first treatment and the lower (worse) audiogram on the right is 60 days after the first treatment. Note the decline in hearing over that period of time, which can be attributed to the drug regimen. The bilateral downward-sloping pattern is common.

Viral and Bacterial Diseases

There are several viral and bacterial infections that can result in sensorineural hearing loss. Infections, such as cytomegalovirus, can be transmitted to the child from the mother in utero. This is a condition known as prenatal. The following diseases are considered prenatal conditions that can result in a congenital hearing loss:

- Syphilis
- Rubella
- Toxoplasmosis
- Cytomegalovirus (CMV)
- Herpes simplex virus

There also are several viral and bacterial infections that occur after a child has been born that can produce sensorineural hearing loss. In most cases these postnatal infections enter the inner ear through the blood supply, which is carrying the infection. The following are some of the most common diseases acquired after birth (postnatal) causing hearing loss:

- Mumps
- Measles
- Bacterial meningitis
- Herpes zoster oticus

Ménière Disease

The Lost City of Atlantis was introduced to the West 2,400 years ago by Plato, who claimed it to be the island home of an advanced society. Legend says it was sunk by an earthquake, with later interpretations as an underwater kingdom protected by mermaids. Its whereabouts are still a mystery.

Ménière disease is named after the French physician Prosper Ménière, who first reported that vertigo was caused by inner ear disorders in an article published in 1861. Ménière's disease, in its "classic form" is used to describe a hearing disorder with one or more of the following characteristics:

1. A hearing loss (usually in one ear) of sudden or rapid onset.
2. A fullness or pressure sensation in the ear.
3. Brief and sudden episodes of severe dizziness (vertigo)
4. A roaring (tinnitus) in the affected ear.

One or all of the symptoms require an immediate referral to a physician. There are many subcategories of Ménière disease beyond the scope of this chapter. Some types of cochlear hearing losses of sudden onset, such as Ménière, although they are sensorineural, may actually return to normal levels.

The exact cause of Ménière disease is not known, but it is believed to be related to *endolymphatic hydrops* or excess fluid in the inner ear. It is thought that endolymphatic fluid bursts from its normal channels in the ear and flows into other areas causing damage. This is called "hydrops." This may be related to swelling of the endolymphatic sac or other tissues in the vestibular system of the inner ear, which is responsible for the body's sense of balance.

There is no standard "signature" audiogram for Ménière, but in general there tends to be more low-frequency hearing loss than observed for most other sensorineural pathologies. That is, the audiogram often appears "flat" or upward sloping rather than the more

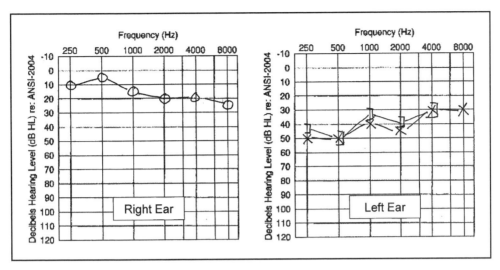

Figure 5–7. Asymmetric left sensorineural hearing loss consistent with Ménière disease.

common downward sloping pattern. Figure 5–7 shows an audiogram of a patient diagnosed with Ménière disease. Note the asymmetric (unilateral) nature of the hearing loss. After this hearing loss has stabilized, and the physician has given authorization, this person might be fit with a hearing aid in the affected ear.

Retrocochlear Disorders

In general terms, retrocochlear disorders or pathology refers to damage to the nerve fibers along the ascending auditory pathways, running from the internal auditory canal to the auditory cortex. In other words, we might be quite certain that the problem does not lie within the middle ear or the cochlea, and therefore, the locus must be somewhere more medial. Commonly, in audiologic practice, retrocochlear is used to refer to the eighth nerve and the

low brainstem, and auditory dysfunction at higher auditory levels is referred to as "central."

In most cases, eighth nerve retrocochlear pathologies involve tumors. Retrocochlear tumors, referred to as acoustic schmannomas, acoustic neuromas, neurinomas, or neurilemomas, typically (but not always) produce unilateral high-frequency hearing loss in their more advanced stages. And, unlike presbycusis and many other types of *cochlear* pathology, it is unlikely that there would be uniform symmetric tumors, so there usually is asymmetry between ears in the audiogram (Figure 5–8).

The signs and symptoms of eighth nerve retrocochlear pathology are subtle and difficult to identify with conventional audiometry. In many cases, in the early stages, there is no significant hearing loss (although there may be a reduction of speech understanding for speech in noise, or other difficult speech tests). Many patients will complain of tinnitus on the affected side,

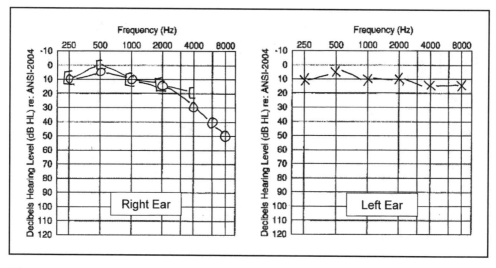

Figure 5–8. A mild, right asymmetric sensorineural hearing loss consistent with possible retrocochlear pathology.

vertigo or dizziness, fullness, or speech not sounding clear. In cases where retrocochlear pathology is suspected, a complete audiologic diagnostic battery and otologic referral is needed. Your job is to refer the patient to a physician or audiologist if a "red flag" for a retrocochlear pathology exists.

Central Auditory Disorders

As mentioned earlier, technically a retrocochlear pathology would include everything medial of the cochlea, but usually we refer to pathology above the low brainstem as "central." When thinking about auditory disorders, it's important to remember the "subtlety principle." That is, as the pathology becomes more central, going from the middle ear to the auditory cortex, the impact of the disorder on traditional

audiologic tests will be more subtle. For example, a cochlear pathology will nearly always cause a reduction in hearing thresholds and speech understanding. A disorder of the brainstem (e.g., multiple sclerosis, tumors, etc.) may cause no hearing loss and no loss of speech understanding (unless a difficult speech-in-noise test is conducted). The bottom line: If the patient's history suggests a problem with the auditory or balance system, even if all the audiometric results are very normal, medical referral is still warranted.

Nonorganic Hearing Loss

Every few years you read reports of Bigfoot carrying someone off. In 2008 there was even a photo taken of a dead Bigfoot. We were skeptical of this finding when we heard the creature was found in the woods next to a busy highway in Georgia! A few weeks later the entire report was found to be a

---

TAKE FIVE: Pure-Tone Hearing Screenings

As more than likely you will be working primarily with adults, you need to know a little about hearing screenings. When it comes to actually conducting a hearing screening, there is no acceptable standard for the identification of hearing loss in the adult population. The term "screening" implies that we are conducting some type of a "pass/fail" procedure to see if the patient needs further testing.

Some experts think that a pure-tone hearing screening should be conducted at 1, 2, and 4 kHz using a 40 dB signal. Others suggest that a 25 dB signal be used. Regardless of the cutoff criteria, the screening would be considered a "fail" if the patient does not respond to the signal at the lowest intensity level tested. Keep in mind that during a screening we conduct testing at a designated intensity level, rather than identifying threshold. When a patient fails a screening, they usually are referred for further testing, which includes a complete auditory evaluation.

There are several tools that can be used to screen older adults. The Welch-Allyn Audioscope is a hand-held device with a built-in audiometer. There are many hand-held audiometers on the market today. There is even an application, called uHEAR, that can be downloaded onto an iPod. If you do a Google search on Unitron uHear you can download it to your favorite MP3 player. Other hearing aid manufacturers have similar screening tests.

---

hoax—the dead Bigfoot body was actually made out of wax! Bigfoot might be a hoax, but we are quite sure you will have a close encounter with someone who presents a mysterious hearing loss that turns out, with careful testing, to be a hoax.

There are cases where a hearing loss may be measured on the audiogram, but there is no organic basis to explain the impairment. Some of the terms used to describe this include nonorganic hearing loss, pseudohypocusis, and functional hearing loss. If indeed the patient knowingly is exaggerating their hearing loss, the term malingering is used.

Aside from the cases of malingering, where with adults, exaggeration of the hearing loss often is related to financial compensation, the reasons for nonorganic hearing loss are not clearly understood. A number of signs can alert you to the possibility, however. These signs may include inconsistent test results, poor test-retest reliability, inappropriate behavior during the test (e.g., exaggerated attempt at listening or lipreading), or poor agreement between test results and real-world communication (e.g., the patient answers your questions in the waiting room, but then demonstrates a flat 70 dB HL hearing loss). Is some cases, there may be an underlying hearing loss, and the patient is simply adding to it.

One reason SRTs should be conducted during routine testing is to cross check the reliability of pure-tone thresholds. If the SRT and pure-tone average differ by more than 10 dB, the reliability of the test should be questioned. If there is a discrepancy, the SRT will nearly always be *better than* the pure-tone average. We recommend conducting the SRT before the pure-tone thresholds, as this will provide you with a general idea of where the thresholds should be falling for the speech frequencies. If there is poor agreement, there is no need to test all the other frequencies, as you would simply assume that the entire exam is invalid. Many other special tests have been developed to detect nonorganic hearing loss, including the Stenger test which is very effective when the "loss" is only in one ear.

Hereditary Hearing Loss

As a professional who primarily fits and dispenses hearing aids, we doubt you will spend too much time thinking about hereditary hearing loss. However, it's good to know a few important things about it. Hearing disorders can be classified into two types of groups: exogenous (outside the genes) and endogenous (within the genes).

■ Exogenous hearing disorders are those caused by toxicity, noise, accident, or injury that damages the inner ear. We have already summarized many exogenous factors of hearing loss in this chapter.

■ Endogenous hearing disorders originate in the genes of the individual. An endogenous hearing disorder is transmitted from the parents to the child as an inherited trait. Hearing losses resulting from hereditary factors comprise a significant number of all hearing disorders.

It is estimated that there are over 400 different genetic syndromes in which hearing loss is either a regular or occasional feature. Unless you are regularly testing children, you are not likely to be commonly involved in the identification of hearing disorders related to genetic transmission. During a routine case history with adults, you may encounter various genetically transmitted syndromes that have hearing loss as one of their characteristics. It's also probable that you will uncover a hearing loss that is genetic that the patient was unaware of because many progress at a very slow rate. As a professional (nonaudiologist) who dispenses hearing aids you don't need to have an in-depth understanding of genetic factors as they relate to hearing disorders; however, it is useful to know a few key concepts that you may even remember from high school or college biology class.

Mendelian Laws

Hereditary hearing loss is based on the Mendelian laws of inheritance. According to Mendelian law, genetic traits may be dominant, recessive, or sex-linked. Genes are located on the chromosomes and with the exception of those genes that are located on the sex chromosomes of males, chromosomes come in pairs. One member of each gene pair is inherited from each parent. Humans have 22 pairs of autosomes, or non-sex determining chromosomes, and one pair of chromosomes that determine sex. The sex chromosomes for females consist of two X-chromosomes, and for males, one X and one Y. During reproduction each egg and each sperm carries half the number of chromosomes from each parent. When the egg is fertilized, the full complement of chromosomes is restored, so that half of a child's genes are from the mother and the other half from the father.

Modes of Transmission

There are three modes of transmission for hereditary hearing loss: autosomal dominant inheritance, autosomal recessive inheritance, and X-linked inheritance. The term autosomal implies that the abnormal gene is not carried on the sex chromosomes. In autosomal dominant inheritance one parent exhibits the inherited trait and this trait has a 50% chance of being transmitted to the child. Examples of autosomal dominant conditions you may encounter include Waardenburg syndrome, branchio-otorenal syndrome, and neurofibromatosis 2 (NF2).

In cases of autosomal recessive inheritance, both parents of a child with hearing loss of the autosomal recessive type are clinically normal. Appearance of the trait in the child requires that an individual possess two similar abnormal genes, one from each parent. Because the laws of probability permit this type of hearing loss to be transmitted without manifestation through several generations, the detection of the origin of autosomal recessive inheritance is very difficult. Usher syndrome and Pendred syndrome are two of the more common types of

autosomal recessive hearing disorders you may encounter in clinical practice.

Another type of genetically transmitted hearing disorders is X-linked or sex-linked inheritance. X-linked inheritance is determined by genes located on the X chromosome. About 2 to 3% of all genetic hearing loss is a result of X-linked inheritance. Alport syndrome is one type of X-linked hearing disorder.

More than 70% of hereditary hearing loss is nonsyndromic, which means the hearing loss is not associated with any other signs or symptoms. The causes of nonsyndromic deafness are complex. Researchers have identified more than 30 genes that, when mutated, may cause nonsyndromic deafness; however, some of these genes have not been fully characterized. Different mutations in the same gene can cause different types of hearing loss, and some genes are associated with both syndromic and nonsyndromic deafness. In many affected families, the gene responsible for hearing loss has not been found.

Regardless of the hereditary pattern of hearing loss, we are not even scratching the surface of this topic. To learn more go to http://www.ncbi.nlm.nih.gov and enter the key words genetics and hearing loss.

Classification of Hearing Disorders by Time of Onset

Hearing loss is also classified by the time in which the hearing loss is acquired. One important reason for knowing when a hearing disorder is acquired is related to language development. When an infant has a hearing loss at birth

---

TAKE FIVE: Hearing Loss Prevalence

Hearing loss is the most common birth defect and the most prevalent sensorineural disorder in developed countries. One of every 500 newborns has a permanent, sensorineural hearing loss. By the time a child reaches adolescence, 3.5 out of 1,000 have this condition. In the general population, the prevalence of hearing loss increases with age. This change reflects the impact between genetics and environment, as well as interactions between the environmental triggers and a person's genetic predisposition. According to the National Institutes of Health (NIH) Web site, more than 50% of pre-lingual deafness is genetic, most often autosomal recessive and nonsyndromic. Approximately 50% of autosomal recessive nonsyndromic hearing loss can be attributed to the disorder DFNB1, caused by mutations in the GJB2 gene and the GJB6 gene. The carrier rate in the general population for a recessive deafness-causing mutation is about 1 in 33.

---

he or she will not develop language normally. On the other hand, a child acquiring hearing loss at say, age 12, would already have normal language development. Hearing loss caused by viral and bacterial infections are most commonly associated with the terms listed below.

Congenital Hearing Loss:
A hearing loss acquired at birth. Common causes include bacterial or viral infection, or ingestion of ototoxic medications.

Prenatal: A hearing loss that has developed before birth in which the mother has passed the hearing disorder onto the child. In other words, the hearing loss was acquired while the baby developed in utero. The most common prenatal hearing disorder are viral or bacterial infections. Many hereditary hearing disorders are acquired prenatally.

Perinatal: The hearing loss develops during or shortly after birth. Many of the same conditions causing a prenatal loss can occur perinatally.

Acquired or Postnatal: A hearing loss that develops later in life. Prelingual hearing loss is a hearing loss acquired during the critical language development years of between birth and about 12 years of age. Postlingual hearing loss is acquired after the most critical language years.

In Closing

During your first few months on the job, you are likely to have a close encounter with several of the hearing disorders mentioned in this chapter. When you do encounter one that seems a little mysterious, it's wise to refer that person to an audiologist or a physician specializing in disorders of the ear. Unlike hearing aid technology, which is rapidly evolving, the subject of hearing disorders changes at a much slower pace. For this reason we recommend that you invest some of your hard-earned dollars into one or two hearing disorders textbooks. The text doesn't have to be all that current to be useful. One we like is, *Hearing Disorders* by Jerry Northern. The third edition, which was published in 1995, is available online for a reasonable price. Another is entitled, *Audiology: The Fundamentals* by Fred Bess and Larry Humes. It has a comprehensive introductory chapter on hearing disorders that expands on this chapter.

6

The Hearing Aid Selection Process

> *It starts with an inspiration, a recipe that may have been passed down to you from a friend or family member, careful planning, and attention to detail. How selecting hearing aids is like making your favorite home-cooked meal.*

The hearing aid selection process is a lot like making your favorite home-cooked meal. For example, making your favorite cake requires selecting the proper ingredients, precisely following a recipe, getting the ideal baking temperature, and just the right amount of tender loving care to ensure a great-tasting outcome.

No matter what type of hearing aid you fit or how much hearing loss a patient may have; there are several concepts we have already covered in this book which contribute to the hearing aid selection process. Some basic knowledge of each of them will help you more smoothly navigate the hearing aid selection and fitting process, and with any luck knowing about them will help you make better clinical decisions when it comes to determining hearing aid candidacy. This chapter takes you

step-by-step through the entire process of selecting hearing aids for a patient. We show you how following several steps during the prefitting selection process will consistently lead to a successful hearing aid fitting.

This chapter has been divided into two main parts: Part 1 reviews all the major components of the prefitting tests, including the tests (think ingredients to your recipe) you'll need to complete prior to selecting hearing aids. Part 2 takes you through several of the most important prefitting considerations you need to address once you have obtained all the prefitting test data outlined in Part 1. Think of the common obstacles you have to overcome to make a dinner party successful.

Before getting started, it's important to remember that the case history is a good time to establish rapport with the patient and really get to know them. Just like great cooks have a fondness for using only the best ingredients, you will need to have affection for patients in need of your services. Taking the time for small talk with the patient in the exam room prior to asking them personal questions about their hearing will help you build a more effective relationship with them.

Part 1—
The Prefitting Hearing
Assessment Battery

The Case History

Conducting a good case history with your patient is akin to asking your guest what their favorite dish might be before you invite them over for dinner. For example, a conscientious host would want to serve a vegetarian dish if a guest doesn't eat meat. The case history is sort of the same way. It's the time when you get to know a little something about your patient that might help you plan and prepare for a successful engagement.

The primary goal of the case history is to identify any problems requiring medical intervention prior to selecting hearing aids. One of your most important professional obligations is an awareness of the eight signs of a medical pathology. The so-called FDA questions are designed to help you identify a possible medical problem relative to the ears and hearing before proceeding with the selection and fitting of any hearing aids. These questions must be asked during the initial case history. As

a hearing care professional you are mandated by the U.S. Food and Drug Administration (FDA) to refer a patient immediately to a physician. In many of these cases the physician will evaluate and treat the patient and refer them back to you for a hearing aid evaluation. A useful term to know is **RED FLAG**.

A red flag is any of the eight signs of a hearing disorder that show up on the audiogram or your case history. Red flags need to be handled immediately by referring the patient to a physician, preferable one that specializes in diseases of the ear (otolaryngologist). Once the patient has been evaluated and given written medical clearance by the physician, you can begin the hearing aid selection process.

Red Flags

Here are the eight red flags related to ear pathology and hearing disorders:

1. Visible deformity to the outer ear
2. Visible evidence of significant cerumen accumulation or a foreign body in the ear canal.
3. Any history of active drainage from the ear within the previous 90 days.
4. Any history of sudden hearing loss within the previous 90 days
5. Any acute or chronic dizziness
6. A hearing loss in one ear of sudden or rapid onset within the previous 90 days
7. Ear pain or discomfort
8. An air-bone gap on the audiogram of more than 15 dB at 500, 1000, and 2000 Hz.

The sample case history form in Figure 6–1 shows the questions that

SONUS. hearing care professionals

_____ Date

Patient Hearing Health Interview

_____   _____
Patient Name   Hearing Care Professional

_____   _____
Companion Name   License #

1. Tell me what prompted you to visit me today   _____

2. What do you hope to achieve from your visit today?_____
_____

3. What have you noticed about your hearing/communication ability? _____
_____

4. How long have you noticed any difficulties? _____

5. What are the people closest to you saying about your hearing/communication ability? _____
_____

6. Have you had your hearing tested before? If so, by whom? _____ Date: _____

7. Check any of the following conditions, and add any comments that may help us understand and treat all hearing concerns.

Yes   No
☐   ☐   Pain/Discomfort in ears _____

☐   ☐   Noises/Ringing in ears _____

☐   ☐   History of hearing loss in your family _____

☐   ☐   Dizziness or balance problems (acute or chronic) _____

☐   ☐   Excessive noise exposure _____

☐   ☐   Surgery or medical problems with ears,
          active drainage within previous 90 days. _____

☐   ☐   Sudden hearing loss in the past 90 days
          (unilateral or rapidly progressive within previous 90 days)_____

☐   ☐   Visible congenital or traumatic deformity of the ear_____

☐   ☐   Audiometric air-bone gaps equal to or
          greater than 15dB at .5, 1 & 2 kHz _____

☐   ☐   Visible evidence of significant cerumen
          accumulation or a foreign body in the ear canal _____

8. What medications, if any, are you currently taking?_____
_____

9. Do you have any other medical conditions that we should be aware of? _____
_____

10. Who is your family physician? Doctor's name: _____

11. How did you hear about Sonus? ☐ TV ☐ Newspaper ☐ Mail ☐ Internet ☐ Doctor referral ☐ Friend/family member

    ☐ Other _____

Figure 6–1. A blank sample case history form. Note the FDA questions are listed in Question 7. Copyright 2009 Sonus USA Inc. Reprinted with permission.

need to be asked during the initial hearing aid evaluation. Notice that many of the disorders discussed in Chapter 5 are addressed during the case history.

After completing the case history, the next step is to conduct a detailed assessment in order to determine candidacy for hearing aids. This includes evaluating the patient's perception of handicap associated with a potential hearing loss, motivation, communication needs, and expectations regarding the use of hearing aids. By using a battery of assessment tools and through proper counseling, hearing aid candidacy will be determined.

Prefitting Questionnaires

Although you probably won't administer a formal questionnaire before serving a meal to your guests, you are likely to ask them exactly how they like their food cooked. Let's say you're grilling steaks on your deck for several people. While the steaks are cooking you might ask each guest how they like it prepared. For those who like their steak rare you pull it off the grill a little early and set it aside whereas you allow the others to cook a few minutes longer.

You can think of prefitting questionnaires in a similar way to food preparation. It is useful preliminary information that helps you customize your fitting a little later in the process.

During the prefitting appointment it is common practice to administer one or more questionnaires to the patient in order to collect some information about the patient's expectations and attitude toward hearing loss and the possible use of hearing aids. Some experts refer to these questionnaires as "income" or "in-take" measurements because they are designed to measure several patient variables before the patient is seen, whereas "outcome" measures are used after the fitting to assess patient results following the hearing aid fitting.

There are several nonaudiologic variables, such as expectations, degree of self-confidence, manual dexterity, and attitude that contribute to the success of the fitting. Administering a prefitting questionnaire enables you to obtain a more accurate appraisal of many of these nonaudiologic variables by measuring them on a scale. There are dozens of prefitting questionnaires that have been developed over the years. We have decided to review two that have practical merit in a busy dispensing practice.

Characteristics of Amplification Tool (COAT)

The COAT was developed at Cleveland Clinic in 2006. The COAT has nine questions that evaluate several important prefitting dimensions, including technology and hearing aid style preferences. The COAT is designed to discover patient preferences and attitudes toward hearing aid use, so that the practitioner can make one firm recommendation at the end of the fitting appointment. The COAT, shown in Figure 6–2, can be downloaded at http://www.audiologyonline.com and conducting a key word search using the term COAT. Look up the article published by Sharon Sandridge and Craig Newman of Cleveland Clinic in March, 2006. The COAT authors even encourage clinicians to customize the questions to fit the needs of their practice.

Hearing Handicap Inventory for the Elderly-Screening Version (HHIE-S)

Hearing handicap is best defined as the patient's perception of a problem or limitation in daily communication associated with hearing loss. In order to learn more about a patient's communication

Characteristics of Amplification Tool (COAT)

Name: _____ Date: _____

CCF #: _____ Audiologist: _____

Our goal is to maximize your ability to hear so that you can more easily communicate with others. In order to reach this goal, it is important that we understand your communication needs, your personal preferences, and your expectations. By having a better understanding of your needs, we can use our expertise to recommend the hearing aids that are most appropriate for **you**. By working together **we** will find the best solution for you.

Please complete the following questions. Be as honest as possible. Be as precise as possible. Thank you.

1. Please list the top three situations where you would most like to hear better. Be as specific as possible.

_____

_____

_____

2. How important is it for you to hear better? Mark an X on the line.

Not Very Important   *Very Important*

3. How motivated are you to wear and use hearing aids? Mark an X on the line.

Not Very Motivated   *Very Motivated*

4. How well do you think hearing aids will improve your hearing? Mark an X on the line.

I expect them to:

Not be helpful at all   *Greatly improve my hearing*

5. What is your most important consideration regarding hearing aids? Rank order the following factors with **1** as the most important and **4** as the least important. Place an **X** on the line if the item has no importance to you at all.

____ Hearing aid size and the ability of others not to see the hearing aids

____ Improved ability to hear and understand speech

____ Improved ability to understand speech in noisy situations (e.g., restaurants, parties)

____ Cost of the hearing aids

Page –2-

6. Do you prefer hearing aids that: (check one)

____ are totally automatic so that you do not have to make any adjustments to them.

____ allow you to adjust the volume and change the listening programs as you see fit.

____ no preference

7. Look at the pictures of the hearing aids. Please place an X on the picture or pictures of the style you would **NOT** be willing to use. Your audiologist will discuss with you if your choices are appropriate for you – given your hearing loss and physical shape of your ear.

[ ] BTE   [ ] Full Shell   [ ] Canal

[ ] Mini BTE   [ ] Half Shell/ Low profile   [ ] CIC

8. How confident do you feel that you will be successful in using hearing aids.

Not Very Confident   *Very Confident*

9. There is a wide range in hearing aid prices. The cost of hearing aids depends on a variety of factors including the sophistication of the circuitry (for example, higher level technology is more expensive than the more basic hearing aids) and size/style (for example, the CIC hearing aids are more expensive than the BTE instruments). The price ranges listed below are for *two* hearing aids. Please check the cost category that represents the maximum amount you are willing to spend. Please understand that you are not locked into that price range. It is just very helpful for us to know your budget so that we can provide you with the most appropriate hearing aids.

____ Basic digital hearing aids: Cost is between $2000 to $2499

____ Basic Plus hearing aids: Cost is between $2500 to $2999

____ Mid-level digital hearing aids: Cost is between $3000 to $3999

____ Premium digital hearing aids: Cost is between $4000 to $6000

Thank you for answering the questions.

Your responses will assist us in providing you with the best hearing healthcare.

Figure 6–2. The COAT questionnaire downloaded from Audiology Online. Posted August, 2006. Reprinted with permission of Audiology Online.

handicap any number of self-assessment tools can be used to measure the degree of the problem (see review in Chapter 11).

One example of a self-assessment hearing handicap scale that can be used in a busy office is the Hearing Handicap Inventory for the Elderly–Screening Version (HHIE-S), originally created by Ira Ventry and Barbara Weinstein in 1983. This is a 10-question self-report that can be administered to both the patient and a significant other during the prefitting appointment.

The HHIE-S allows the patient to evaluate the emotional and social impact their hearing loss has on communication. The HHIE-S is scored by having the patient answer yes, sometimes, or no to 10 questions. Four points is assigned if the patient answers yes, 2 points are assigned if the patient answers sometimes, and 0 points are awarded if the patient answers no to any of the questions. The point totals are calculated and a degree of handicap is determined using the published norms listed in Table 6–1.

Table 6–1. The Published Normative Data for Interpreting the HHIE-S score.

0–10	No significant perception of a hearing handicap
12–22	Mild to moderate perception of hearing handicap
>22	Severe perception of hearing handicap

from your office. As mentioned previously, an added benefit of the HHIE-S is that it can be administered to both the patient and a companion. Before you actually have conducted the hearing test, valuable insights about motivation and the patient's perception of the problem can be obtained when scores for both people are compared. For example, if the patient has a low score of 4 to 8 (little perception of the problem) and his or her companion has a higher score of 18 to 22 (moderate perception of problem) this is an indication that the patient is denying a hearing loss or has no motivation for receiving help—and conversely, the patient's companion is noticing that the patient has a significant degree of difficulty in everyday listening situations (Figure 6–3).

TIPS and TRICKS:
Different Versions Available

We'll go into this in more detail in Chapter 11, but the HHIE also has a companion version for adults under 65 years of age called the HHIA (A = adults). Both the HHIE and the HHIA have a 25-question version and a 10-question version —the latter called the "Screening," or "S" scale.

The score from the HHIE-S helps determine the patient's perception of hearing handicap and to some extent their motivation to receive services

Communication Needs Assessment

The next component of determining hearing aid candidacy is conducting an assessment of the patient's communication needs. There are several self-reports available that can measure the patients many of which are reviewed in Chapter 11. During the prefitting appointment it is important to not only measure the extent of any handicap related to

Intake Questionnaire

Thank you for visiting us today. To help us provide you with the best possible care, please take a few moments to complete the following questionnaire. Your responses will help make your hearing evaluation and fitting appointment more efficient, effective and successful.

Instructions

• Please read the following statements.

• Beside each statement, mark the circle that *best* describes your experience in each situation.

Name: _____ Date: _____

Always | Sometimes | Never

1. I have to ask people to repeat themselves even when I am in a quiet conversation with one or two other people.

2. My family members complain that I need to turn the television volume louder than they do.

3. When I talk on the telephone or cell phone, I miss some of what is being said.

4. During a card game (or other game) around a table, I have difficulty hearing the conversation.

5. When I am in a busy public place, such as a shopping center, I have difficulty communicating with others.

6. In meetings, I have to strain to make sure I hear everything.

7. When I'm eating in a restaurant, I have to ask my dining companion to repeat things.

8. I miss a lot of information during church and/or classroom lectures.

9. When I'm listening to music/concerts, I miss parts of the performance.

10. If I'm in the car with others who are talking, I can't hear what they're saying.

Figure 6–3. An example of the HHIE-S used in clinical practice. Reprinted with permission of Unitron.

hearing loss, but to target specific listening situations where the patient struggles with hearing, and that are also important to the patient.

Getting COSI

An example of a useful communication needs scale is the Client Oriented Scale of Improvement (COSI). It is a popular, open-ended communication needs assessment tool that allows the patient to nominate two to five or six specific areas in which communication is a problem. These specific situations, put forward by the patient, can be targeted

as goals to improve with hearing aid use. Figure 6–4 gives an example of a COSI that has been completed during the prefitting appointment. Notice that the five listening situations targeted for improvement are specific and measurable. Shortly after the fitting these five situations will be reviewed by you and the patient to measure hearing aid benefit.

Great Expectations?

Another important part of determining hearing aid candidacy is patient expectations. If you think about it,

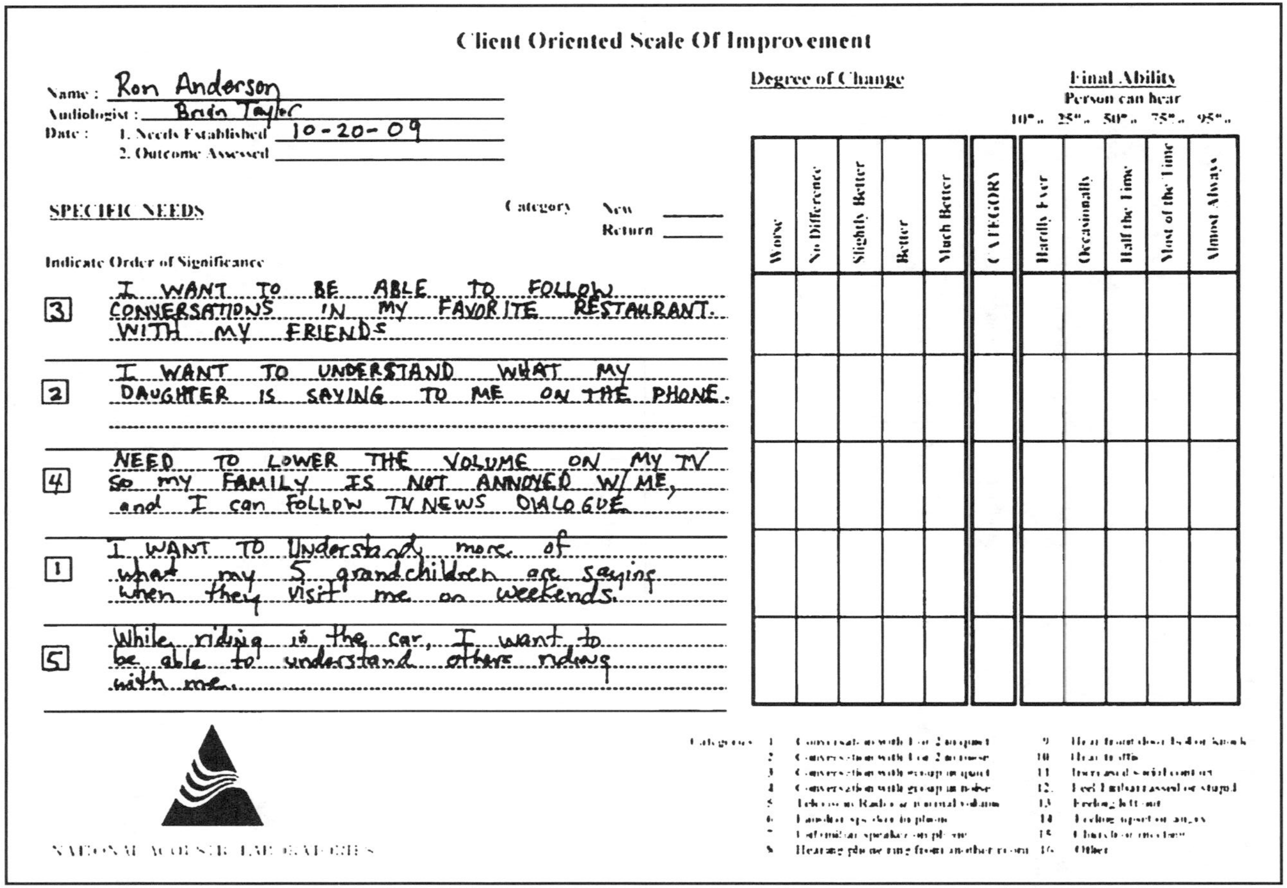

Client Oriented Scale Of Improvement

Name: Ron Anderson
Audiologist: Brian Taylor
Date: 10-20-09   1. Needs Established
                  2. Outcome Assessed

Category: New _____
             Return _____

SPECIFIC NEEDS

Indicate Order of Significance

[3] I WANT TO BE ABLE TO FOLLOW CONVERSATIONS IN MY FAVORITE RESTAURANT. WITH MY FRIENDS.

[2] I WANT TO UNDERSTAND WHAT MY DAUGHTER IS SAYING TO ME ON THE PHONE.

[4] NEED TO LOWER THE VOLUME ON MY TV SO MY FAMILY IS NOT ANNOYED W/ ME, AND I CAN FOLLOW TV NEWS DIALOGUE.

[1] I WANT TO UNDERSTAND more of what my 5 grandchildren are saying when they visit me on weekends.

[5] While riding in the car, I want to be able to understand others riding with me.

NATIONAL ACOUSTIC LABORATORIES

Degree of Change

	Worse	No Difference	Slightly Better	Better	Much Better	CATEGORY

Final Ability
Person can hear
10%, 25%, 50%, 75%, 95%

	Hardly Ever	Occasionally	Half the Time	Most of the Time	Almost Always

Categories
1 Conversation with 1 or 2 in quiet
2 Conversation with 1 or 2 in noise
3 Conversation with a group in quiet
4 Conversation with a group in noise
5 Television/Radio at normal volume
6 Familiar speaker on phone
7 Unfamiliar speaker on phone
8 Hearing phone ring from another room

9 Hear front door bell or knock
10 Hear traffic
11 Increased social contact
12 Feel embarrassed or stupid
13 Feeling left out
14 Feeling upset or angry
15 Church or meeting
16 Other

Figure 6-4. An example of a completed prefitting COSI. Notice that the patient has nominated 5 specific prefitting goals to target with amplification, and they have been recorded on the COSI for by the hearing care professional. COSI form downloaded from http://www.nal.au .

144

TAKE FIVE: BRINGING A FRIEND TO THE PARTY

Most professionals who have fitted hearing aids for a while say that it's important to have the patient who is seeing you for the first time to bring a companion with them. The companion, sometimes called the third party, is someone with a familiar voice who can make the consultative appointment more comfortable for the patient. Research has shown that new patients are twice as likely to purchase hearing aids from you if they bring a companion to the initial appointment. Five reasons a significant other should be present during the prefitting appointment:

1. Provide details about the general health of the patient

2. Give a second opinion (so-called third ear) about how the patient is communicating in daily living.

3. Facilitate discussion during the needs assessment and testing phase of the appointment

4. Help the patient remember what was said during the evaluation

5. Assist in making treatment and purchasing decisions

---

expectations are an important part of any transaction. For example, when you purchase a new car your attitude and outlook is different compared to when you buy an old beater to run around town for $1,000. Of course, we are not saying any patient will ever be fitted with second-hand hearing aids, but price is certainly an important part of patient expectations. The take-home point is that every patient has certain expectations about hearing aid use, and you will need to address those expectations on an individual basis.

Given the relative cost of hearing instruments, and consumer marketing surrounding modern hearing devices, some patients might even have inflated expectations. An important part of the initial conversation you have with patients regarding hearing aid use needs to focus on their expectations of the benefits that they expect from the use of hearing aids. Fortunately, there are some tools to help you more care-fully address expectations with your patients. A couple of self-assessment questionnaires have been developed to measure patient expectations. One is called the ECHO (expected consequences of hearing aid ownership. It's a short questionnaire that is easy for patients to complete and simple for you to score. If you are interested in measuring patient expectations, the ECHO is a good tool to administer. To learn more about using the ECHO and to download a copy go to Robyn Cox's Web site: http://www.ausp.memphis.edu/harl

The Hearing Test Battery

If you're planning on trying out Patti LaBelle's mac and cheese recipe, you better have a good supply of cheese on hand. You need two kinds of cheddar, muenster, Monterey jack, and some Velveeta (this isn't really cheese, but you get the idea). We like

to kick it up a notch will some bacon and jalapeño peppers, but don't tell Patti.

Just like there are several key ingredients to your favorite mac and cheese dish, there are several components to the hearing test battery used for the purpose of selecting aids. These tests include measuring the threshold of audibility (the basic hearing test), loudness discomfort level (LDL) testing, speech-in-noise testing, and measuring the acceptable noise level. Although it's a little more complicated than most recipes, when you meticulously combine the key ingredients of the hearing test battery you are very likely to end up with a successful final outcome. The results of a hearing test battery will be used to program the hearing aid and to counsel the patient about realistic expectations and use.

Hearing Thresholds

The bread and butter of the prefitting evaluation is the pure tone audiogram. Speaking of bread and butter, when it comes to home cooked meals we can think of nothing more satisfying than the smell and taste of freshly baked bread. People from all cultures around the globe have their own variations of home-made bread. Although the type of flour and yeast as well as the shape and texture may vary, fresh bread is enjoyed by everyone. Regardless of your cultural background, when high quality flour is combined with water and yeast and baked at the proper temperature the end result is a real delicacy. When earphones are placed on a patient and a calibrated audiometer is used by a professional to conduct an audiogram, it doesn't matter what type of hearing aids you are likely to recommend, your final result is a test that is used the world over to make important diagnostic and hearing aid selection decisions.

Recall from Chapter 4 that the primary goal of threshold testing (the X's and O's on the audiogram) is to identify the type and degree of hearing loss. This, of course, remains the primary goal of pure-tone threshold testing. When it comes to selecting hearing aids, however, threshold testing has a slightly different purpose. What you have plotted on the audiogram serves as the lower end of the patient's residual dynamic range.

The residual dynamic range is the auditory area in which hearing aids will provide amplification. Because each patient's thresholds of audibility and discomfort are different, residual dynamic ranges vary from patient to patient. Before you can fit hearing aids, you need to know the patient's residual dynamic range. Right now, you should have the first step of this process mastered: measuring the threshold of audibility using a "bracketing" procedure, like the one described in Chapter 4.

The threshold of audibility will largely determine the amount of gain (volume) the patient will require from the hearing aid. Gain is the difference between the input level of the sound going into the hearing aid and the output after this sound has been amplified. Generally speaking, for any given threshold on the audiogram expressed in dB HL, only about half of that value typically is need-ed for gain, although this varies significantly depending on the level of the in-put signal. For example, if the threshold on the audiogram is 60 dB HL at 2000 Hz, only about 30 to 35 dB of gain is required to reasonably restore audibility.

You might be wondering why you need to restore gain by only 50 to 60% and not the full amount. This is because there is a balance between audibility and comfort of sound. In other words, if we took that patient mentioned above with the 60 dB hearing loss, and re-stored his thresholds with hearing aids back to around 0 dB HL; it is very probable that this patient will complain that many sounds are uncomfortable.

The tradeoff between providing enough amplification to make soft speech audible while maintaining comfort is a constant challenge you need to be prepared to tackle. Fortunately, researchers have developed many prescriptive formulas that will help you more precisely juggle audibility and comfort. Because prescriptive formulae are really not needed until you actually order the hearing aid, we will table our discussion on that topic for a later chapter.

Loudness Discomfort Level (LDL) Testing

Conducting accurate (LDL) testing is similar to a good meatloaf dinner. Meatloaf, of course, is a classic comfort food and LDL testing is also sort of a classic, as the procedure has been used by most professionals fitting hearing aids since the 1940s. Hopefully the LDL test procedure also will lead to "comfort."

The second step in the hearing test battery is to measure the patient's threshold of discomfort. This step will establish the top end of the dynamic range. This test goes by a host of names, including uncomfortable listening level (UCL), threshold of discomfort (TD), and loudness discomfort level (LDL). No matter what you call it, this is an important step to get right

because the results of the test (and related hearing aid adjustments) will help prevent the loud sounds the patient encounters from being uncomfortably loud. The results of unaided LDL testing can be entered into the hearing aid fitting computer software. Most manufacturers use LDL information to establish the hearing aid's maximum power output (MPO).

TIPS and TRICKS: Tones Not Speech

Historically, LDL testing has been conducted most commonly using a speech stimuli, rather than tonal stimuli. For a number of reasons, the use of a speech signal is *not* the preferred method. Because tones can be delivered to the ear in a precise manner compared to speech, results of testing using this stimuli is more accurate. More importantly, you will need to use the results of this testing for programming the hearing aids, which requires frequency-specific information.

One of the most common characteristics of a sensorineural hearing loss is an abnormal growth in loudness, sometimes referred to as recruitment. LDL testing determines how sensitive your patient is to loud sounds.

Research has shown that taking the time to accurately measure LDLs actually contributes to the success of the hearing aid fitting. This is because the LDL values allow you to adjust the MPO so that loud sounds are loud enough, but not too loud. When you can more accurately repackage sound into the patient's residual dynamic range, they will be more satisfied.

As with measuring hearing thresholds of audibility, there is a standard protocol for measuring LDLs. When you follow this standard protocol, you can be sure you have a precise idea of the upper limits of the patient's residual dynamic range.

LDL Procedure

1. Patient completes the test with ear phones. Testing is conducted in each ear separately.
2. Review the Cox contour loudness anchors (Figure 6–5) with the patient. The Independent Hearing Aid Fitting Forum (IHAFF) loudness anchors need to be posted on the wall in the test booth, or printed on a sheet of paper that the patient can easily see (laminate the sheet on cardboard, and have them hold it).
3. Instruct the patient (see the Uncomfortable Loudness Level section of Chapter 4) in a practice run to ensure the patient understands the instructions.
4. Testing should be completed at two discrete frequencies using pulsed pure tones; 500 Hz and 2000 Hz are the two most commonly used frequencies.
5. Begin testing at 55 dB HL. Increase in an ascending (increasing the intensity level of the audiometer) order using 5 db steps
6. Complete two test runs for each frequency in each ear. If the #7 value is within 5 dB for both runs, use the average of the two.
7. If the two runs are more than 10 dB apart, a third test run is recommended. Take the average of the three.
8. Record the calculated average value for the #7 rating from the Cox countour loudness anchors on the patient's audiogram.

Speech Audiometry

Speech audiometry is a bit like apple pie. Everyone loves it, but there are several variations of it. Although the basic ingredients are found in every recipe, the type of apples, crust and extra ingredients, like raisins or cheddar cheese, varies with the inclination of the baker. In our speech audiometry recipe (we covered the basics in Chapter 4) we are going to be purists and stick with proven ingredients that are supported by research.

One of the primary goals of amplification is improving speech intelligibility. Speech intelligibility is directly related to audibility. This means that if you can restore audibility chances are very good that speech intelligibility will be improved. In other words, when you turn up the volume for speech so that

7 = Uncomfortably Loud

6 = Loud, but Okay

5 = Comfortable, but Slightly Loud

4 = Comfortable

3 = Comfortable, but Slightly Soft

2 = Soft

1 = Very Soft

0 = Can't Hear

Figure 6–5. The loudness anchors of the Cox Countour Test.

the patient can hear more of it, you greatly improve the chances of them understanding it.

The relationship between audibility and intelligibility actually is quite complex—a bit more than we can explain here. However, to better appreciate the relationship between the two you can read the Take Five devoted to the concept later in the chapter.

Traditionally, speech audiometry has been conducted using single words in quiet. The NU-6 and W-22 word lists are two commonly used single-word speech tests, usually conducted under earphones or in quiet listening conditions. When these tests are conducted properly (i.e., recorded voice, a full 50 words per ear at multiple intensity levels) they actually are quite sensitive. In fact, many states still require that speech audiometry be conducted using this specific word lists during the hearing aid selection process.

Keep in mind, however, that the purpose of speech audiometry during the hearing aid selection process is to get a better idea of how the patient might understand speech when sound is made more audible with hearing aids. For this reason, we suggest the use of speech-in-noise testing. For no other reason than it provides a more true to life idea of how well the patient understands speech in noisy listening conditions.

Speech-in-Noise Testing

Chicken and dumplings are a favorite home cooked meal of both authors. Many chicken and dumplings recipes call for rutabagas, which are a type of turnip found in many chicken and dumpling recipes, especially if you hale from the Midwest. Uncooked rutabagas have a distinctly different taste than when they are cooked in placed in

dishes like chicken and dumplings. This is similar to what happens when you add noise to speech testing. Depending on the "flavor" of the noise, the results of the speech test can be dramatically different than results obtained on the same patient for speech testing conducted in quiet.

There is an abundance of data suggesting that speech-recognition performance in background noise cannot be predicted from speech recognition performance in quiet. For this reason, it is recommended that speech intelligibility testing be conducted with background noise. There are two issues unique to speech recognition in noise testing compared to similar testing in quiet. The first is the type of noise used to mask the signal. The second is the procedure used to obtain speech-in-noise scores; either an adaptive or fixed signal-to-noise procedure can be used.

Type of noise. The first issue surrounds the type of background noise used during the test. Historically, developers of speech-in-noise tests have chosen either multitalker babble, or some type of bandpass filtered noise that approximates the energy of speech. Multitalker babble is a collection of two or more speakers reading passages recorded at the same time. When these passages are mixed and presented to the listener they sound like noise. Another type of noise commonly used in speech-in-noise testing is speech spectrum noise, a type of broadband noise that has been filtered to resemble the long-term average speech spectrum. An alternative to speech spectrum noise would be white noise from the audiometer. Environmental noise including traffic and industrial noises also have been employed.

Many studies have indicated that the various types of random noise are less effective maskers than are certain environmental sounds. Because multitalker babble is such a common noise that virtually everyone is exposed to on a daily basis, most speech-in-noise test developers have made the decision to use some type of speech-spectrum or multitalker babble.

Determining the best SNR. The second issue as it relates to speech-in-noise testing is the type of procedure used to generate results. There are two methods of obtaining scores when conducting speech-in-noise testing. The fixed procedure means that the intensity level of the speech, and the intensity level of the noise, remain the same, or fixed throughout the procedure, or until a percent correct score have been obtained for a certain predetermined number of words. The pitfall of using a fixed procedure is that the clinician does not know if he or she is testing the appropriate signal-to-noise ratio (SNR). If the fixed SNR is too easy a ceiling effect is encountered, and if the SNR is too difficult, the opposite occurs. Whenever floor or ceiling effects are present, it is difficult to observe change over time, unaided versus aided differences, or differentiate among different instruments. In order to ascertain the SNR that communication breakdowns begin to occur using a fixed procedure would require the use of several presentation levels. This often is not clinically feasible.

The other procedure is referred to as the adaptive procedure. The adaptive procedure allows the clinician to change the SNR within a list of words or sentences. That is, the background or

---

TAKE FIVE: The Audibility Index

If we think in terms of the audiogram, the dynamic range of average conversational speech is between 20 to 25 dB HL for the softer components, and 50 to 55 dB HL for the louder components. The audibility index (or articulation index) or Speech Intelligibility Index (SII) is a prediction of what percent of average speech is audibile for a given individual. It can be quite complicated to calculate, however, a simplified version of it exists, called the Count-the-Dots Audiogram. The original purpose of the Count-the-Dots Audiogram was to measure audibility of speech during hearing aid use and to demonstrate the benefit of amplification. The thinking being that the more dots you make audible with hearing aids, the better speech intelligibility would be. Although not used too much clinically, these days, the Count-the-Dots Audiogram is an excellent teaching tool. For one thing it shows you the relative importance of high-frequency sounds to speech intelligibility. Notice how there are more dots in the high-frequency region relative to the lower frequencies. The take home point is that the more dots you can restore with hearing aids, the more likely your patient will understand speech (Figure 6–6). **Important Point:** The percent of audibility *is not* the same as the percentage of speech understanding. There is a conversion chart, however, which allows you to estimate speech uderstanding from the audibility index.

speech is systematically altered until the patient is performing at a predetermined level (often 50%). The advantage of an adaptive procedure is that it allows the clinician to quickly identify the SNR where communication breaks down.

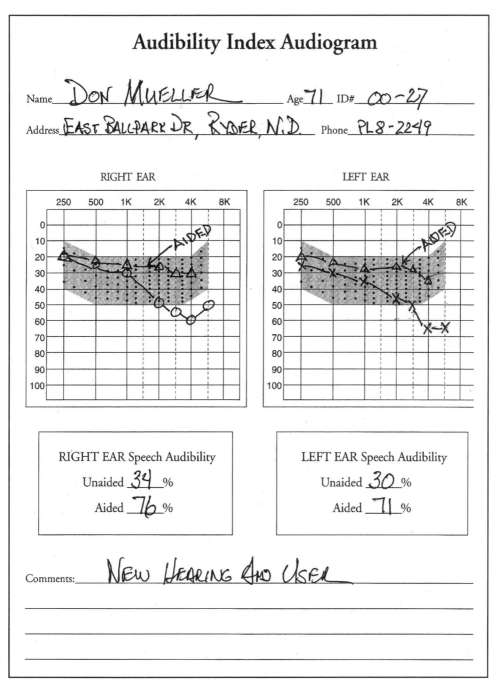

Audibility Index Audiogram

Name *DON MUELLER*   Age *71* ID# *00-27*

Address *EAST BALLPARK DR, RYDER, N.D.*   Phone *PL8-2249*

RIGHT EAR   LEFT EAR

RIGHT EAR Speech Audibility

Unaided *34* %

Aided *76* %

LEFT EAR Speech Audibility

Unaided *30* %

Aided *71* %

Comments: *NEW HEARING AID USER*

Figure 6–6. A Count-the-Dots Audiogram for the left and right ear. Unaided and aided sound-field thresholds have been plotted, and the AI (audibile dots) calculated.

Speech-in-noise tests traditionally have been conducted like speech in quiet tests, with the results expressed as a percent correct score. However, reporting the signal-to-noise ratio (SNR) required for 50% words/sentences correct can be a reliable alternative scoring method. Both the WIN (Words in Noise) and QuickSIN procedure outlined here rely on calculating the SNR.

Finally, we remind you that there is a clear clinical advantage for conducting speech-in-noise tests. For the most part, these results are independent of speech recognition scores obtained in quiet, and therefore can provide new insights regarding the patient.

Clinical applications. When using speech-in-noise tests as part of your prefitting selection test battery, it's important to have a good understanding of signal-to-noise ratio (SNR). SNR is simply the difference between the intensity level of the speech and the intensity level of the ambient noise. If speech stays constant, the larger the SNR, the weaker the background noise, and the more likely the patient is to understand speech. SNR can be calculated for both the listening situation (e.g., a noisy restaurant usually will be about +3 dB SNR) and for the actual patient (determining how a given patient's speech understanding in noise varies from "normal"). Let's turn our attention to how we can calculate a patient's SNR loss.

There are a many different speech-in-noise tests that you can use to assess speech intelligibility in the presence of background noise. One of these commonly used in research is the Hearing-in-Noise Test (HINT), which allows you to measure the SNR threshold, defined as the lowest SNR that a listener can recognize 50% of the speech material. The HINT is an excellent tool for differentiating small differences among people or products, but seldom is used in clinical practice.

The speech-in-noise test that clinically is most commonly used is the Quick Speech-in-Noise test, known simply as the QuickSIN. We've mentioned this before, but here are a few more details. Like the HINT, the QuickSIN measures SNR threshold, which is the signal-to-noise ratio that the listener is able to recognize 50% of the speech material. This value is then compared to the performance of people with normal hearing, and the patient's "SNL Loss" is calculated. This calculation provides a dB level showing how the SNR would need to be changed in order for the patient to perform as someone with normal hearing. For example, if a patient had an SNR Loss of 6 dB (which is common), this would mean that either the speech would need to be 6 dB louder, or the noise would need to be 6 dB softer, for the patient to perform as someone with normal hearing.

The QuickSin test was developed in the early 1990s at Etymotic Research in Elk Grove Village, Illinois. Using the Institute for Electrical and Electronics Engineers (IEEE) sentences as the target signal, and four-talker babble as the masker, the QuickSIN is a variable SNR test. Additionally, the QuickSIN employs a female talker at one presentation level (loud MCL, at or near "Loud, But Okay"), and six signal-to-noise ratios (0, +5, +10, +15, +20, and +25). The QuickSIN requires that five key words per sentence be scored. A sample score sheet is shown in Figure 6–7. We believe that the QuickSIN should be a routine part of the prefitting battery. Therefore, we have provided you with the steps for conducting the QuickSIN.

QuickSIN Procedure

1. Place the ear phones on the patient,
2. Zero the VU meter with the calibration tone presented from the CD.
3. Instruct the patient on the required task (see the QuickSIN manual for details).
4. Present the sentences at 70 to 75 dB HL, or at the patient's "Loud, But Okay" level, which usually is 5 to 10 dB below their LDL.
5. Familiarize the patient with the procedure by presenting 1 block of 6 six sentences.
6. Present the first list . Note that the correct SNRs are recorded on the CD, so you do not need to move the audiometer dials or buttons to change the SNR.
7. Score the number of key words correct for each sentence and total.
8. Conduct two lists of the six sentences per ear and calculate correct responses for each ear by averaging the scores obtained on both lists.
9. Record the SNR Loss (25.5 minus the total # of key words correct) for each ear.

The QuickSIN results have been categorized based on the degree of SNR Loss. After you measure the QuickSIN in the unaided condition, you might want to look at Table 6–2 to see where your patient falls in relation to normal hearing in noise. The higher the SNR value, the more likely the patient will have significant communication problems in noise.

List 1   **Score**

1. A white silk jacket goes with any shoes.   S/N 25   _5_
2. The child crawled into the dense grass.   S/N 20   _5_
3. Footprints showed the p**X**th he took up the beach. S/N 15   _4_
4. A w**X**nt near the edge brought in fi**X**sh air.   S/N 10   _3_
5. It is a band of s**X**el t**X**ee in**X**hes wide.   S/N 5   _2_
6. The w**X**ght of the pa**X**age was s**X**n on the h**X**h sc**X**e. S/N 0 _0_

   25.5 - TOTAL = __**6.5**__ SNR Loss   **TOTAL** _19_

Figure 6–7. A example of how one list from the QuickSIN is scored during prefitting testing. The red X's denote words repeated incorrectly by the patient.

Table 6–2. Degrees of SNR Loss as Measured on the QuickSIN.

0 to 2 dB SNR loss	Normal
3 to 7 dB SNR loss	Mild
8 to 14 dB SNR loss	Moderate
<14 SNR loss	Severe

TIPS and TRICKS: Getting Started with QuickSIN

We recommend adding the QuickSIN to your battery of pretests. In order to get started with it, you will need a two-channel audiometer, insert ear phones, CD player and the QuickSIN CD and manual. Once your have all the necessary equipment, you can start conducting the test. By calculating the SNR loss for each ear you can more carefully counsel your patients about their ability to communicate in realistic situations. Rather than going over all the details of how to conduct the test here, we will refer you to the QuickSINs instruction manual and score sheets. With the right equipment and a little bit of hands-on practice, you will be able to conduct SNR loss measurements using the QuickSIN. You can order a copy of the test at http://www.etymotic.com or call them at 847-228-0006.

Acceptable Noise Level Test

Another speech test which can be implemented into your prefitting battery is the acceptable noise level (ANL) test.

Although it's been around for several years, it has been shown in some recent research to be a good predictor of hearing aid use (which we hope leads to benefit and satisfaction). The ANL does not measure speech intelligibility; rather it measures annoyance to sound. It does this by comparing the unaided most comfortable listening level (MCL) and comparing it to a second measure, called the background noise level (BCL). The difference between these two measures is referred to as the acceptable noise level, or ANL. The average ANL is around 6 to 9 dB. That is, people say that they can "put up with the noise for an extended period" when the noise is 6 to 9 dB *below* the speech signal. If someone simply isn't bothered by background noise, his ANL could be 2 to 4 dB. If someone finds background noise to be very bothersome, his ANL could be 12 to 15 dB or higher. You'll want to put a "star" by the high ANL patients, as research suggests that they may need more hand-holding to become successful hearing aid users.

The ANL test, which can be conducted in just a few minutes, allows you to talk intelligently with the patient about issues related to noise annoyance during the prefitting appointment. Because annoyance from background noise is such a prevalent problem among hearing aid users, taking the time to measure a potential problem with noise annoyance during the prefitting appointment is a wise use of your time. The ANL test, complete with background noise, is available on CD. To obtain a copy of the ANL test, along with istructions on how to conduct the test, go to Fry Electronics (not the electronics superstore, but the audiology equipment superstore) Web site http://www.frye.com .

Explanation of Results

A complete set of prefitting tests are like a homemade cake. Several ingredients have been combined to yield something far greater than the sum of their individual parts. What makes a freshly baked cake even more delicious, however, is a first class frosting. The explanation of the test results are like the frosting on a great cake.

After you have completed the battery of prefitting tests reviewed here, the next step is to clearly explain the results to the patient. Just like a cake is not finished unless it has been frosted, your hearing aid selection test battery is not complete without properly explaining the results to the patient. Although it's easy to overlook, this part of the hearing aid selection process cannot be emphasized enough. Patients expect to leave this appointment with a thorough understanding of the test results, along with treatment options.

During your explanation of the audiogram be sure to describe the type and degree of hearing loss. One way to do this is to use something called the "speech banana audiogram" shown in Figure 6–8. This counseling tool is an effective way to relate the patient's hearing thresholds to the speech sounds being missed. Notice that the sounds of speech are clustered in an area on the audiogram resembling a banana. Vowel sounds are in the lower frequencies and consonants sounds are in the mid to high frequencies.

There actually is a company based in Evanston, Illinois that sells a Web-based report writer and template counseling audiogram. This company, called CounselEAR, allows you to generate customized reports for patients and physicians. To learn more about their system go to http://www.CounselEAR.com .

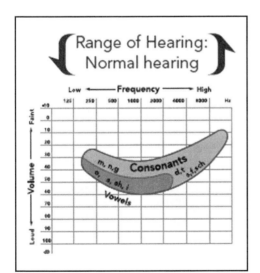
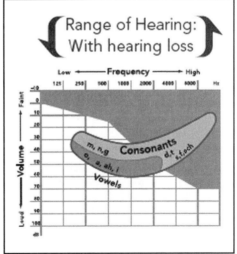

Figure 6–8. An example of an audiogram that can be used to explain results to the patient. The patient's thresholds can be placed on the audiogram shown here. The shaded audiogram on the right shows the missing sounds of speech for a downward sloping hearing loss. Copyright ©2009 Sonus USA Inc. Reprinted with permission.

TIPS and TRICKS: Be More Memorable

All of us have experienced that puzzled feeling after an interaction with a highly technical expert who used language we didn't completely understand. After the elaborate explanation we likely left the appointment confused and full of more anxiety than before we arrived. It's important to keep that in mind when you are about to explain test results to one of your own patients. Here is a tactic that will help you avoid overwhelming patients with information they don't completely understand.

Start by asking the patient if they would like a relatively brief review of the results, or if they would like to go into the details. By asking the patient how to proceed you are providing them more ownership of the visit. You are communicating on their terms rather than your own.

Once you have been given permission to proceed, it is important that you use language that the patient understands. Also, it's important to relate the test results to the communication difficulties the patient is experiencing on a daily basis. When reviewing results always use visual aids like the one shown in Figure 6–8 to reinforce your message. Studies have shown that visual aids and other educational tools help patients remember your explanation of results and your follow-up recommendations.

Prefitting Considerations

After you have enjoyed your favorite home-cooked meal with friends, there are a lot of things to consider. Did your guests like the meal? Did they get enough to eat? Are you willing to share the recipe with them? Would you modify the recipe next time you make it? Will they stay and help you do the dishes?

The prefitting considerations we discuss here are like some of these questions you might have after your meal. After you have taken the time to complete all the prefitting tests, what are the common considerations you will need to think about with your patient?

So far we have talked about prefitting tests we need to do during the initial appointment with a hearing aid candi-

date. In addition to these pretests there are several considerations we need to think about during the selection process. You will need to think about each of these considerations every time you sit down with a patient after conducting the pretests outlined in this chapter.

Bilateral Versus Unilateral Fitting

Assuming most patients you will see have a bilateral hearing loss, the first consideration is whether your patient needs two hearing aids or can get by with just one. There are several proven advantages to bilateral hearing, which we'll soon review. Using one or two hearing aids is an important question because patients want to know if the advantages of restoring bilateral hearing with two hearing aids outweigh the extra financial costs of purchasing an additional device. The majority of dispensing professionals, at least in North America, seem to believe two hearing aids are preferable to one, as the bilateral fitting rate is about 80%.

TAKE FIVE:
Binaural or Bilateral?

You may have noticed in other chapters that the words binaural and bilateral have been used in reference to hearing with two ears. There is an important difference between these two terms. When we refer to the auditory system we use terms binaural hearing and monaural hearing. When we are talking about hearing aids, we use the terms bilateral fittings and unilateral fittings. In general, you can presume a bilateral fitting improves binaural hearing.

Given that two hearing aids cost more, and create more work for you and the patient, another important question is, are bilateral hearing aid fittings worth the time? After all, if a patient is just as satisfied with one and it's less work for both of you, why not simply fit all your patients with one hearing aid.

Fortunately, there are several proven advantages to fitting nearly all patients bilaterally. It's important to have a basic understanding of each advantage, as you will want to explain this to your patients. Here is a summary of the primary reasons why two hearing aids might be better than one for most of our patients.

Loudness Summation

This refers to the auditory system's ability to integrate sound from each ear. When a patient wears two hearing aids, he needs between 2 and 8 dB less gain (depending on individual variances and input level) to achieve an equal amount of loudness compared to the person wearing only one hearing aid. For this reason, bilateral hearing aid users are less likely to encounter problems with acoustic feedback or squealing from their hearing aids because they can keep the overall gain lower on each individual hearing aid when they are worn bilaterally. Think of it as "free gain" from the brain..

Improved Auditory Localization

Reverberation causes sound to arrive at diffuse angles around the human head. The timing of the sounds arrival at each ear to a large extent helps humans determine the location of sound. There is evidence to show that many patients fitted bilaterally have localization ability rivaling that of those with normal hearing.

Another advantage related to localization is the reduction of something called the "head shadow effect." Sounds arriving from one side of the head, particularly high frequency sounds, are reduced or attenuated 10 to 15 dB. Assuming a relatively symmetrical hearing loss, a bilateral fitting will eliminate the head shadow effect. This of course also has an impact on speech understanding, as the patient no longer has a "bad side.".

Improved Speech Understanding

When sound is combined in both ears, there usually is a minimum of 3 dB improvement of the signal to noise ratio for soft and average intensity levels of speech. For this reason, in typical listening situations with background noise, two hearing aids are preferred over one. Given the fact that many patients report significant trouble understanding speech in noise, it makes good sense to make the most of the binaural advantage by fitting two hearing aids. In fact, for some patients, the benefit of bilateral will exceed the benefits of directional technology and digital noise reduction. While a 2-dB advantage does not sound like much, as we've mentioned before, this can improve speech intelligibility by 10 to 20%, which can be significant.

TIPS and TRICKS: Why the Improvement?

Why do most people understand speech better in background noise when wearing two versus one hearing aids? It appears to be due to two factors. One is redundancy. By hearing the same speech message in two ears, they get two chances to get it right. The second factor involves noise squelch. The central system, to some degree, can suppress things we don't want to hear, and this works best when there are two signals to compare at the low brainstem.

Improved Sound Quality and Better Spatial Balance

The stereo analogy probably best explains why new bilateral users previously fitted unilaterally often report an improvement in both spatial balance and overall sound quality. This im-provement in sound quality when listening in a noisy situation with two ears is referred to as the squelch effect. It appears as if the listener is able to selectively attend to a particular sound and suppress unwanted sounds when listening with two ears. Just like your favorite music sounds better through a pair of speakers than through only one, sound is perceived to be of higher quality and more balanced with two hearing aids compared to only one.

TIPS and TRICKS: Be More Memorable, Part 2

You will need to clearly communicate the reasons two hearing aids are better than one. Using the information we've reviewed in this chapter, you might say something like, "Mr. Smith there are three good reasons proven by research to use two hearing aids, rather than one. First, you will be able to locate the direction of sound easier with two instruments. Second, speech understanding in background noise is improved with two hearing aids. Third, patients wearing two hearing aids report better sound quality and spatial balance compared to those wearing only one device. In a recent study of listener preference, in which the subjects with hearing loss in both ears were able to compare bilateral to unilateral fittings for an extended period of time, over about 90% of the subjects preferred the bilateral arrangement."

Preventing Auditory Deprivation

An indirect advantage of bilateral amplification for a patient with a relative bilaterally symmetrical hearing loss, is the prevention of auditory deprivation, more appropriately called the "unaided ear effect." This refers to a decrease in speech understanding (without a change in pure tone thresholds) in the unaided ear resulting from the use of unilateral amplification. Of course, any hearing loss causes a reductioin in audibility in the auditory centers of the brain. But there is considerable evidence suggesting that patients with a symmetric hearing loss fitted unilaterally lose their ability to understand more rapidly in the unaided ear.

We also know that when a hearing aid is fitted to the unaided ear after two or three years of nonuse, there can be significant recovery in speech understanding ability in the newly aided ear for some patients. These recovery effects can be measured within a year of the fitting of the second hearing aid. Unfortunately, some patients show no recovery. It is also worth noting those patients with normal hearing in one ear and an "aidable" loss in the other also experience auditory deprivation and sometimes recovery upon amplification. Regardless of the hearing loss, overcoming the "unaided ear effect" is possible through bilateral amplification.

Why Unilateral?

You have now heard four or five good reasons to routinely fit your patients with two hearing aids. At this point you might be thinking that there is no reason for your patients with hearing loss in both ears to ever consider one hearing aid. There are, however, some reasons a unilateral fitting might preferred for those with a bilateral hearing loss. Besides the nonauditory factors, like cost and inconvenience we mentioned, there are some other reasons related to the auditory system that might warrant a unilateral fit.

The most obvious cases in which a bilateral fitting would not be warranted would be a profound unilateral hearing loss in one of the ears. In these cases, there is so much damage to the structures of the inner ear, that a hearing aid has very limited benefit. Even in such cases, a conventional hearing aid or special device (e.g., CROS or BICROS, which are covered in Chapter 7) may restore a sense of balance that is lost due to the head shadow effect resulting from the severe unilateral

---

TAKE FIVE: The Unaided Ear Effect

There appears to be two reasons why the unaided ear effect happens. First, when a person starts wearing a hearing aid on one ear, their world becomes softer (people don't have to talk to them as loud, the TV is softer, etc). Hence, there is less audibility for the unaided ear. Secondly, the use of amplification in one ear leads to a mismatch in central timing. The aided ear wins, and signals from the unaided ear are given less priority. Over time, the brain could start to ignore the signals from that ear. We know, that's rude, but it could happen.

TAKE FIVE:
The Binaural Preference Demonstration

Rather than simply discuss the benefits of binaural hearing provided by bilateral hearing aids, it is a good idea to demonstrate it. The Binaural Preference Demonstration is an informal way for patients to experience the advantages of binaural hearing. Best of all it just takes a few minutes.

Step 1. While the patient is seated in the test booth with earphones, in place, begin talking to the patient and find a comfortable volume level. The presentation level should then remain the same throughout the test.

Step 2. Present your voice (best to just start having a conversation at their MCL) in one ear only. Talk to the patient for 10 to 20 seconds.

Step 3. Now, talk to the patient in both ears.

Step 4. Then talk to the patient in the opposite ear only.

Step 5. Go back and talk to the patient in both ears.

Step 6. Ask the patient to tell you which condition had the best sound quality and balance. You may have to repeat steps 2 to 5 a few times. The majority of patients with a bilaterally symmetrical hearing loss will prefer the bilateral presentation.

---

hearing loss. These patients also may be considered for a cochlear implant, depending on the status of the "good" ear.

Binaural interference. Although rare, some patients suffer from something called binaural interference. This condition, which is difficult to measure in your clinic, prevents patients from using two hearing aids successfully. This is because, as the name indicates, the signal from the second ear actually reduces, rather than improves the signal from the first ear—this is happening within the central auditory mechanisms. As it appears to be a relatively rare condition, you might be able to "catch it" through counseling during the postfitting follow-up appointment—for unexplained reasons, a patient says that things get worse when he wears his second hearing aid. For now, just file away

that binaural interference exists, but it appears to be rarely encountered.

Cochlear Dead Regions

Recall from Chapter 3 that, in most cases, hearing aids are designed to replace the function of the previously healthy outer hair cells in the cochlea. When you are selecting and fitting hearing aids, however, there is a specific type of damage to the cochlea, called cochlear dead regions, that may need to be considered. No one knows exactly how common these dead regions really are. For example, some recent research in this area suggests that as many as 80% of patients with steeply sloping, severe hearing loss have a dead region, whereas other reports suggest the prevalence is closer to 30%. Regardless of the exact number, it is good to know what the audiogram of a patient with dead region typically may look like, and how this could impact your hearing aid fitting.

Cochlear dead regions are areas of the cochlea where the inner hair cells have been destroyed and no longer function optimally. In rare cases, when high-frequency amplification is provided by the hearing aids, and the dead region is located in the lower frequencies, patients actually experience a reduction in speech understanding when audibility is applied.

There is some evidence indicating that cochlear dead regions are relatively easy to identify by simply looking at the audiogram. In fact, it appears that *experienced* clinicians examining the shape of the hearing thresholds on the audiogram are nearly as good at spotting cases of cochlear dead regions as a clinical test designed to identify dead regions. An example would be a steeply downward sloping loss, the thresholds of 90 dB or worse in the 3000 to 4000 Hz range.

Typical Audiogram?

Experts believe that if the audiogram drops by more than 40 to 50 dB per octave, and the hearing loss is greater than 70 dB at any given test frequency, cochlear dead regions should be suspected. Even if you suspect your patient might have a cochlear dead region, they still are a good candidate for hearing aids. Figure 6–9 shows an example of an audiogram from a patient with a suspected cochlear dead region in the right ear based on the results of the TEN test.

Another possible characteristic of a dead region is when a patient perceives a hiss or buzz, instead of a pure tone during a routine hearing test. During audiometry, if the patient mentions that

---

TIPS and TRICKS:
Why Dead Regions Usually Don't Alter Your Fitting

It's easy to get excited about high frequency cochlear dead regions, but the fact is that they usually don't alter your hearing aid fitting. There are two primary reasons for this:

1. They typically are only present when the hearing loss is severe-to-profound (e.g., >80 dB HL). With these patients (downward sloping losses), it would be difficult to obtain audibility regardless, so your fitting strategy doesn't really change.
2. Research has shown that even when there is a dead region, we should amplify about an octave or so above the edge of the dead region. So if the dead region was at 2000 Hz, we would still amplify up to 3500 Hz or so. If at 3000 Hz, we'd amplify up to around 5000 Hz. That's about what we would do if there wasn't a dead region, so nothing really changes.

Note: The rules are different for dead regions in the lower frequencies, but these are far less common.

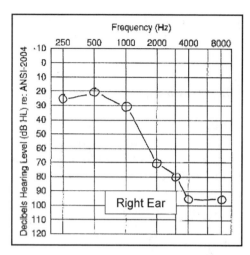

Figure 6–9. The audiogram for a patient suspected of having a high frequency cochlear dead region in his right ear (based on configuration and TEN test results). Notice how the audiogram drops to 95 dB in the high frequencies and slopes more than 40 db per octave.

the pure tone sounds like a hiss, buzz, or crackle, make a note of it, as it might be an indication of a dead region.

Rule of Thumb

A good rule of thumb is only to provide amplification to about one octave above the suspected dead region. Given that most hearing aids we fit today are programmable with multiple memories, providing the right amount of gain to maximize speech intelligibility can be achieved for those with these dead regions. If you do suspect a cochlear dead region, you might want to use the multiple memories of the hearing aids to see what frequency response is most acceptable to the patient, as there is always a tradeoff between intelligibly and comfort for amplified sounds for patients with suspected dead regions. In one memory, fit the hearing aid to NAL-NL2 targets through 4000 Hz. In a second memory, roll off the gain in the higher frequencies.

You can learn a lot more about how to test for dead regions by conducting a Web search on Brian C. J. Moore and the TEN (HL) Test.

TAKE FIVE: "Good-to-Know" Market Statistics

Fitting hearing aids is hard enough, but the challenge is compounded when you are often fitting a medical device on a person who does not really want to use it. There is a strong stigma associated with hearing aid use, which we mentioned in Chapter 1. In fact, many experts believe this stigma is mostly responsible for the low (20%) market penetration, even though the segment of the market that needs hearing aids (so-called aging Baby Boomers) is growing quickly. The Better Hearing Institute (www.betterhearing.org), under the direction of

Sergei Kochkin, Ph.D. has been capturing and analyzing consumer market data for over 20 years. Here are some of the more interesting facts you need to remember from a recent survey.

- Average age of first-time user: 69 years old
- Percent of purchased hearing aids not used regularly: 16%
- Percent of hearing aids in the drawer (not used at all): 15 to 18%
- Additional percent of patients who use their hearing aids but are dissatisfied: 17%

Auditory Processing Disorder (APD)

In Chapter 4 we addressed the function of the central auditory pathways and their relationship to speech understanding. An auditory processing disorder (APD), at least to a mild degree, is a relatively common condition in patients over the age of 70 to 80. Some estimates suggest that about half of all patients over the age of 65 have APD to some degree (based on difficult speech-in-competition testing). Undoubtedly, APD can affect the outcome of the hearing aid fitting; therefore, it is important to know what to look for.

In essence, in order to understand speech in difficult listening situations, the auditory centers of our brain must be functioning properly. As a result of aging, this central processing system may not be functioning optimally. The end result is that persons with auditory processing problems cannot understand speech as well as you would predict based on their audiogram, or even the speech-in-quiet performance.

Their complaints typically are similar to someone with a much more severe hearing loss. The mystery wrapped inside an enigma as it relates to APD is that the patients with APD often have audiograms suggestive of a much milder problem than you might think based on the complaints of the patient.

The first important question for the hearing professional is, "How do I know my patient is suffering from APD?" Unfortunately, there is no simple answer to this question. There currently is some debate about the value of screening for APD during the prefitting appointment. There are some procedures available that are designed to screen for APD; however, they do take about 10 or 15 minutes to conduct. Rather than relying on an APD screening, some simply look at some basic test information, particularly the results of sentence-length speech-in-noise testing, like the QuickSIN, to see if APD might be part of the hearing problem.

If you're interested in screening for APD, a test we recommend is the Dichotic Sentence Identification (DSI). The DSI test can be used to evaluate

---

TIPS and TRICKS: Patient with APD

Here is the typical profile of a patient with suspected APD

Age: 72 years

Audiogram: Mild to severe, bilateral downward sloping SNHL

Speech in quiet: PBmax of 88%

Speech-in-Noise Results: Poor speech understanding ability, especially in relation to the threshold results. QuickSIN Loss of 12 dB.

Patient Complaint: Simply can't understand in background noise, even when the noise is something as minor as the television in the background.

Treatment Recommendations: Conventional hearing aids to treat the threshold loss with the use of wireless technology and an FM system to improve the signal-to-noise ratio.

possible APD in patients during the pre-fitting appointment. The DSI is available on CD and employs the dichotic presentation of sentences. Dichotic means that two different items are presented bilaterally. To obtain a copy of the DSI, along with instructions and age-appropriate normative data, go to http://www.auditec.com .

Patients with APD remain good hearing aid candidates in most cases, but plan on additional counseling. Your primary responsibility will be to fit them with devices that substantially improve the signal-to-noise ratio of the listening environment (e.g., FM systems), offer aural rehabilitation exercises, and perhaps lower their expectations with regard to hearing aid benefit.

Because APD can afflict a patient of any age, and although rare, can be caused by a space-occupying lesion, there are times when it is important to refer the patient to an audiologist who specializes in the evaluation and treatment of APD.

Auditory Acclimatization

Believe it or not, not everyone has always liked sushi. But you know what happens? After urging from friends (and a few bottles of cold sake), they try something that looks a little daring but is cooked, like a crunchy shrimp roll. Then, on their next visit to the sushi bar, they move on to a California roll. A few weeks later, a rainbow roll, and then, after only a couple months—some tuna sushi. Before long, they are happily dining with the rest of us on five different kinds of sashimi bathed in wasabi. Isn't acclimatization great?

We end this chapter discussing auditory acclimatization. Although acclimatiza-

tion doesn't happen until your patient starts wearing hearing aids, we bring it up here because it definitely is something that you need to talk about with your patients during the prefitting appointment.

"Don't worry, you'll get used to it after a while" is a counseling phrase that has been used by nearly everyone who ever has fitted hearing aids. In the phrase, "Getting used to it," the "it" could mean hearing aid noise, ambient noise, environment sounds, unwanted high-frequency gain, too much gain for loud sounds, or a number of other things. The assumption made when this counseling statement is employed is that the hearing aids have been programmed correctly, and the patient will experience some degree of *acclimatization* to the bothersome acoustic signal(s). After a month or two of hearing aid use, this fitting and counseling technique usually results in one of four outcomes:

1. The hearing aid user acclimatizes or adapts to whatever it was that was bothersome, and he or she might not even remember what it was that was bothersome during the first week or so of hearing aid use. All is well.
2. The hearing aid user is still bothered by the annoying acoustic feature(s) (maybe a little less than initially), but the benefits of using hearing aids outweigh the nuisance, so he or she is a fairly happy full-time hearing aid user.
3. The hearing aid user is still bothered by the annoying acoustic feature(s). So much so that he or she reserves hearing aid use for isolated listening situations, and is a fairly unhappy part-time hearing aid user.

TAKE FIVE: A Fletcher-Killion Story

Whenever we think of auditory acclimatization we're reminded of a frequently told anecdote about one of the great hearing scientists of the 1900s, Harvey Fletcher. The following version of the story was kindly provided by Mead Killion, although we've added a few of our own embellishments:

Back in the 1940s, wideband high-fidelity phonograph consoles were just becoming available. Because of his interest in high-quality audio, Harvey Fletcher bought one for his home. Harvey enjoyed listening to this new high-fidelity system but, unfortunately, the enjoyment was not shared by his wife. After listening to an old 78 rpm record, with the surface noise made particularly

prominent by the extended bandwidth of this new high-fidelity system, she said: "That sounds awful. I don't really like having that screechy sound in my home." Always the creative thinker, the next day, when his wife was out of the house, Harvey went into the living room and soldered 20 1 uF capacitors across the loudspeaker terminals, rolling off the high frequencies. (Remember that amplifiers were high impedance back then, so the trick worked.) That evening, when the music played, his wife was now happy.

One night each week, while his wife was sleeping, Harvey would sneak downstairs and clip one capacitor. After 20 weeks, when the music played, they were both happy.

---

4. The hearing aid user is still bothered by the annoying acoustic feature(s) and either has returned the hearing aids, or keeps them in his or her possession, but never uses them.

It's obvious that choices #3 and #4 are undesirable for the manufacturer, the dispenser, and most importantly, the patient. As you will learn in later chapters, today we program hearing aids according to an established prescriptive fitting method (e.g., NAL-NL2, etc.). In many cases, in fact, the hearing aids are programmed to a prescriptive fitting strategy by the manufacturer before the instruments are shipped. The reason for programming the hearing aids to a given prescriptive method is that substantial research has indicated

that this fitting philosophy is most appropriate for the *average* patient, given that patient's specific audiometric characteristics. "Most appropriate" can mean maximizing speech intelligibility, obtaining superior speech quality, restoring normal loudness perceptions, or some combination of these and other factors. Additionally, given the multiple settings required in today's hearing aids for gain, output, and compression, which need to be determined in several channels for varying input levels, it's necessary to have an automated "starting point" for the hearing aid fitting. The question then becomes, are these prescriptive fitting targets a reasonable "starting point" for the average patient? Whether there should be a difference between "first-fit" and "final-fit" is related, in part, to the manufacturers' and dispensers' beliefs concerning the patient's acclimatization, adaptation, adjustment, and auditory learning to hearing aid use.

Sorting Out the Terms

To complete our discussion of acclimatization, it might be useful to review some of the terminology related to the topic, which often is used interchangeably to describe hearing aid adjustment.

Acclimatization: adapting to a new environment (in this case, auditory) or as defined by Darwin, the process of inuring to a new climate, or the state of being so inured. This seems to be a reasonable term, as it also is used to describe how the human body acclimates to temperature, altitude, and other environmental conditions.

Adaptation: the process of adapting to something, such as environmental conditions (in this case, auditory); the responsive adjustment of a sense organ. This too is a reasonable term, as it has long been used in reference to the eye, for example, *adaptation* to varying light conditions.

Adjustment: making or becoming suitable; adjusting or accommodating to circumstances. This term also describes the process quite well; however, we make so many adjustments to hearing aids that it might be best to avoid this term just to reduce confusion, for example, an "Adjustment Module" in the fitting software probably would be viewed as a fitting assistant by most audiologists.

Auditory learning: acquiring new auditory skills or abilities related to perception, cognition, and memory. Although learning does not account for all the factors of hearing aid adaptation, "stimulus learning" probably is related to some of the acclimatization effects.

So, we have several terms that can be used to describe the patient's experience of adjusting to sounds processed through hearing aids. Although it may be the most difficult to pronounce and spell, we nevertheless prefer the term acclimatization.

TAKE FIVE: Original Definition

From an auditory standpoint related to hearing aids, a researcher from the United Kingdom by the name of Stuart Gatehouse was one of the first to use the term acclimatization, explaining the speech processing capabilities of a group of people aided monaurally. In later research Gatehouse used the term acclimatization to describe an improvement in speech recognition over time. Today, the term is used widely to explain adaptation to hearing aid use in general, and is not limited to the Gatehouse definition. In fact, as you will note in your readings, there is little evidence that a significant amount of change occurs for speech understanding.

Why Acclimatization Happens

Today, when we refer to "acclimatization," we tend to combine various things that the patient may have trouble adjusting to, ranging from low-level ambient noise to louder-than-usual soft sounds to the newly acquired audibility of high-frequency speech signals. The underlying mechanisms that allow for acclimatization to occur may not be the same for all of these conditions.

Related to acclimatization associated with the re-introduction of high-frequency signals, researcher Catherine Palmer uses the term "space allocation." That is, if only a small portion of the speech signal has been present over time, the space allocation for processing this signal has been reduced. Conversely, if the patient is fitted appropriately, and a wide range of speech signals are now present, we would expect that eventually more space would be allocated for the processing of these new signals.

Hearing Soft Sounds Again

Since the introduction of wide dynamic-range multiband compression (WDRC) processing, which is now routine, we frequently have been faced with a new acclimatization issue concerning the re-introduction of audibility for soft inputs for the patient, including speech, noise, and environmental sounds. While patients are usually happy to hear the soft voices of their grandchildren, they are not as happy to hear the refrigerator running, the tick of a clock, and all those other environmental sounds they had not been hearing for many years.

This adjustment process often requires several counseling sessions. We suggest you send that patient home with a large printout of the following phrase:

> *"You have to hear what you don't want to hear to know what you don't want to hear."*

It hopefully will serve as a reminder to them that it takes considerable time for the auditory system to get adjusted to new sounds again. As you will soon find out, this is a point that is very difficult to get across to many new hearing aid users.

In Closing

As we've related the hearing aid selection process to cooking a meal, we leave you with a recipe for your first successful fitting. Table 6–3 comes from our "cookbook" of hearing aid selection. Feel free to re-create this recipe with every patient and to share it with your colleagues.

Now that you've read this chapter you should know the essential steps of a routine prefitting appointment. As you might have gathered, there is a balance between interviewing the patient to identify their individual communication needs and carefully measuring their residual auditory function with various pretests. Both of these components, interviewing and measuring, along with several considerations outlined here will help you get started with fitting your first set of hearing aids, and undoubtedly make you think of a nice home-cooked meal.

Table 6–3. The Hearing Aid Selection Recipe

Combine effective communication skills with the following ingredients:

1. Administer at least one prefitting questionnaire to the patient as they wait in the reception area to see you. The COAT and/or HHIE-S are prime choices and always in season.

2. One case history done face-to-face with the patient for at least 15 minutes.

3. A comprehensive communication needs assessment conducted with empathy and respect for the patient and third party for at least 15 minutes.

4. After 20 to 30 minutes of gathering this information, proceed to the routine audiologic test battery.

5. Combine the findings from the following tests:
   - LDL, QuickSIN, and Acceptable Noise Level, along with the pure tone results to better understand the residual auditory capability of the patient

6. Fold the information from step 5 with the information obtained in steps 1 to 4 and carefully explain the results to the patient.

7. After an in-depth discussion, add flavor to your recommendation by considering the following:
   - Bilateral or Unilateral hearing aid use
   - Auditory Deprivation issues
   - Cochlear Dead Regions
   - Acclimatization Factors

8. Combine all the information, simmer in your head for a few minutes, and serve up a hearing aid recommendation to your patient with confidence.

7

All About Style:
Hearing Aids and Earmolds

Is this really a topic that is related to wine tasting?

If you've ever been to a wine tasting event, you know there usually are several different varieties of wine that might revolve around a common theme. For example, you could be tasting wines from a certain country or region, like South Africa or Napa Valley. Or perhaps you taste various types of Pinot Noirs or Sauvignon Blancs from around the world and decide on a favorite region. Whatever wine you taste, chances are each person has a favorite vintage or variety they enjoy the most. Believe it or not, hearing aids styles are similar to a wine tasting event, although less cheese is involved.

With hearing aids, some clinicians might prefer fitting an open-canal mini-BTE over a custom-made CIC, depending on the audiogram and lifestyle of the patient. Or, another dispenser might

prefer to use large vents, while another likes to keep the fitting pretty "closed-up." Think of it this way: a well-stocked wine store has a tremendous range of varietals at several price points, and a well-stocked hearing aid practice has a wide range of form factors and price points that accommodate all types of patients.

Traditionally, we refer to hearing aid "styles" when we are talking about how hearing aids look—"She was wearing a cute "ABC" model," or "He had a pair of large clunky "XYZs." Recently, however, the term "form factor" has become popular; a term borrowed from the computer industry, and historically used to describe mother boards, which basically means "geometry of an object."

No matter what you call them, it's important to know the advantages and disadvantages of each form factor or style. Obviously, in many cases the style is selected because it provides the best acoustic solution to the problem. But, believe it or not, beauty also is part of the equation because many patients are more likely to wear their hearing aids if they think they're not ugly (or noticeable). Sometimes, you will need to strike a compromise with your patient.

In addition to hearing aid styles, this chapter also addresses other important aspects, such as earmolds, that are often needed to successfully customize hearing aids. And, if we are talking about earmolds, it's important to detail the process of taking ear impressions, which is a critical component. Let's get started by looking at the various types of hearing aid styles or form factors available. Yes, some of them might even be considered fine vintages.

Behind-the-Ear (BTE)

We like to think of BTEs as the Merlot of hearing aid styles. If you saw the movie Sideways *several years ago, you may recall that they bashed Merlot wines, and for good reason. Inexpensive Merlot tastes bad and, after it was mocked in* Sideways*, sales plummeted. However, since 2008, vintners have gotten their act together and produced a high quality Merlot at a reasonable price. Since this time Merlot has experienced a bit of a comeback among wine enthusiasts. The rise in popularity of the BTE is similar to the rise in higher quality Merlots. Hearing aid manufacturers have managed to produce a wide variety of cosmetically appealing mini-BTEs and the result as been a surge in popularity. You don't have to be a fan of Merlot to appreciate the comeback of the BTE.*

The behind-the-ear (BTE) hearing aid is worn over the pinna and typically is coupled to tubing with an earmold that fits in the ear canal and directs the amplified sound to the tympanic membrane. Traditionally, BTEs have been known to have more power, more features, more flexibility and a longer battery life then their custom-made cousins. In some cases, the BTE may only be connected to tubing that is inserted directly in the ear canal for a more open fitting. An advantage of the BTE hearing aid is that it requires no special modifications to the shell case and thus can be manufactured completely in advance of the order placed for a specific patient. Many hearing aid dispensers actually keep a stock supply of BTE hearing aids in their office for same-day fittings with a temporary earmold. In contrast, the circuitry for custom-made products must be inserted and attached to the hearing aid shell casing that is made from an earmold unique to each patient. For these products, the fabrication of the hearing aid shell casing and wiring of electronic components is performed at a manufacturer's product assembly plant prior to shipping.

According to the Hearing Instrument Association (HIA), the BTE model constituted over 60% of the hearing aid market in 2010. Concomitantly, the BTE was the most often returned hearing aid for credit (16%). The next highest return rate for other hearing aid styles was less than 13%. Presumably, this higher return rate can be attributed to patients' dissatisfaction with the size of the hearing aid, as the larger BTEs lack cosmetic appeal, particularly for those patients with shorter hair. It should be noted that in spite of the fact that BTEs have became smaller and more cosmetically appealing in the past few years, BTE hearing aids still seem to carry a negative connotation associated with their size. This is changing, however, with the increased popularity of mini-BTE open-canal (OC) products, a subcategory of BTEs.

BTEs for Children

BTEs are still the favored and most appropriate choice for fitting children. With a BTE fitting, only the earmold needs to be replaced as the child grows. This is much less costly than re-casing a custom-made hearing aid. In addition, because BTEs are the most powerful hearing aid style in terms of gain and output, they remain the premier choice for fitting severe-to-profound hearing losses. The larger sizes of BTEs allow a larger battery, which in turn provide a longer operating life before a battery change is necessary. This also is important for the elderly, as it can be quite difficult for people with limited manual dexterity and visual impairments to change a battery. In addition, larger user controls may be placed on the BTE-style hearing aid, making them easier to see and manipulate (these controls often are blocked for children).

Other advantages of using larger BTE instruments with children (and some adults) include:

■ Stronger telecoil
■ Flexibility for direct audio input

■ Better durability
■ Easier to adjust controls.

Receiver in the Canal (RIC) Instruments

In recent years a modification of the traditional BTE has been introduced. In this hearing aid, the receiver is placed in the ear canal rather then in the hearing aid, while the microphone/amplifier remains located at the upper portion of the hearing aid behind the pinna. With this style of hearing aid, the tubing routed to the ear canal does not transmit sound via air conduction, but rather via electrical wiring. By moving the receiver out of the hearing aid, more options are available regarding the size of the BTE, and usually RIC products are the smallest of the mini-BTE category. In the canal, the receiver can be loosely fitted in a tip (open fitting), or embedded in a large ear mold, useful for more severe hearing loss (more on this in the next section).

Before continuing on about form factors we include Figure 7–1 as a handy overview of the most popular styles or form factors.

Open Canal (OC) Fittings

A style (which really isn't a style) that actually has been around a long time, but has gained popularity over the past few years is the open canal (OC) style (fitting). Many think of the OC style as a subcategory of the BTE—it's usually considered a mini-BTE, although you can have an OC fitting with any BTE, large or small.

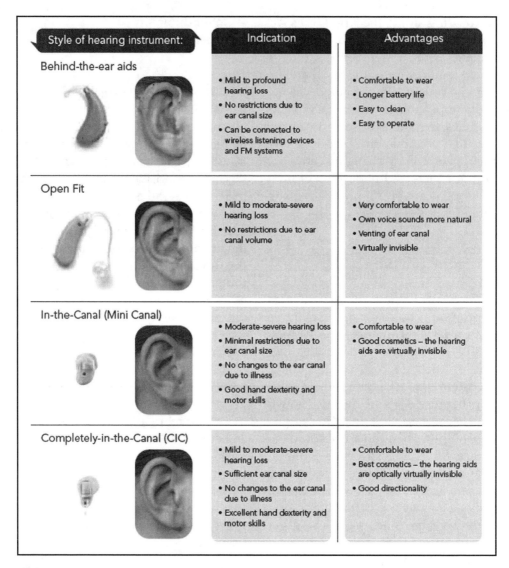

Style of hearing instrument:	Indication	Advantages
Behind-the-ear aids	• Mild to profound hearing loss • No restrictions due to ear canal size • Can be connected to wireless listening devices and FM systems	• Comfortable to wear • Longer battery life • Easy to clean • Easy to operate
Open Fit	• Mild to moderate-severe hearing loss • No restrictions due to ear canal volume	• Very comfortable to wear • Own voice sounds more natural • Venting of ear canal • Virtually invisible
In-the-Canal (Mini Canal)	• Moderate-severe hearing loss • Minimal restrictions due to ear canal size • No changes to the ear canal due to illness • Good hand dexterity and motor skills	• Comfortable to wear • Good cosmetics – the hearing aids are virtually invisible
Completely-in-the-Canal (CIC)	• Mild to moderate-severe hearing loss • Sufficient ear canal size • No changes to the ear canal due to illness • Excellent hand dexterity and motor skills	• Comfortable to wear • Best cosmetics – the hearing aids are optically virtually invisible • Good directionality

Figure 7–1. Four common hearing aid styles or form factors, along with typical candidacy requirements and advantages. Copyright 2009, Sonus USA, Inc. Reprinted with permission.

Because they usually are smaller and couple to the ear using a noncustom mold that fits into the ear, micro-BTE devices offer several potential advantages to the end user compared to customized instruments. There are two general types of OC devices. One type, which we discussed earlier, has the receiver in the ear canal, separated from the rest of the electronic components by a thin wire. This sometimes is referred to as a "thin wire," receiver-in-the-canal (RIC) or a receiver-in-the ear (RITE) device.

The other subcategory of OC device has the receiver in the hearing aid case itself (like all other types of BTEs). This subcategory of OC product is often called a "thin tube" or receiver-in-the-aid (RITA) device. The terminology here becomes quite confusing, as RIC devices also have a "thin tube" that has a wire in it.

Although there are no significant differences in performance between a "thin tube" and a "thin wire" fitting, there are some small differences worth mentioning. Because a RIC uses a wire rather than a tube to deliver the amplified sound to the ear, there are no tubing resonances that might affect sound quality, and no thin tubing that could roll off high frequencies. In addition, as mentioned earlier, RIC products have a smaller case, and are perceived by some patients as more cosmetically appealing than RITA devices. On the other hand, the thin tube RITA device doesn't have an electronic component suspended in a waxy ear canal. For this reason, it is less prone to mechanical failure due to cerumen and moisture. If you are a fan of RICs, you will quickly learn how to replace plugged receivers!

RIC products are currently popular, and make up about 50% of the market of the mini-BTE style. Figure 7–2 shows the differences between the two different subcategories of OC devices on the market today. Regardless of which one you may prefer, given the popularity of these two types of OC fittings, we encourage you to keep up with the published reports comparing these two products. Both http://www.audiology online.com and http://www.hearing journal.com frequently publish studies, survey data and market reports.

With the RIC and RITA discussion put aside for the moment, we now focus on the general category of OC fittings. There are advantages of leaving the ear canal partially open. First, OC devices usually are mini-BTEs, and are coupled to the ear canal with a dome or tulip-shaped tip. Therefore, they make minimal contact with the tissues of the ear canal. Because they do make minimal contact and leave room for sound to leak out of the ear canal, wearers of OC devices are less likely to complain of problems related to using an occluding earmold, such as the occlusion effect (see Chapter 10 for a

TIPS and TRICKS: RIC Myths?

Some have suggested that placing the receiver in the ear canal improves sound quality, and many dispensers seem to believe this; however, there is little research to support this claim. Others have suggested that the RIC approach reduces feedback problems; but research has shown that this claim is false. More high-frequency gain with the RIC? It's hard to compare apples to apples—this seems to vary among manufacturers. In general, surveys have shown that dispensers beliefs about the RIC benefits are significantly higher than what the patient will likely experience. For the typical mini-BTE OC fitting—expect performance to be very similar between an RIC and RITA.

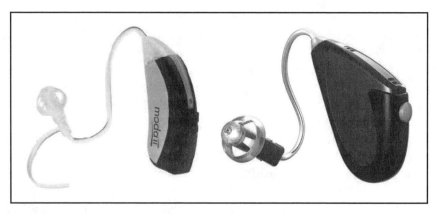

Figure 7–2. An example of a receiver-in-the-aid "thin tube" device (*left*). An example of a receiver-in-the-canal "thin wire" device (*right*). Reprinted with the permission from Unitron, all rights reserved.

complete description of the occlusion effect). Second, OC devices have thin tubes connecting the fitting tip in the ear canal to the case of the BTE. The case of most OC products is relatively small and can easily be hidden behind the pinna. Thus, OC devices are cosmetically appealing. Today, most OC products are of the OC mini-BTE variety. To expand the fitting range, a customized earmold, called a sleeve mold, can be snapped onto the tubing. By adding a closed mold to the mini BTE more low and midfrequency gain can be provided to the patient. Of course, it then would no longer be an OC fitting, as the ear canal would be closed.

A balanced wine is one whose sugars, acids, tannins, and alcohols are evident but do not mask each other. You can think of OC mini-BTEs as balanced in the sense that they combine many of the advantages of a small custom-made product in that they are well hidden in the ear, along with some of the advantages of a traditional BTE with a large vented earmold. When fitted, they also provide a reasonable balance between

natural low-frequency sounds (entering the open ear canal) and amplified high-frequency sounds, with no aftertaste!

In-the-Ear (ITE)

The in-the-ear (ITE) hearing aid resides in the concha portion of the pinna with the receiver portion extending into the ear canal. The ITE style became commercially available in the 1960s. Recent HIA reports show that the ITE style accounts for approximately 30% of all hearing aid sales in the United States. Currently, there are three variants of the ITE style: the full shell, low profile, and half shell.

The full-shell ITE fills the entire concha portion of the outer ear. The low-profile ITE fills the inner portion of the concha from top to bottom, but does not protrude outward as much as the full shell ITE. The half-shell ITE style only fills the lower half of the concha.

The full-concha ITE usually is used when more gain and output is required, although not usually producing as much gain as that obtained with the larger BTE styles. In general, the ITE and smaller styles are easier to insert and remove in comparison to the BTE: there is only one piece rather than two. Additionally, ITEs and smaller styles are less susceptible to wind noise, which can be quite annoying when hearing aids are worn outside.

Sticking with the wine jargon, full-shell ITEs are robust and flavorful, something akin to an Italian Barolo. Like a good Barolo it might take your patient some time to fully appreciate the somewhat boxy and astringent features of the full-shell ITEs.

In the Canal (ITC)

The in-the-canal (ITC) hearing aid only partially fills the lower one-half/one-quarter of the concha. It accounts for about 20% of custom hearing aid sales. Currently, it also is the smallest style of hearing aid that can contain directional microphone technology, as a directional microphone needs port spacing of several millimeters on the faceplate to function effectively. Because it represents a compromise between amplification power and size, the ITC hearing aid may be appropriate for patients that have cosmetic concerns about hearing aids, less severe hearing losses, and/or a moderate loss of dexterity.

A middle-of-the-road choice for patients interested in custom products. The ITC is like a bottle of $20 Cabernet Sauvignon from Sonoma Valley, California. It's a well-balanced compromise between a full-shell ITE and a CIC.

Completely in-the-Canal (CIC)

As its name implies, the completely in-the-canal (CIC) hearing aid is completely contained within the ear canal. Ideally, the face plate does not extend into the concha (although in many cases it does, often because the ear impression wasn't taken deep enough, or the ear canal is simply too small). This product accounts for about 10% of the hearing aid sales. This low percentage of total sales for the CIC is somewhat surprising, as most patients typically ask for the smallest hearing aid possible. One explanation for this may be that hearing professionals are counseling patients away from this smallest of the hearing aid styles toward larger styles that have many advantages over the CIC.

CICs may not offer the gain/output appropriate for patients with moderate to more severe hearing losses. Another disadvantage of the CIC is its lack of a directional microphone, which usually is advantageous for improving understanding performance in the presence of background noise. CICs also require more frequent repair than other hearing aid styles. The electronics contained within the CIC shell are more susceptible to perspiration and cerumen as the CIC is placed deeper in the ear canal of the patient. Moreover, although a volume control is not desired by all patients (or hearing professionals, for that matter), the face plate of the CIC often is too small to accommodate one when it is wanted or needed. Research indicates that 78% of all hearing aid consumers want a volume control, and 33% of those consumers without a volume control on their present hearing aid would like to have one. Finally, because the microphone port opening of the CIC is so close to the area where sound is leaking out of the ear, these products are more prone to feedback.

There are some advantages associated with CIC use, including ease of use with telephones. And, because they come equipped with a removal string, for many patients they are the easiest product to put in and take out. How-ever, given its small size, the CIC is not an appropriate product for all candidates, as primarily its intended fitting is for mild and moderate hearing loss.

Often difficult to fit, thought of by some as delicate and prone to break down, but with tremendous user advantages for exactly the right candidate, the CIC is to hearing aid form factors what the Pinot Noir grape is to wine.

TAKE FIVE: Smaller CICs

Hearing aid circuitry keeps getting smaller, which of course allows for smaller products. In the last few years, there has been somewhat of a "rebirth" of the CIC, as manufacturers are introducing products that fit deeper in the ear canal. Some are recessed considerably in the canal, and indeed are "invisible." Some are even "extended wear." Look for this product area to keep expanding. The flurry over "mini-thin-tube-BTEs" has pretty much run its course, and we all need something new, right?

Other (Rarely Used) Hearing Aid Styles

Body Aid

Given that the body aid was the style of the 1920s, it may come as a surprise to you to learn that this type of hearing aid is still manufactured. In rare cases, body aids are sometimes recommended today for:

- Profound losses where considerable gain is needed
- For some patients in which there are severe physical limitations (the controls on the body aid are very large and easy to use)
- Anatomic conditions in which an air conduction hearing aid is not practical (such as atresia; a bone conduction receiver can be attached to the body aid).

The parts of the body hearing aid are the same as with other hearing aids, except that the receiver is external to the aid. The body aid was at least 20% of the hearing aid market until 1964, and at least 10% of the market until 1972.

Although body aids do not represent much of the current hearing aid market in the United States or Europe (less than 1%), they have found a place in many developing countries. Because of their larger size and standard construction they can be manufactured much less expensively. Additionally, they are popular in countries where hearing aid batteries are a rare commodity and can be very expensive relative to earned salaries. Body aids utilize larger, cheaper batteries such as the AA size, whereas other styles of hearing aids use less commonly available battery sizes. Some body aids even utilize alternative energy sources such as solar cells. Fully charged, some solar-powered body aids can last up to two weeks without recharging. However, users generally are advised to charge them one hour each day during midday direct sunlight. An example of a solar-powered body-worn hearing aid may be found at http://www.com careinternational.org .

Eyeglass Hearing Aids

Although still relatively popular in some European countries, the eyeglasses/hearing aid combination (Figure 7–3) device has almost disappeared from the North American market. We include it under available hearing aid styles because it was an innovative concept in its day during the 1960s.

Conceptually, the combination of eyeglasses and a hearing aid unit sounds like a good idea. After all, if a person

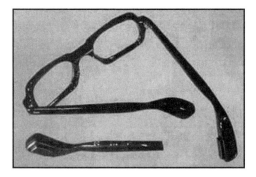

Figure 7–3. An example of a bone-conduction eyeglass hearing aid. Reprinted with permission of Audiology-Online, www.audiologyonline.com .

has to wear both, why not put them all in one apparatus? In practice, however, there are several drawbacks. First, adding the hearing aid technology to the eyeglasses makes them considerably heavier, and less comfortable to wear. The fitting process also is a problem. A prescription from an optometrist for the eyeglasses must be included along with a hearing evaluation to order an appropriate device. This introduces the problem of a considerable amount of inconvenience for the patient, as they would be required to go back and forth for follow-up visits to both an audiologist and an optometrist. Moreover, who should order and sell the device, the optometrist or the audiologist? In cases where the hearing aid or the eyeglasses component needed to be modified in some way or needed a service repair that required the entire device to be mailed back to the manufacturer the patient would be without both. These circumstances do not nearly encompass the times that the patient may not need or want to wear the eyeglasses, for example, at social events or after a long day of work that required large amounts of reading, but if the eyeglasses come off, the hearing aids must come off as well. As an added inconvenience, the need to remove the eyeglasses to change the hearing aid batteries make the already daunting task of removing and inserting small hearing aid batteries even more challenging. Much of the elderly population already has difficulty with changing hearing aid batteries due to poor manual dexterity, even when wearing eyeglasses. Last, because so few eyeglasses/hearing aid combination devices are ordered, there is a very narrow selection of products, which often contain outdated technology.

Slightly out of fashion, sometimes difficult to find, but a great value for the select few refusing to use conventional styles, eyeglass and body hearing aids are the boxed wines of the industry.

Special Applications

Although these are not hearing aid styles per se, or form factors, there are times when we fit individuals with a severe to profound hearing loss in only one ear. One approach is to use a contralateral routing of the signal (CROS) design. These products are commonly used with patients having severe-profound unilateral hearing loss, which is also referred to as single-sided deafness(SSD).

CROS and BiCROS Designs

Because CROS devices are not really styles, rather they are applications of different styles, our wine analogies don't really work as well. But consider this: As much as wine is great to drink, there are times when you might want to use a given wine to make a great sauce. Noted examples would be Madeira (great with roasted chicken or turkey) and Bordelaise (served with red meat). If you'd like a nice wine sauce for your fish, try a Beurre Blanc. So yes, special applications of wine, just like hearing aid styles, can be quite beneficial to the consumer.

For the individual who has an unaidable hearing loss in one ear, and normal hearing or an aidable hearing loss in the other ear, contralateral routing of sound (CROS) or bilateral contralateral routing of signal (BiCROS) amplification may be the most appropriate hearing aid arrangement (Figure 7–4). A CROS hearing aid is used when there is nor-mal or near-normal hearing in one ear and the opposite ear cannot benefit from amplification. This device places a microphone on the side of the poor ear and its receiver directed to the normal ear, so the good ear can receive sound from the opposite side of the head. Using CROS amplification will make a person a "two-sided" listener, but importantly, *not* a "two-eared" listener.

Somewhat different from the CROS fitting, BiCROS hearing aids are used in cases where one ear is unaidable but there is some degree of aidable hearing loss in the other (that is, the signal needs to be amplified even when it is originating from the "good" side). This device has two microphones, one near the better ear and the other near the poorer ear. The acoustic signals from both sides are delivered to a single amplifier and receiver, and the output is then directed into the best ear.

For both the CROS and BiCROS, sound is transmitted either via wire or radio frequency (RF) signal, which is called a wireless system. In the *wired* system, the signal is carried from one side of the head to the other by wires concealed within an eyeglass frame or a cord around the back of the neck in the ITE and BTE styles. If a wireless system is utilized, signals are transferred across the head by an RF transmitter and picked up by an RF receiver positioned near the better ear. The signal is then converted back to acoustic energy and presented to the better ear.

The CROS was developed several decades ago for unilateral hearing loss, patients who complain of an inability to understand speech and localize sounds as a result of the head-shadow effect. The head-shadow effect occurs because traveling to the good ear of a unilateral user is blocked by the skull. The head

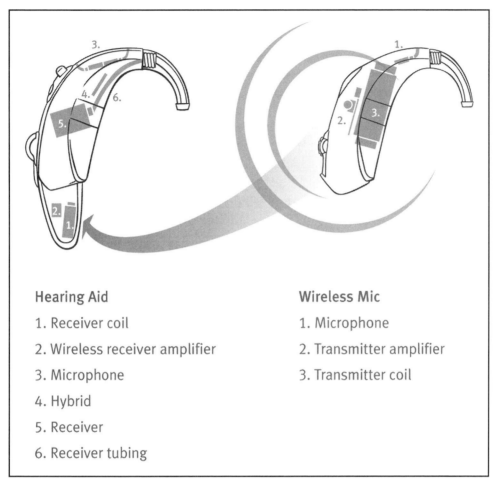

Hearing Aid

1. Receiver coil

2. Wireless receiver amplifier

3. Microphone

4. Hybrid

5. Receiver

6. Receiver tubing

Wireless Mic

1. Microphone

2. Transmitter amplifier

3. Transmitter coil

Figure 7–4. The essential components of a wireless CROS system. Notice that amplified sound is being transmitted from the wireless microphone on the right-hand side of the figure to the receiver on the left. Reprinted with permission from Unitron, all rights reserved.

shadow effect reduces speech by about 7 dB, and the higher frequency components of speech (>2000 Hz) by up to 15 dB. The CROS is designed to minimize the effects of head shadow and improve speech understanding and localization.

The application of the CROS is shown in the upper panel of Figure 7–4. In most applications of the CROS, a traditional hearing aid cannot be worn on the poor ear side because the loss is too severe. In some unique cases, however, a CROS fitting approach is used that is termed "transcranial." In this application, a bone conduction signal from the bad side is transferred to the good side, either through the use of a high-output air conduction signal (deep fitted in the bad ear), or a direct bone conduction stimulation, which can be accomplished in a coupler different ways. In these cases, the contralateral *routing* of the signal is through skull vibrations, not a signal traveling around the head. Here are some examples:

Traditional CROS

■ Transmission of signal from bad side to good side using wiring; going behind the head or through eyeglasses.

■ Transmission of signal from bad side to good side using FM signal. This could involve BTE or ITE on good side, and can be implemented with DAI.

Transcranial CROS

■ A high-intensity air conduction signal is delivered to the bad ear via a power BTE or CIC instrument.

■ A bone conduction input is delivered to the bad ear via a bone conduction receiver placed in the ear canal (e.g., the Trans Ear from United Hearing Systems).

■ A bone conduction input is delivered to the bad ear via an implantable device in the mastoid (e.g., the Baha from Cochlear Corporation).

**TAKE FIVE:
Treatment Options for
Single-Sided Deafness**

There are many styles and approaches to choose from when considering a CROS fitting for your patient. Moreover, there are special techniques needed for fitting and verification. For example, you can use your probe-mic system to develop targets for a transcranial fit. For a complete review of the fitting options and verification techniques, see the excellent article from Valente and colleagues: audiologyonline.com/articles/article _detail.asp?article_id=1629

Choosing a Form Factor

When you are sitting "knee to knee" with a prospective hearing aid user, an important consideration is choosing the best form factor or style to match the hearing loss and communication needs of the individual. The choice of style is based on several factors, including the patient's manual dexterity (can they change the small batteries?), degree of hearing loss (does the smallest hearing aid have enough power?), cosmetic needs, ease of use, and the need for special features, among other issues. Part of addressing each patient's hearing problem requires us to arrive at a cosmetically appealing solution without sacrificing critical auditory needs by choosing the most appropriate form factor.

Figure 7–1 reviews the four most popular and cosmetically appealing hearing aid styles, along with the advantages associated with each of the styles. Before you sit down with your first patient, get to know the advantages and disadvantages associated with each form factor. Although the patient ultimately will be responsible for the selection, in many cases they will be greatly influenced by your recommendation, so it's important that you "get it right." Today, we know of dispensing offices that are located a few blocks apart in a metropolitan area, where one office might dispense 80% BTEs and the office down the street only 30% BTEs— the patients entering these two offices are all pretty much the same.

Before you enjoy a glass of wine, there is a labor-intensive process in which grapes are crushed, destemmed, pressed, and allowed to ferment for an extended period of time.

Before a patient walks out the door of your office with a new set of hearing aids something similar happens.

Earmolds and Earmold Impressions

This section reviews issues related to earmolds and the ear impressions needed for earmolds and custom instruments. In this section of the chapter we review some of the important acoustical and mechanical details of hearing aids styles, including the earpieces that help them work effectively.

Much of our attention will be devoted to earmolds and ear impressions. You can think of the earmold as the plumbing system of the hearing instrument. Earmolds couple the hearing aid to the ear. Their size and shape help fine tune sound, and in many cases might determine the success or failure of a hearing aid fitting.

Impressions of the external ear are needed for two primary reasons: making a customized earmold (to be fitted to a BTE instrument) or making a hearing aid shell for a custom in-the-ear product. The ear impression process is the same, however, so we simply refer to it as an "ear impression" in the following sections.

After grapes have been crushed and destemmed there is a lengthy process in which the liquid is separated from the skins of the grapes, yeast is added, and the mixture is placed in a fermentation tank. Several of these steps are akin to the ear impression process. A couple of different silicone-based chemical compounds are mixed together, injected into the ear canal, and allowed to cure. The end result of ear

impression process may not be as tasty as the wine making process, but when executed properly it results in a perfectly fitting earmold or shell nearly every time.

Ear Impressions

There are two reasons that taking a high quality ear impression is important:

1. The earmold impression procedure is mildly invasive. It is the procedure that you conduct routinely that is the most likely to result in physical harm to the patient's ear if it is not completed using the proper techniques. Even when the procedure is conducted with skill and precision, you can still possibly harm the eardrum or tissues of the ear canal.

2. A poor quality ear impression will result in a custom hearing aid or earmold that fits poorly. You cannot rely on the earmold manufacturer to fix mistakes you made in the impression taking process. It is possible, perhaps even probable that a poor impression (and resulting poor fitting earmold/hearing aid) could cause an otherwise eager hearing aid candidate to reject amplification.

The ear impression (EI) process is relatively straightforward when you follow some standard rules. Similar to the hearing test, EI taking needs to be completed in a step-by-step process every time. Failure to follow a routine procedure will result in either a poor quality impression or a painful, even traumatic experience for the patient. The first rules of proper EI taking are follow the procedures methodically and always take your time. Never rush through this process.

Procedures

Step 1. Gather necessary materials

There are several items you will need when taking EIs. It is a good idea to gather these materials, organize them and place them in one place, like a drawer or carrying kit. Here is what you need:

1. Otoscope
2. Head light (penlight/ear light can be used, but will reduce ear canal visibility and increase risk)
3. Foam or cotton ear dams (ear blocks)
4. Impression material
5. Antimicrobacterial wipes
6. Impression gun or syringe
7. Extra batteries for otoscope and penlights

Step 2. Explanation of procedure

Use a schematic diagram of the external ear anatomy to show the patient what you are about to do. Inform the patient that you gently will be placing the ear dam into the ear canal about 5 mm from the eardrum. Tell the patient that this might feel somewhat uncomfortable. It often will make the patient cough or even gag (this is because there is a branch of cranial nerve X [the vagus] in this part of the ear canal, and an associated branch in the throat). This is a completely normal response. In almost all cases the coughing or gagging only lasts a couple of seconds. Let them know that the next step is to slowly inject the impression material. This may feel a little cool and it will stay in the ear for about 5 or 6 minutes. It is possible that the patient will feel some pressure while it sits in his or her ear. The patient will also feel some discomfort when the material is removed by you.

When you explain the procedure to patients it is important to calmly review the entire process and ask if they have any questions. You want to be sure the patient understands the aversive nature of the procedure, while you put them at ease about it. Also, remember that the earmold material will act like an ear plug, and will give the patient further hearing loss (temporary), so it is important that you give all your instructions, and answer all their questions *before* inserting the material.

Step 3. Infection control

Because this procedure involves the possibility that skin could be broken and some light bleeding could occur, infection control strategies must be employed at all times. Antimicrobacterial wipes must used to disinfect the all instruments that come in contact with the ear. In addition, all nondisposable equipment must be disinfected, using proper infection control techniques following each use.

A detailed description of the many issues related to infection control are beyond the scope of this book. The interested reader is encouraged to visit http://www.oaktreeproducts.com for more information on infection control practices and products. Dr. A. U. Bankaitis of Oaktree Products is an authority on infection control practices and

---

TIPS and TRICKS: A Series of Unfortunate Events

An improperly placed or wrongly sized otoblock easily can result in something called "blow-by." This simply means that EI material has run past the otoblock. "Blow-by" often results in EI material that adheres to the eardrum. Although a blow-by doesn't automatically mean you need to refer to a physician, your patient likely will experience some significant discomfort when you remove the EI. This sometimes happens in a surgically altered ear, and a surgically altered ear may have a perforated or partial eardrum, which then would allow the impression material to go into the middle ear cavity. Although uncommon, there have been reports of this happening. Again, a reminder concerning the importance of a good otoscopic examination.

---

has authored a practical book on the subject.

Step 4. Otoscopic examination

Otoscopic techniques were outlined in Chapter 4. It will take practice, with supervision, to recognize red flags that need medical referral. As you examine the ear prior to taking any EI, take note of the following key landmarks and/or pathologic characteristics:

- Length and course of the external ear canal
- Any foreign objects in the ear canal
- Excessive or impacted cerumen
- Intactness of tympanic membrane (no perforation)
- Surgical modifications or changes (e.g., mastoid cavity)
- Cone of light emanating from eardrum
- Size of concha bowl and texture of ear

Step 5. Bracing the otoscope

Whenever you conduct an otoscopic exam or EI, you need to support the patient's head by using your "off" hand (the hand not holding the instrument). This technique is called bracing. Bracing is used to avoid injury to the ear canal if the patient moves suddenly during the otoscopic exam or EI procedure.

Step 6. Placing the otoblock or ear dam

Following the otoscopic exam, an otoblock is gently placed beyond the second bend of the ear canal. Before placing the otoblock into the ear canal a drop of water-based lubricant should be placed on the otoblock to help guide it into place with minimal discomfort. The otoblock protects the sensitive tissues of the eardrum from being damaged during this process. Otoblocks come in several diameters. You will need to select the correct size that matches the diameter of the ear canal. The otoblock is in place when the outer edges of the otoblock make contact with the ear canal wall. There should be no gaps between the otoblock or ear canal wall. The penlight is used to guide the block into the ear canal around the second bend. Always check the final placement of each otoblock with an otoscope.

TAKE FIVE: Video-Otoscopy

In Chapter 4, we discussed how to conduct otoscopy using a hand-held otoscope. Another popular method is video-otoscopy. By connecting an otoscope to a television screen, the patient can actually see how their ear canal looks. Not only does this make the otoscopic evaluation more interesting to the patient, but many video-otoscopy units allow you to record the image. A recorded image of the ear canal can be sent to a physician or placed in the patient's chart notes. Many hearing care professionals rely on video-otoscopy before and after the ear impression process. There are several video otoscopy units on the market. Your local independent equipment distributor can help you sort your options.

Step 7. Mixing the impression material

There are two common methods used for inserting impression material into the ear canal:

- Injection gun—This method utilizes premixed cartridges of EI material
- Syringe—This method requires you first to mix the EI, place the material into the syringe, and then to inject it into the ear canal.

Both methods have advantages and disadvantages. Today, the injection gun and premixed EI cartridges are more popular than the syringe method. Before going any further you should check to ensure that the EI has an expiration date that has not expired. The expiration date should be clearly labeled on the package.

Step 8. Injecting the material

This step requires the utmost attention. Take your time and do it right. You should follow this order:

1. Pull the pinna up and back gently to straighten out the ear canal

2. Place the tip of the injection gun or syringe into the aperture of the ear canal. The tip should always be visible to you.
3. Squeeze the syringe or injection gun smoothly allowing the material to flow freely up to the otoblock. Never inject the material with force.
4. Once the entire concha bowl has been filled with EI material, let go of the pinna with your other hand.
5. Keep the tip of the injection gun or syringe in the material until it flows back around it.
6. Make sure you have filled the entire concha and helix area with material before removing the tip from the ear.
7. Allow the material to sit 5 to 10 minutes.

There is considerable debate about taking the EI with the patient's jaw open versus closed. There is no clear consensus in the industry regarding which procedure is preferred. Therefore, it is best to stick to one procedure and become extremely proficient with it.

TIPS and TRICKS: Two Methods for Taking an Ear Impression

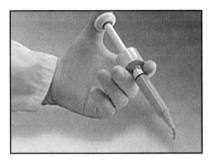

A standard syringe used to made ear impressions.

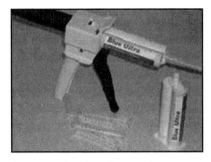

An example of an impression gun or pistol.

Silicone with syringe: The impression base and accelerant should be measured with the tools provided by the manufacturer. The ratio should not be changed. A spatula should be used to mix the material on a splead pad for 20 to 30 seconds until the color is uniform. Form into a cylinder then quickly load into the syringe. Insert the plunger and gently push some material through the tip out onto a tissue. Put the syringe tip deeply into the ear canal. Fill the deepest portion of the canal first, and then gradually work your way out, keeping the syringe tip in the material until you have finished filling the concha and helix. Let impression material sit in canal 5 to 8 minutes until pressing a fingernail into the impression material does not leave an indentation. The syringe has the advantage of more easily filling in voids because of its higher viscosity material. The downside to this higher viscosity is the tendency to expand the ear canal resulting in an oversized impression. This is less concern for children who have very soft cartilage. This artifact of overestimating the volume of the ear canal could be problematic for older adults who have bonelike cartilage and a severe hearing loss.

Impression gun with silicone: Attaching a mag light mounted on the syringe greatly enhances visualization of the ear canal during impression taking. After attaching the mixing tip to the cartridge and positioning the plunger, release a small amount of impression material onto a tissue. Place the tip deep in the canal until almost touching the otoblock and gently squeeze the impression gun handle, slowly releasing material into the ear canal always leaving the tip in the impression material; building from the bottom up then withdrawing the gun slowly building out until the ear canal is filled, then filling the concha bowl and helix. Let the impression material sit in the ear canal for 5 to 8 minutes until a fingernail pushed into the impression does not leave a mark. The thinner viscosity of this material poses more of a challenge to ensure that no voids are present in the impression. However, this lower viscosity results in an impression that does not overestimate the volume of the ear canal and may produce better results for older adults.

There is some consensus that an open jaw impression should be taken when one of the following is observed:

- A significant mandibular displacement is observed during jaw movements
- Changes in the auditory canal can be detected during the otoscopic inspection
- The patient complains of feedback related to jaw movement
- The hearing aid lacks retention and slides out of the ear
- The patient reports a noticeable loss of hearing aid gain associated with jaw movement.

Step 9. Removing the EI

The EI is ready for removal from the ear canal after at least 5 minutes of waiting. To ensure that the EI is ready for removal, use your fingernail or the corner of a credit card to lightly push on the EI. If the indention you made does not leave a lasting mark on the impression, it is time to remove the EI. Follow this process:

- Gently pull the pinna up and out to loosen the seal.
- Pull the helix portion (top part) of the EI out slightly away from the ear canal. Gently rock the EI back and forth further loosening it.
- If the patient is not in too much discomfort, carefully and slowly continue to gently pull the EI out of the ear canal. Usually, the otoblock will adhere to the material and come out at the same time. If not, you will need to conduct an otoscopic evaluation and remove the remaining otoblock from the ear canal with the proper instrumentation.

Step 10. Inspect the ear canal and the EI

As soon as you remove the EI from the ear, use the otoscope to inspect the ear canal. Look for any trauma in the ear canal or on the eardrum. A red ear canal and maybe even some slight bleeding are quite normal. Inform the patient that there should be no discomfort within a few hours.

Next, carefully examine the ear impression to be sure that it is a proper image of the ear. EIs that have voids or underfillings, especially in the canal area need to be remade. Industry experts say that about 20% of all ear impressions arriving in the shell lab are of poor quality. It should seem obvious that a poor quality ear impression will lead to a poor quality fitting, but don't expect manufacturers to call you when they receive a poor quality ear impression. They don't want to risk putting some professionals on the defensive by calling them and asking for another EI; therefore, they will do the best they can with the impression you send them.

> **TAKE FIVE:**
> **Take a Reading Break and Watch This Video**
>
> If you want to see how an earmold impression is made from start to finish, there is a good example of the entire procedure on a video at this Web site: http://www.ear impressions.com

Step 11. Send the information to the manufacturer

Once you have completed otoscopy and an inspection of the ear impression, you will need to send the information to the manufacturer.

Currently, there are two methods for doing this. The traditional method is to simply place the EI in a shipping box, include the order form, and express mail it to the manufacturer. Another method is to electronically scan the EI and send the scan via e-mail to the manufacturer. Regardless of the method you use, the bottom line is that using a consistent ear impression process is more likely to result in a high-quality ear impression, which in turn will lead to a well-fitted hearing aid.

Earmolds

Wine glasses are used to hold wine and earmolds are designed to hold (or couple) the hearing aid to the ear. Just like there are different types of wine glasses for different types of wines, there are different types of earmolds for various types of hearing loss. All wine glasses have three essential components: the base, the stem, and the body, which holds the wine. All earmold coupling systems have three essential components: the tubing, the vent, and the earmold itself. But the similarities don't end there.

Like earmold styles, there literally are dozens of different types of wine glasses. Wine connoisseurs say there are three general types of wine glasses. Red wine glasses are taller and wider so the complexities of the wine can be appreciated. You can think of the red wine glass as being similar to a full-shell earmold. White wine glasses are smaller in order to keep the wine cool. For a young, crisp white wine you need a glass that's slightly larger than the body of the glass. The thinner and sleeker skeleton mold is the equivalent of the white wine glass. The third type of essential wine glass is the Champagne flute, which is extremely

tall and thin, thus allowing the bubbles of the Champagne or sparkling wine to build up properly. The extremely small canal or sleeve mold is the earmold equivalent of the Champagne flute.

Most earmolds are custom made in a laboratory, and are designed to couple the hearing aid to the patient's ear. Because they are part of an acoustic system, earmolds play a significant part in shaping the amplified sound before it reaches the tympanic membrane. When selecting the best earmold to couple to any BTE instrument, there are several considerations. The earmold style typically is selected based on the configuration and degree of the hearing loss, although in some cases, the physical dexterity of the patient also must be weighed. As we discuss in detail, some earmolds leave most of the ear canal open, others close the canal completely. But even those that completely occlude the canal have an air hole, referred to as a vent. The size of the earmold vent usually depends on the degree of hearing loss, especially for the lower frequencies.

TAKE FIVE:
More on Earmolds

One of the most comprehensive earmold manuals is available for free. It can be ordered at this Web site: http://www.earmolds.com/manual.html

All the major earmold manufacturers have instructional Web sites, including Great Lakes Labs, Westone, Emtech, EDI, and others. One Web site that is particularly useful is from a Canadian earmold company named Emsee. Their Web address is http://www.emsee.ca .

Earmold Style

The names given to earmold styles are relative to the National Association of Earmold Labs (NAEL). Figure 7–5 shows common earmold styles. As a general rule, the greater the hearing loss the more material is used to fill the ear canal.

We learned in Chapter 3 that the ear has specific landmarks, and like the ear, an earmold also has landmarks. Landmarks are important because they bring consistency to the dialogue we might have with other professionals. For example, let's say a recent patient you fitted with new a earmold has a pressure sore (a relatively common occurrence with a new earmold that causes the skin in the ear canal to be irritated). You have tried to modify the earmold in your office, but your modifications have been ineffective. To fix the problem, you have to take a new ear impression with exact instructions on where the earmold needs to be made looser or smaller. Using a common terminology for earmold landmarks allows you to communicate more effectively with the earmold lab. In this example, perhaps you have to tell the lab to make the crural groove more narrow. Figure 7–6 depicts the most commonly used terms for the important landmarks on an earmold. In a matter of a few months, chances are good you will have these memorized. If you use the scanning procedure, you also can go back and draw on the image itself and make comments, which will add helpful information. The take home message is that common terminology for landmarks facilitates the communication between you and other professionals.

The next section provides a general overview of some of the mechanical changes you can make to earmold and their plumbing, such as tubing, venting, sound bore, and so forth. Even though we make many adjustments to hearing aids electronically with our cable and software, mechanical changes to the plumbing are still important.

Venting

In simple terms, a vent is a hole or trench in the earmold or custom hearing aid that allows communication (air and sound) from the residual ear canal space to the outside world. There are three major types of vents found in a

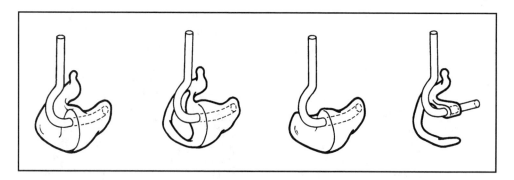

Figure 7–5. The four most common earmold styles from left to right; shell, skeleton, canal, and free-field/CROS. Reprinted with permission from Unitron, all rights reserved.

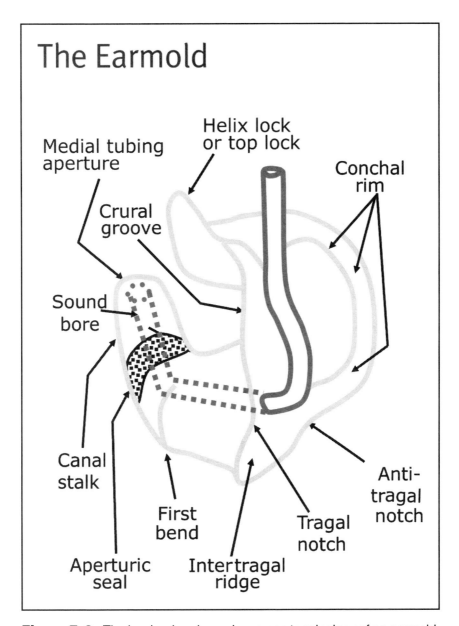

Figure 7–6. The key landmarks and common terminology of an earmold. Reprinted by permission from Dillon (2001) "Hearing Aids."

hearing aid shell or earmold. They are parallel, side branch, and trench. (Figure 7–7 shows the two most common types). All three types are designed to accomplish the same thing, which is to provide some reduction of amplified low frequency sound; allow low-frequency sounds to leak out of the ear. Venting also allows for some pressure relief, which results from bone conducted sound getting trapped in the closed off ear canal when a tight-fitting hearing

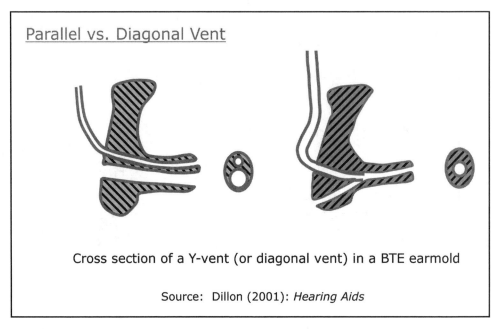

Parallel vs. Diagonal Vent

Cross section of a Y-vent (or diagonal vent) in a BTE earmold

Source: Dillon (2001): *Hearing Aids*

Figure 7–7. The two most common types of vents: parallel on the left and side branch on the right.

aid is inserted into the ear canal (the sound is generated from the condyle area of the mandible, which is located close to the ear canal). This additional low-frequency energy is especially a problem when patients talk or chew. We talk more about this in Chapter 11 when we discuss the occlusion effect and how to treat it.

The most commonly used vent is the parallel type. It comes in a variety of sizes. Although earmold and hearing aid manufacturers are sized according to the vents internal diameter expressed in millimeters, we'll keep it simple. There are five major vent sizes: pressure, small, medium, large, and IROS. Figure 7–8 shows the size of the vent recommended for the degree of low-frequency hearing loss on the audiogram. When selecting a vent size use this information to determine which size is most appropriate.

When the most appropriate size vent is not known, or when it's expected that vent adjustments might be needed, it's common to order what is called a "select-a-vent." For this fitting application, a large bore is placed in the earmold, and then plugs can be added to create a complete closed earmold, or a pressure, small, or medium vent size.

How Big Should the Vent Be?

As shown in Figure 7–8, the size of the vent usually relates to the desired gain (or "release of gain") for the lower frequencies. Figure 7–8 provides a general guideline regarding low-frequency gain reduction for five different vent sizes. Let's say that you have a patient with a 50 dB loss at 500 Hz and 1000 Hz. According to the chart you need to order the hearing aid with a small vent. You are probably wondering, "What

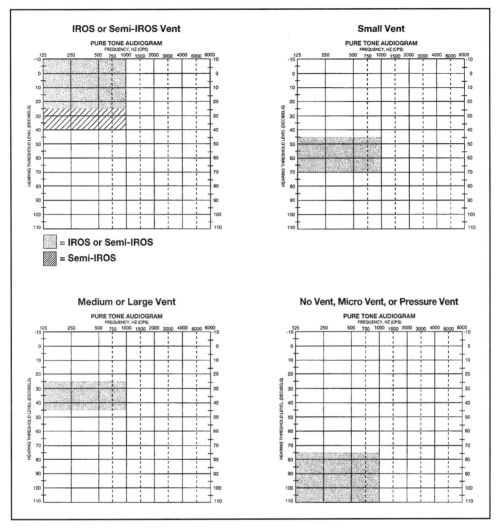

Figure 7–8. Vent size guide. If the low-frequency thresholds on the patient's audiogram fall in the shaded area request the most appropriate vent size for one of the four audiograms. Reprinted with the permission from Unitron, all rights reserved.

exactly is a small vent?" In our opinion, it is less than 1 mm in diameter. Granted there is some subjectivity when it comes to differentiating between small, medium, and large vents. Generally, large would constitute a vent larger than 2 mm, medium 1 to 2 mm, and small is less than 1 mm. Because it's not an exact science, and you will need to balance vent size based on patient comfort and adequate gain before feedback, we suggest you order a select-a-vent (SAV) whenever possible. With SAV you can change the vent size in your office depending on the specific needs of your patient. The only downside of an SAV is that it might be slightly more visible on some products.

Vent selection is an important aspect of the hearing aid selection process,

---

TIPS and TRICKS: A Few Additional Tidbits About Venting

- Many earmolds do not fit extremely tight, and there is sound leakage around the rim of the concha, which indirectly is "venting." This is referred to as "slit leak."
- When fitting someone with a profound hearing loss, where a very tight seal is required, it's good to order a "tight seal." (or whatever terminology you earmold manufacturer uses), along with a very small pressure vent or slit leak vent.
- With custom products, it's common to create or enlarge vents in the office. One simple-to-do vent approach is to run a small trench along the bottom of the custom

product, called a trench vent. It's also simple to drill through the case of the hearing aid using this procedure, so be careful!
- If you cannot increase the size of the vent, shortening the vent length by several millimeters will have the same effect, which is a reduction in low-frequency amplification.
- Some manufacturers automatically calculate the vent diameter and vent length based on the audiogram you send with the order. There is some evidence that an automatic calculation of venting parameters leads to less occlusion-related problems.

---

and its effect on the success of the fitting is sometimes overlooked. If you provide too much venting, the hearing aid might not be delivering enough low and mid-frequency information. (This is especially true in open-canal BTE products, which have maximum venting). If the vent is too small, the patient is more likely to complain of the occlusion effect, which we mentioned earlier. If a patient has normal hearing in the lower frequencies, a large vent will make average speech sound more "natural." But a large vent will make the fitting more prone to feedback, and perhaps the patient will not be able to obtain the needed gain for audibility in the high frequencies.

Figure 7–9 gives you an idea of effects of venting on gain. Notice in the low frequencies how much low-frequency attenuation occurs as a result of increasing the vent size from 1 to even 2 mm. For patients that have more than a 30 to

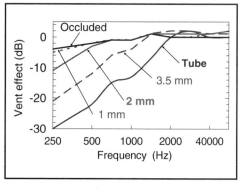

Figure 7–9. The expected low-frequency gain reduction for five different vent sizes. Reprinted with the permission from Unitron, all rights reserved.

35 dB hearing loss in the low frequencies, too large a vent can compromise audibility. We hope you are beginning to see the balancing act needed for proper vent selection and how it contributes to improved audibility and proper sound quality.

Earmold Materials

Although earmold manufacturers may use different trade names, when it comes to selecting the most appropriate material to use for the earmold, there are three primary choices: acrylic, silicone, and soft silicone. Acrylic is the most popular and thought to be the most versatile. Each material has distinct advantages and disadvantages reviewed in Table 7–1. The old adage is "soft earmolds for hard ears and hard earmolds for soft ears" but it's not quite that simple.

Finishes and Color

Earmolds also are available in two types of finishes: glossy (shiny) or satin (matte). In addition to the finish, you need to request the color of the earmold. At the minimum, the following three colors are available for any one of the three types of earmold material you select:

- Clear
- Translucent pink
- Translucent brown

There are other subcategories of earmold material available to you. In cases of allergic reactions, it makes good sense to consult your preferred earmold manufacturer for advice on which ones work well. Use Mediflex or Frosted Flex silicone earpiece material if allergies are a concern. However, earpieces made from silicone can be abrasive to

Table 7–1. The Three Primary Earmold Materials (plus advantages of each material)

Name	Characteristics	Advantages
Acrylic	Hard	Extremely durable
		0 cytotoxicity (hypoallergenic)
		Easily modified in office
		Appropriate for mild to severe loss
		More easily inserted
Silicone	Semisoft	More soft than acrylic
		May expand to reduce slit leaks
		Appropriate for mild to severe loss
		0 cytotoxicity (hypoallergenic)
Soft silicone	Very Soft	Flexes to accommodate TMJ movement
		Better seal for profound loss
		Good choice for sports
		Good choice for children
		0 cytotoxicity (hypoallergenic)

Source: Reprinted with permission from Unitron, all rights reserved.

delicate skin, particularly in elderly patients. Select acrylic or vinyl earpiece materials have been boiled in saline solution as an alternative to Mediflex or Frosted Flex. Polyethylene earpiece material is available for extreme allergy situations. Keep in mind that there are several reputable earmold labs around the world, and each uses slightly different names for the same material.

Tubing Modifications

Part of the total BTE "plumbing" is tubing, which is needed to couple most earmolds to a BTE device. You might think that tubing is simple; however, there are many variables that have an effect on the frequency response, and hearing aid sound quality. Like earmold styles, there are some considerations that must be made when selecting the right tubing for the device and patient.

Tubing length and internal diameter can have a pronounced effect on the frequency response of the hearing aid. Tubing diameters are standardized according to the internal diameter.

The most commonly used tubing with conventional BTE instruments is #13. Table 7–2 summarizes the different tubing sizes and diameters.

As mentioned, the length and internal diameter of the tubing can impact the frequency response. When the internal diameter of the tubing becomes smaller, there is a gradual reduction in the hearing aid's gain in the frequencies above 2000 Hz. There are times when earmold tubing might become crimped during the production process (or maybe when you replaced a patient's tubing). It's important to keep this in mind when you are conducting probe-mic verification, and are wondering why you are not seeing much gain in the high frequencies. A quick check would be to see if the gain is present in the 2-cc coupler. If it is, then conduct some troubleshooting measures with the plumbing.

Changing the tubing length results in a slightly more complicated result, as the peak of the frequency response shifts as the length changes. (Remember our discussion of resonance in Chapter 2). As the length of the tubing is usually dictated by how the hearing

Table 7–2. Dimensions for Common Hearing Aid Tubing

Tubing Size	Inner Diameter (mm)	Outer Diameter (mm)
#12 Standard	2.16	3.18
#13 Medium	1.93	3.10
#13 Thick	1.93	3.31
#13 Super Thick	1.93	3.61
#15 Standard	1.50	2.95
#16 Standard	1.35	2.95

aid is coupled to the wearer's ear, we don't need to concern ourselves too much with how changes in tubing length affect frequency response. That is, you won't be changing tubing length to alter the frequency response.

Tubing customarily is glued into the sound bore of the earmold, and needs to be replaced 2 to 4 times per year on average. It's important that you tell your patient not to remove the earmold by pulling on the tubing, but they'll probably do it anyway. Something called a continuous flow adaptor (CFA) is a handy alternative to traditional tubing using glue. Because the CFA does not require glue there is less mess when periodically changing it. The CFA also can be combined with a large sound bore to create a horn effect, which slightly increases high-frequency gain—more on horn tubing shortly.

As discussed earlier in this chapter, OC fittings with a mini-BTE have become popular. Some of these products use an RIC fitting. These products impact on "tubing" in two different ways:

■ With the RITA, the tubing has a very small internal diameter. You will need somewhat more high-frequency amplifier gain to account for this.

■ With the RIC, there is no tubing! This small receiver is placed in the ear canal (usually fitted in a silicone dome or custom-made earpiece). This would be an example when "tubing" is not a determinant in the frequency response of the hearing aid.

The Horn Effect

Recall from your earlier reading on acoustics that flaring out the end of tubing (in a systematic fashion) results in an increase in high-frequency gain. Because high-frequency sound is so important to understanding speech, even a few extra dB of sound between 2000 and 5000 dB can results in significant improvement is speech intelligibility for the patient. Optometrist Cy Libby is credited with taking advantage of this phenomenon commercially, using the basic research of Mead Killion, and creating the Libby Horn (Figure 7–10). There are two types of Libby Horns. The 3-mm Libby Horn, which is the more common of the two, increases the high frequency response 4 to 6 dB in the 2000- to 5000-Hz range. The 4-mm Libby Horn (which is too big for many ear canals) increases the high-frequency

---

TAKE FIVE: Tubing for Custom Products?

You've perhaps noticed that our discussion about tubing relates to BTE products. But custom products use tubing too, and this tubing does impact the frequency response. It is often "tweaked" by the manufacturer to alter the frequency response, just like with BTEs. The difference is that you won't be directly involved in changing the tubing for custom products, as it's enclosed in the case.

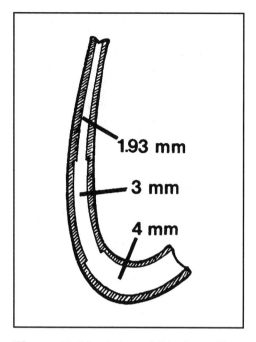

Figure 7–10. A 4-mm Libby horn. Note how the internal diameters increases over the distance of the horn.

Bore Modifications

The sound bore can also be modified to change the frequency response of the hearing aid. The standard sound bore is 2 to 3 mm diameter. When the sound bore is increased to 4 mm at the end of the sound channel, a horn effect may be achieved and high frequency gain is increased 2 to 4 dB. A smaller bore (1 to 2 diameter) can be used to slightly enhance low-frequency sound. Below are four types of common sound bores.

Damping

Damping is another method for altering the frequency response of a hearing aid. The most common use is to put dampers in the tone hook of the BTE instrument, and many manufacturers offer tone hooks with different size dampers (typically dampers in tone hooks are placed by the manufacturer, not the dispenser).

response by 6 to 8 dB in the 2000- to 5000-Hz range. Because of the size of the "horn," it only can be used effectively with smaller vents, for example, there would not be room for tubing this large and also a large vent. It is possible, however, to fit the tube as an "open" fitting with some instruments.

If you're ordering a larger ear mold, talk to your ear mold manufacturer about the option of including horn technology. It's actually "free" gain in the frequency region where gain usually is at a premium. The only downside would be size, and possible cosmetic concerns.

There have been attempts to duplicate the "horn effect" in custom instruments. This doesn't work very well, as the space and dimensions needed for "step-bore" technology simply aren't available. It probably does no harm, however.

We haven't talked much about tone hooks, but for many BTE instruments, the hook is an important part of the overall plumbing. Tone hooks tend to have a resonant frequency around 1600 Hz, which cannot always be eliminated through tuning the frequency response. This resonant peak can be flattened with dampers. It also is possible to insert filters or dampers into the tubing or sound bore. For example, lamb's wool can be used to smooth the frequency response of the hearing aid. This approach, however, often leads to moisture collection: the damper can become "plugged" which causes significant attenuation of the amplified signal. Damping usually has the biggest affect of frequencies between 750 Hz and 2000 Hz. The downside of dampers

TAKE FIVE: Four Common Types of Sound Bores

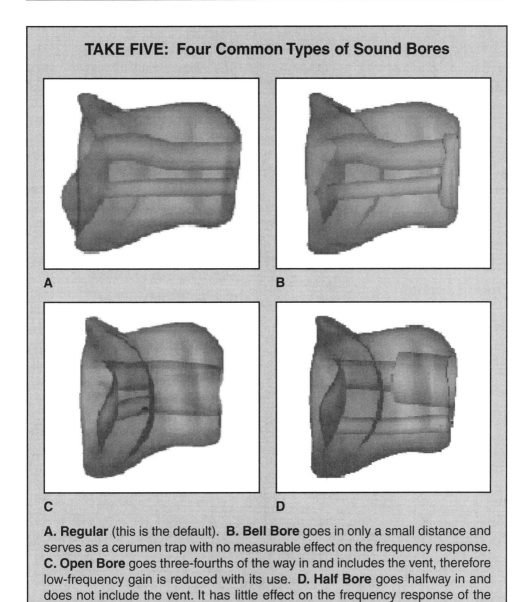

A. Regular (this is the default). **B. Bell Bore** goes in only a small distance and serves as a cerumen trap with no measurable effect on the frequency response. **C. Open Bore** goes three-fourths of the way in and includes the vent, therefore low-frequency gain is reduced with its use. **D. Half Bore** goes halfway in and does not include the vent. It has little effect on the frequency response of the hearing aid.

is that they do reduce the overall output, which might be undesirable for severe to profound hearing losses.

Overall Effects

When it comes to mechanical modifications to the hearing aid and its plumb-ing, there are a lot of options. The physics are fairly straightforward, but you might want to reread Chapter 2 to get a deeper understanding on how these changes to the hearing aid or ear-mold mechanics actually work. For now, we provide a handy reference that summarizes what happens when you modify the venting, damping, or horn of any hearing aid system. Figure 7–11 shows how changes to each part of the system effects sound quality. For example, changes in the horn effects of the earmold or tube effect the perceived "brilliance" of sound because we know that increasing the horn of an earmold and tube increase high-frequency energy, which is perceived by the patient as sounding more "brilliant." One of the pioneers of "hands-on" hearing aid fitting is Cy Libby, and we acknowledge his work in this area.

Open Earmold Effects

So far, we have focused on the acoustical effects of a closed ear canal system, with venting added in some cases. Given the popularity of OC products, however, we now review effects of open earmold systems in comparison to their closed earmold counterparts. Unlike a closed system, OC fittings (the ones that are truly open) maintain most of the resonance of the unoccluded ear canal. Because the ear canal is open, rather than partially closed, the volume of air in ear canal is much greater. This changes the way sound arrives at the tympanic membrane.

There are three major benefits associated with open earmold systems:

- If the ear canal is truly open, the patient's natural ear canal resonance will remain. This means that less amplifier gain will be needed to obtain the same SPL at the eardrum (studies have shown about a 5 dB free-gain advantage for open vs. closed in the 2000–3000 range)
- With an open earmold system the amplification below about 1500 Hz is greatly reduced, while leaving

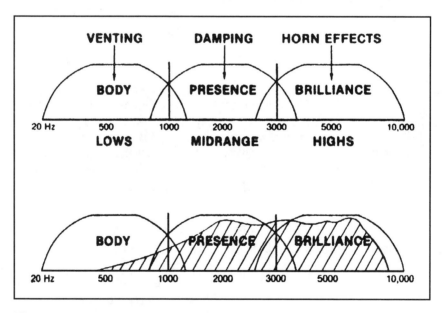

Figure 7–11. The effects of venting, damping, and acoustic horns on the frequency of a hearing aid based on the work of Cy Libby. Note on the bottom schematic a typical frequency response is superimposed on the figure.

the high frequencies much as they would be with a closed mold system. For this reason, open mold systems are an excellent choice for patients with normal hearing up to 1000 Hz and then a drop in threshold in the higher frequencies. Unamplified low-frequency sounds will be heard naturally. Because of this, most patients will say that things sound "more natural."

■ The third positive outcome of the open earmold system relates to

patient comfort with their own voice. With a closed earmold system, sound pressure builds up in the ear canal when the patient talks. This is a normal consequence of closing off the ear canal, and it is generated by bone conduction of vocalization. Even though vents reduce the annoyance of this phenomenon to some extent in closed earmold systems, it still can be quite annoying for some patients. In an open earmold system, the sound pressure buildup in the ear

---

TIPS and TRICKS: Open or Closed?

Why an Open Fitting Can Be Good

■ Allows for unwanted amplification of low-frequency sounds to leak out of the ear.

■ Reduces or eliminates the occlusion effect (related to the low-frequencies leaking out of the ear—the occlusion effect usually has its maximum peak at 600 Hz or below).

■ Allows for low-frequency speech and environmental sounds to pass naturally to the eardrum (natural low frequency sounds typically are rated as having higher quality than amplified sounds for individuals with normal hearing in the low frequencies).

■ If the fitting is very open, some or most of the natural ear canal resonance will be preserved. This reduces "insertion loss" and less amplifier gain is needed to obtain the desired ear canal output.

■ For a BTE fitting, the natural low-frequency occurring sounds will improve localization, when compared to amplified sounds.

■ Some external or middle ear pathologies require an open earmold to allow for appropriate aeration.

Why an Open Fitting Can Be Bad:

■ Sound leaking out of the ear will be picked up by the microphone, resulting in acoustic feedback, causing annoyance and limiting maximum gain.

■ Sound leaking out of the ear will prevent obtaining significant low-frequency gain.

■ The effects of special features such as directional technology and digital noise reduction will be reduced when low-frequency signals can pass directly to the ear.

■ The direct and amplified signals can have unexpected summation and cancellation effects when the two signals are similar in intensity.

■ If the hearing aid has a long processing time (referred to as "group delay"), the patient may hear a slight "echo" because of the different arrival time of the direct versus the amplified signal.

canal of bone conducted sound is allowed to escape normally.

In daily practice, there is often a compromise regarding the "openness" of the fitting. Both closed and open fittings have their own advantages, and for each patient the pros and cons of vent style (degree of openness) must be weighed carefully.

In Closing

Some people prefer Chardonnay from California over Chardonnay from France. Or, if you're into Burgundy wines, you might prefer the 1985 vintage over the one produced in 1995.

Usually, having choices is a good thing. Both dispensers and patients have preferences regarding hearing aid styles; sometimes they mesh, other times they don't. We hope you've learned a little about these hearing aid styles, and all the different fitting options. And you now know the term "form factor." It's important to know the advantages and disadvantages of each form factor or style. In many cases, the style is selected because it provides the best acoustic solution, but you also must consider "appearance," as the patient must accept the looks. A compromise is sometimes necessary. You know that the RIC product will have more repair problems, but the patient wants the cutest mini-BTE available. What to do?

After reading this chapter, you should be better versed on how earmold style and plumbing contribute to the hearing aid selection and fitting process. A perfectly programmed hearing aid can produce the "wrong" output in the earcanal, if the appropriate plumbing isn't used. An uncomfortable earmold may be all it takes to convince a new user that he really doesn't need hearing aids.

And, finally, you might be a bit more knowledgeable about wine. After you have taken a few ear impressions, changed some tubing, and selected the best hearing aid style for a few patients, sit back and enjoy a complex Spanish Roija or an earthy French Bordeaux. You might even know what type of glass to use!

Hearing Aids:
How They Work!

Want to understand how a hearing aid works?

Just think about cars and their operation!

Anyone who has driven a car for the past 25 years knows how much automobiles have changed over that period of time. Just about every aspect of the driving experience today is computerized and automated. You can even start your car on a cold January morning from the warmth of your home, which is a very positive technology advancement if you live in Minnesota or North Dakota. Even though cars have become more automated, many of the basic parts have not changed over the years. You still have to put gas in it and change the oil and spark plugs every so often. In many ways, hearing aids are like cars in the sense that many of the internal operations have become computerized, but the basic components have remained unchanged.

To remind you how comprehensive the overall profession of dispensing hearing aids has become, it's taken us until Chapter 8 to get to the topic of how

hearing aids work! And, moreover, when it comes to learning how hearing aids work, this chapter is only the beginning of the journey. We're giving you the training wheels for what you will learn in subsequent chapters, but knowing the material in this chapter really is an investment in your future success. That's because this chapter lays the foundation for further knowledge concerning all aspects of hearing aids. The better you understand the basics, the better you will understand advanced features found in modern hearing aids.

It is commonly speculated, that the very first hearing aid was the hand cupped over the ear. You didn't know that cavemen used hearing aids? Until the electronic era that was pretty much all a hearing-impaired person could do to improve his hearing. Yes, there were cow horns, ear trumpets, and speaking tubes, but they didn't work much better. We have come a long way. In today's digital electronic era, the number of calculations and acoustic manipulations a hearing instrument can make in a single second is truly staggering. In this chapter you will be introduced to the inner workings of a hearing aid, and some of the terms surrounding hearing aid performance.

You already know that a hearing aid is an electronic sound amplifier. Simply stated, it is designed to take sounds that are too soft for those with a hearing loss to hear appropriately, and make them louder. Basically, we usually want the hearing aid to make soft sounds audible, average sounds comfortable, and loud sounds loud, but not too loud. A modern hearing aid accomplishes this feat through microphone, amplifier, receiver, and a series of electronic calculations. As you will soon learn, there are many hearing aids for you to choose from, and the way in which you program (fine tune) them makes a tremendous difference in how they work for the patient. The good news is that all hearing aids have some common components. We start by discussing the common function of all modern hearing aids.

What Is Amplification?

A hearing aid performs an electronic sleight of hand. It takes sounds that occur naturally in the real world, borrows energy from an outside source (a battery), changes it into a electrical current (microphone), makes it a digital signal, digitally manipulates the signal (processing algorithms), boosts it up (amplifier), changes it back to an acoustic signal (receiver), and sends the sound to the person's ear canal. And, it does all this is a few milliseconds while immersed in a hot and humid environment (behind the ear or in the ear canal).

The important point is that all hearing aids perform these tasks in a very similar way. When selecting and fitting hearing aids, there are two general ways to categorize things. One is by style, or the way the hearing aids look when they are being worn, we just discussed in Chapter 7. The other way is by how the hearing aid actually operates, or the electronics within the device. Figure 8–1 shows the manner in which sounds travel through a simple electronic hearing aid.

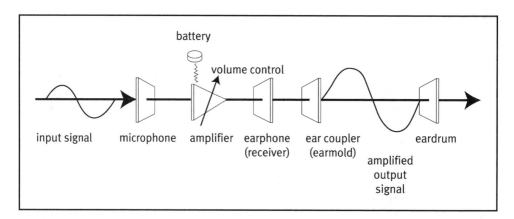

Figure 8–1. Basic components of a hearing aid. From Berger, *The Hearing Aid: Its Operation and Development.* 1984. National Hearing Aid Society.

TAKE FIVE: Hearing Aid History and Overview

The hearing aid dispenser of today carefully measures the patient's hearing thresholds using an audiometric test battery. If the results of testing and the patient's lifestyle deem a hearing aid fitting necessary, a relationship begins. Part of that relationship involves amplification. When it comes to selecting what what's best, both the patient and fitter have many options.

Pre-electronic hearing aids date back centuries, and include such systems as hearing horns, or trumpets. If we were to describe amplification in physical measurement terms, the pre-electronic horns were capable of delivering around 10 to 20 dB of acoustic gain, for a narrow frequency region.

The electronic era of hearing aids began with inventions initially appearing in other innovations of the day. An era sometime called the "carbon era" began around 1900, and is characterized by the use of carbon material behind the diaphragm of the carbon style microphone. The carbon style era hearing aid was capable of providing about 20 to 30dB of amplification (also with a limited frequency bandwidth). This was appropriate for mild to moderate losses. This era lasted into the 1940s. Some "shaping" of the frequency response, selectively amplifying certain frequencies to match hearing loss, was possible. Filtering, or limiting of the hearing aid response was not feasible.

When the vacuum tube triode amplifier was invented in 1907, the "vacuum tube" era was born. Vacuum tubes appeared in some hearing aids during the 1920s, and emerged more fully during the 1930s. They were very large requiring multiple tubes and batteries. Power, however, did increase substantially to near 70 dB gain and 130 dB output. This would be appropriate for much more severe losses. During this era, filtering, shaping, and limiting were electronically possible. The first one-piece hearing aid was not introduced until around 1944. The wearable body aid was born. The vacuum tube era ended in the 1950's with the acceptance of the transistor style hearing aid.

The "transistor era" began in 1947, and hearing aids began to use the technology in the early 1950's. In the transistor era, hearing aid components became smaller, yet more efficient. Hearing aids could now be worn on the head via eyeglass, or postauricular aids. Eventually, (1964) transistors became small enough to be put on a small integrated circuit chip, allowing for in-the-ear custom hearing aids. In 1960, body aids accounted for approximately 25% of sales, eyeglass aids, 45%, and BTEs, 30%. In-the-ear sales were reported as 2% in 1961, and did not reach 10% until 1967, not 30% until 1977.

Programmable analog hearing aids become commercially available in the mid to late 1980s. In the mid-1990s digital hearing aids were introduced. Digital signal processing (DSP) enables sound to be shaped by the hearing aid in an infinite number of ways. For example, DSP allows the hearing aid to separate certain types of noise from speech based on the timing of sound, and how it is calculated by the hearing aid. Today, in the United States, digital hearing aids comprise over 95% of the market. Even though DSP is a significant technologic breakthrough, it does not replace the skill of the hearing care professional when it comes to making hearing aid selection and fitting decisions.

Basic Components

It doesn't matter if you own a brand new Lamborghini Gallardo LP560-4 or a 1984 Yugo hatchback, some of the basic parts are the same. A $100,000 sports coupe and a $1000 jalopy both allow you to get from point A to B, but we know there are obvious differences in style and performance. Hearing aids are the same way. All hearing aids, no matter how sophisticated, have the same basic electronic components assembled together in a series. This section reviews those basic components and how they work.

Hearing Aid Batteries

Hearing aids are electronic devices. They need energy to work. This energy comes from a dry cell battery. Hearing aid batteries commonly have a reserve amount of storage of 1.4 volts. Batteries come in a variety of sizes. Commonly used battery sizes include the 1.4-volt AA battery for a body aid, the #675 for power BTEs, #13 for smaller BTEs and ITE aids, #312 for canal aids, #10 for small canal and CIC aids, and the #5 for very small CICs. The size of the battery determines its life, i.e., hours of use. Figure 8–2 shows the most common

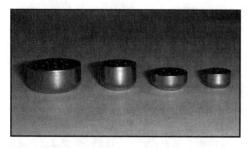

Figure 8–2. The four most common battery sizes from left to right, 675, 13, 312, and 10A/230.

size hearing aid batteries on the market today.

The composition material for most all hearing aid batteries is zinc/air. Although batteries need to be disposed of in an environmental conscious way, zinc-air batteries are considered non-toxic. These batteries are not activated until a tab is removed, exposing the "air holes." For convenience, these tabs are color coded to help identify the size of the battery. The associated colors are as follows:

Blue Tab	Size 675
Orange Tab	Size 13
Brown Tab	Size 312
Yellow Tab	Size 10 (or 230)
Red Tab	Size 5

If you see the television ads for "Lee Major's Bionic Rechargeable Hearing Aids," it indeed is true that some hearing aids have a rechargeable battery (we're not sure about the bionic part). With these instruments, both BTE and custom, it's necessary to charge them after each day's use: a charge lasts around 12 to 16 hours. Some patients prefer this, whereas others consider it a nuisance and prefer to stick with the traditional batteries.

Transducers

Transducer is a technical term for any device that changes energy from one form to another. A gerbil running on a wheel powering a light bulb is a transducer because it is changing mechanical energy into electrical energy. In the case of hearing aids, sound is changed

---

TIPS and TRICKS: How Long Does a Hearing Aid Battery Last?

This is probably the most common question patients ask after purchasing hearing aids. So, you need to be able to give them an accurate answer. Calculating battery life is a fairly straightforward process. You need a few pieces of information to come up with a reasonable estimate. First, you need to know the capacity of the battery in milliamp hours. The milliamp hours is usually listed on the battery package, but as a handy reference we have included some approximate values in the following chart.

Battery Size	Milliamp Hours
675	600 mah
13	260 mah
312	130 mah
10A	70 mah
5A	35 mah

Another piece of information needed to calculate battery life is battery drain. Battery drain is listed on the hearing aid "spec sheet" or it can be measured on a hearing aid test box, both of which we discuss in Chapter 10. A typical battery drain measure is somewhere around .70 to 1.3 milliamps. The smaller the battery the lower the number.

Next, you need to make an assumption for how many hours per day a patient wears his hearing aids. A good number to use is 16 hours per day, but keep in mind that many patients wear their devices far less than that on a daily basis.

Let's say your last patient of the day wanted to know how long his batteries will last on his new hearing aids. You have fitted him with a pair of OC mini-BTEs that use 312 batteries. The calculation looks like this:

Battery Capacity (130 mah) / Battery Drain (.75 ma) = 173.33 hours

Total Hours (173.33 hours) / Hours worn per day (16) = 10.8 days

Pretty simple. This value will vary somewhat depending on what special algorithms are running. That is, with our present example, if the feedback suppression algorithm is running continually, the battery will not last as long as when it is only running in certain listening conditions. This is important for counseling, as often patients will want to know why the batteries are not lasting as long in their new instruments as they were in their old ones (the old ones probably didn't have as many special features).

---

from an acoustic signal to an electric one and back again to an acoustic signal. There are two transducers we need to be concerned about the microphone and the receiver. The sound quality of a hearing aid largely is determined by the effectiveness and integrity of these two components (despite what advanced digital technology is in between).

Microphone

The first electrical component in a hearing aid is an input transducer, most commonly, the microphone. Its duty is to pick up the acoustical sound in the wearer's environment and change it into an electrical form that the amplifier can use. The microphone changes the acoustic input into an analog electrical waveform, similar to a sine wave, of greater and lesser electrical voltages. These changes in voltage eventually are transformed into changes in sound coming out the hearing aid into the wearer's ear. As the microphone changes energy from acoustical to electrical, it also is termed the "input transducer."

A microphone has a diaphragm. When sound strikes the diaphragm, its movement causes changes in the material behind the diaphragm. The diaphragm of a microphone is made of metalicized plastic which holds a permanent electric charge. This means that microphones do not need a power supply, and they are relatively tough and cheap to produce. Microphones also can be "directional" and many of today's products have two microphones, which can be used to accomplish "directional processing." Just file that away for now; we'll talk more about this in Chapter 9.

A few more things about microphones:

■ Microphones used in hearing aids today are quite small, and range in size from around 5 mm × 4 mm × 2 mm, to a cylinder microphone that is 2.5 (diam) × 2.5.
■ Microphones have different frequency response and are "tuned" for different applications.
■ Microphones have a resonant frequency that can be shifted during their production.
■ Microphones have internal noise because of the resistances and semi-

conductors of the electrical circuit. Expansion circuits assist in reducing microphone noise (more on that in Chapter 9).
■ When directional microphones are used, there is a natural roll-off in the low frequencies. If this is compensated with increased amplifier gain, the hearing aid may sound "noisy" in quiet listening environments.
■ When wind strikes the hearing aid microphone noise results. This tends to be worse with BTE instruments.
■ Like receivers, microphones are easily damaged by debris. Even a small amount of debris in the microphone port can alter the frequency response, or turn a good directional instrument into an omnidirectional one.

Telecoil

Another type of input transducer is a telecoil, which certainly is worthy of special mention. As the name suggests, this transducer was originally designed for use with the telephone. Many hearing impaired people have trouble talking on the phone while using their hearing aids. This is either because the telephone signal is not loud enough to be audible, because there is too much background noise, or because placing the phone by the ear causes acoustic feedback. You've probably all heard hearing aids whistle while the person is trying to talk on the phone.

An effective solution to this is the use of a telecoil (Figure 8–3). A telecoil uses the electromagnetic energy present around all phones and turns it into an electrical signal the hearing aid can amplify. The magnetic field, which is

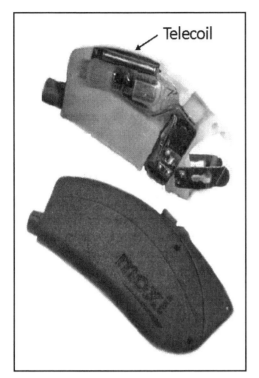

Telecoil

Figure 8–3. The telecoil mounted in the case of an open-canal BTE device. Reprinted with permission from Unitron, all rights reserved.

picked up by the telecoil, is generated by an electrical current that has the same waveform as the audio signal. The effectiveness of a telecoil is determined by the size of the magnetic field that is generated. The strength of the magnetic field is directly related to the ferrite rod size and the number of coil turns. By increasing the size of the ferrite rod, the telecoil becomes more sensitive, thus more effective.

Many devices such as loudspeakers, telephones, and other common electrical gadgets produce a magnetic field. The process of an electrical current inducing a voltage in the coil some distance away is called induction. An induction loop system is intentionally generated by looping a wire around a room or small area.

Routine Use of Telecoils? A telecoil is not always a standard option on hearing aids today; this primarily is because of the size requirement needed to accommodate the coil, or because the user does "Okay" on the telephone by simply using the standard fitting (common with OC fittings). However, the telecoil is a popular and effective extra feature on many devices, and in general is probably underutilized. A telecoil switch is often placed on the hearing aid, or this could be a separate memory, accessed with a memory button or remote control. With some hearing aids, the switching is triggered automatically when the telephone receiver nears the ear.

Other Uses. In addition to use on the telephone, the telecoil can be used to pick up electromagnetic fields generated by electric currents traveling though wires, such as induction loop system used in public facilities (e.g., auditoriums, places of worship, etc.). With a properly functioning telecoil (or t-coil as some refer to it as), patients can take advantage of "looped rooms" by switching the regular microphone setting over to the telecoil setting. A "looped room" or induction loop allows the patient to listen at a much more favorable signal-to-noise ratio when their hearing aids are on the telecoil setting. There is a concerted effort to increase the looping of public facilities in America, which is far behind many other countries in this regard. It's important to instruct your patients regarding this, and have them look for the symbol shown here when they are in public facilities. You can also refer them to the Web site: http://www.loopamerica.com/

HEARING LOOP INSTALLED
Switch hearing aid to T-coil

One of the only disadvantages of telecoils (other than the size requirement) is that they are prone to electromagnetic interference from other electronic devices, like computer screens and security systems. These types of electronic device emit a great deal of electromagnetic energy and telecoils are designed to pick up that type of signal. This type of interference is harmless to the patient and the hearing aid, however, it is relatively common for your patients to encounter it on a temporary basis when in the presence of certain types of electronic devices.

Recently, manufacturers have developed devices utilizing wireless transmission to route the signal from the telephone, including cell phones, to the hearing aids. Such devices offer some potential advantages over telecoil use, including the ability to receive the telephone signal in both ears. We discuss wireless connectivity and hearing aids in Chapter 10.

Receivers

Have you ever put something in the "boot" of your car? We suspect you've done it many times. Some people call it a "trunk."

The same thing can be referred to by different names.

If you are on your back deck listening to a little Tom Petty from your stereo, your receivers are called loudspeakers. In hearing aids, we call them receivers. What they do is the same: they change the amplified electrical signal from the amplifier back into an acoustic form. The wearer then hears an amplified "sound" once again. The term for what comes out of the receiver is "output" or "acoustic output." As the receiver transduces electrical information into acoustical information (or vibratory, in some cases when a bone conducted signal is used—more on that later), the receiver is called the "output transducer." Most hearing aid companies use receivers from Knowles Electronics, and in case you think it's a simple process, this company alone produces around 20 different receivers that can be used with hearing instruments.

Receiver Style. Air conduction receivers operate on a magnetic principle. Magnets on the speaker react to current coming from the amplifier, which makes a diaphragm move back and forth recreating acoustic sound much the same as the speakers of a stereo system.

A few things about receivers:

- The size of the receiver determines is output: larger parts can carry a greater magnetic field.
- The receiver is a major consumer of the hearing aid battery, ranging from around 40 to 50% for a low power instrument, to as much as 80 to 90% in a high power instrument that is normally operating at a high output.
- There is an increased interest in extended high-frequency amplifi-

cation, which means that receivers will have to be designed for this, but the net effect will only be as effective as the accompanying amplifier gain.

- Receivers are damped, just as we discussed in Chapter 7 for earmold plumbing. This helps eliminate undesired peaks.
- Receivers are easily plugged, and this is the number one hearing aid repair problem. For decades, industry has looked for workable solutions—wax traps, wax guards, and wax screens—the problem continues.
- Receivers easily can be damaged from minor shock (dropping). It may continue to work, but have distortions. Always check a hearing aid for distortions if a hearing aid has been dropped.
- Receiver vibrations can lead to vibratory feedback (different from acoustic feedback), because of their proximity to the other components. This is one potential advantage of RIC products.

TAKE FIVE:
Transducers 101

Knowles Electronics and Sonion are two of the leading manufacturers of miniaturized electronics components. A Knowles microphone even made it to the moon! To learn more about the various transducers used in hearing aids as well as to see some examples, you can visit their respective Web sites.

- http://www.knowles.com
- http://www.sonion.com

Amplifiers

An amplifier increases the electrical signal that it has received from the microphone. Many amplifiers have three stages: the preamp, which increases the weak electrical signal created by the microphone, the signal processing stage, and the output stage. An amplifier thus supplies "acoustic gain." An amplifier can be either analog or digital. In today's digital world of electronics it is the amplifier that is the most sophisticated electronic component of a hearing instrument. Because you don't have to be a DSP engineer to fit hearing aids, we are providing you with just a couple of things to remember about hearing aid amplifiers.

- **Integrated Circuit (IC) design:** The common design for integrated circuits is on a circuit board, which has an electrical pathway already etched. Transistors and resistors can then be wired into the electrical pathway. Integrated circuits consist of many transistors and resistors, and other electrical components on the circuit board. Both analog and digital amplifiers use IC technology.
- **Analog amplifiers:** Analog amplifiers reproduce output waveforms that are similar in shape to the incoming electrical waveforms coming from the microphone. As sound pressure increases or decreases in the environment, the electrical waveform from the amplifier also increases or decreases.
- **Digital amplifiers (or digital signal processors):** Digital amplifiers have an analog-to-digital converter that digitizes the electrical waveforms into strings of

mathematical bits. A digital amplifier can manipulate bits of information at great speed, allowing for less internal noise and distortion, great shaping flexibility, and ability to perform changes in the frequency response (noise suppression, feedback management). DSP must convert the digital waveform back into an analog output via a digital-to-analog converter.

■ **Amplifier signal processing stage:** The second stage, after the preamp, the signal processing stage is either linear or nonlinear. A linear signal processor provides constant (the same amount of) gain on an input/output graph until saturation. Analog hearing aids can be either linear or nonlinear.

Basic Descriptors of Hearing Aid Performance

Automobile performance can be evaluated several different ways. If you're a fan of fast cars you might be interested in horsepower. If you're concerned about saving money you're likely going to look closely at the miles per gallon. If you want to be "green" you spend some time comparing emissions ratings. If you have children, you might be interested in safety ratings. Like automobiles, hearing aid performance can be measured across several dimensions. The performance dimension you focus on might vary depending on the problem you're trying to solve.

Recall from Chapter 2 the concepts of intensity and frequency. Intensity relates to how much energy a sound possesses. In the hearing aid world, the terms gain and output quantify the intensity level of amplified sound. On the other hand,

frequency is related to pitch and timbre of sound. Frequency response is the term used to describe this concept in hearing aids.

Gain

Gain is the amount of sound pressure difference between the input of sound as it enters the hearing aid and the amplified sound as it leaves the hearing aid receiver. Gain is always expressed in dB (note that the plural for dB is dB, not dBs). For example, if the input signal is 50 dB SPL and the final output is 120 dB SPL, the gain is simply the difference between the input and output, or 70 dB. Even though this example was in SPL, *gain* is not expressed using any reference, as it is a relative measure.

If we want a given signal to be audible to the hearing aid user, then the gain, added to the level of the input signal, must exceed the users threshold (in ear canal SPL). For example, let's say that a patient had a 60 dB HL hearing loss at 2000 Hz. We need to convert that to ear canal SPL, which is a correction of around 10 dB, so for simple math, we'll say that his hearing loss is 70 dB SPL (re: ear canal). If a soft speech signal at 2000 Hz is around 40 dB SPL (which is very possible), this patient would then need 30 dB of gain to make that signal just barely audible (70 minus 40 = 30 dB). We just worked through some of the basic fundamentals of a "prescriptive fitting," but let's save that discussion for Chapter 10.

Because the input of speech is different for different frequencies, and the patient's hearing loss usually is different for different frequencies, it shouldn't surprise you that the programmed gain of the hearing aid also will be different at different frequencies. As the input signal goes up, the gain that is necessary usually goes down, as most patient's have a nonlinear loudness growth function. The exact amount of gain that is necessary for different inputs for various frequencies is related to the degree and slope of the hearing loss, which we explore more fully later.

As gain does vary for the different frequencies, we often measure average maximum gain to describe the overall gain of the hearing aid using a single number. Peak gain (sometimes called full-on gain) is the maximum amount of gain when the volume control of the hearing aid is full-on. We also need to remember that we usually will want some "reserve" gain, as most individuals hearing loss becomes worse over time. They may develop a mild temporary conductive hearing loss and, also, there may be some listening situations where greater gain is needed. So, if we're thinking that a patient probably will "use" around 25 to 30 dB gain, we'd want an instrument with 35 to 40 dB of gain.

Output

Although gain is simply a difference measure (output minus the input), output is an expression of the overall sound power. Output is expressed in dB SPL and is referred to as maximum power output (MPO) or saturation sound pressure level (SSPL) or output sound pressure level (OSPL). For some measures (e.g., 2-cc coupler), a 90 dB input is used, and the term would then be "OSPL90; previously called SSPL90)." When probemic measures are used, the maximum

output can be measured in the real ear. In this case it is referred to as the real ear saturation response, or RESR.

Nearly all of today's hearing aids allow the fitter to select the maximum output (within a 15 to 20 dB range). This could be controlled by peak clipping, but usually it is adjusted using output compression, something we'll get to later in this chapter. Using compression to set the MPO correctly on a hearing aid is important because this keeps loud sounds from becoming uncomfortably or painfully loud. If loud sounds are too loud, the patient will turn down gain, and not obtain benefit for conversational speech. In extreme cases, if the MPO is left to be too high, making sounds too loud, it even can result in further hearing loss. Patients with severe-profound hearing losses are not always a good judge of when things are dangerously loud, especially if they have become accustomed to listening to very high-level outputs.

On the other hand, if the MPO is too low, and louder components are unnecessarily reduced, the dynamics of speech will be altered, which can result in poor speech quality and reduced speech understanding ability. In other words, the MPO can't be too low or too high, it has to be "just right." For review, check out the LDL measures we described in Chapter 6. They are designed to assist you in setting the MPO on a modern hearing aid.

Frequency Response

A curve depicting the relative gain of the hearing aid over the entire range of amplified frequencies is called a frequency response curve. A hearing aid does not amplify all frequencies uniformly, and hence the frequency response of a hearing is not "flat" like you might expect from a high-end stereo system. It is not intended to be.

The shape of the frequency response of any hearing aid depends on the frequency response of the microphone and the receiver, and the settings of the amplifier. The frequency response on a modern hearing aid can be altered significantly by using the programming software (i.e., adjusting amplifier gain). Just like output and gain, the fine tuning of the hearing aid's frequency response is determined by several factors, including the patient's audiometric thresholds and LDLs. Most hearing aids provide significant low-frequency gain down to 200 Hz or so, although this only is possible with a relatively tight fitting in the ear canal (remember that low frequencies easily leak out of the ear canal if there is venting). High-frequency gain usually extends out to 5000 Hz or so, and then rolls off. In recent years, there have been efforts to extend this high-frequency gain. This has been shown to have some benefit for children learning speech sounds. For adults, the true benefit of extended high frequencies has yet to be determined, and depends on the slope of the audiogram and the degree of the high-frequency hearing loss—look for emerging research in this area.

Contrasting Key Components

Lee and his wife Yvonne are buying a new car. Lee likes a convertible, Yvonne would like a hard top. Lee likes a two door, Yvonne likes four doors. Lee likes a stick, Yvonne likes automatic. By contrasting these options, they'll maybe reach a reasonable decision (or maybe not).

The study of hearing aid terms is really the study of contrasts. This means that if you want to know the meaning of one concept it often helps to contrast that concept to something different. In order to gain a better understanding of these important concepts, let's look at some key hearing aid descriptors in contrasting pairs.

Output Versus Gain

Output: Output is the overall amount of sound energy expressed in dB SPL of the hearing aid for any given input.

Gain: Gain is the difference between output and input. We don't really *measure* gain; we calculate it by knowing the output and input values.

Figure 8–4 compares an output curve to a gain curve. Notice the differences in the metrics used on the *y*-axis for the upper and lower graphics in the figure.

Frequency Response: Smooth Versus Distorted

As mentioned earlier in this chapter, frequency response refers to the range of frequencies a hearing aid will amplify. Most hearing aids have a frequency response ranging from 200 Hz to 5000 Hz. A peaky response represents a poor sounding hearing aid. A smooth frequency response result is a hearing aid of good sound quality. Figure 8–5 provides a comparison of a smooth frequency (top two curves) to a distorted or peaky frequency response. You never want to fit a patient with hearing aids having a peaky response, as it is a char-

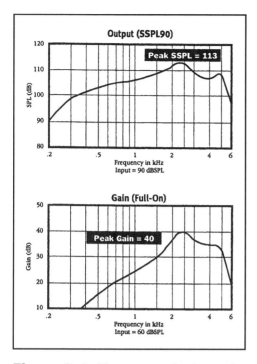

Figure 8–4. The top graph shows the output for a single hearing aid, whereas the bottom graph shows the full-on gain for the same hearing aid. Notice that the vertical axis is different for the two graphs.

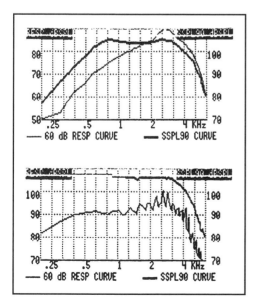

Figure 8–5. Comparision of a smooth and peaky frequency response.

acteristic of a technical problem with the device. All audio devices with a smooth frequency response, including hearing aids, are judged to have superior sound quality than devices with a peaky or distorted frequency response. When fitting hearing aids, you will learn that the hearing aid's frequency response should generally follow the pattern of the audiogram. In other words, if a patient has normal hearing in the lows and a severe loss in the high frequencies, the frequency response of the hearing aid needs to peak (have maximum output) in the high frequencies, and little or no gain in the low frequencies. Importantly, however, you do not want to simply "mirror" the audiogram, which is why we have detailed prescriptive fitting approaches. And remember that what you see in the coupler is not the same as what happens in the real ear!

Channels Versus Bands Versus Handles

Modern hearing aids are almost always multichannel and multiband. It's easy to think that channels and bands are referring to the same thing, but usually they do not. Both refer to how the frequency response of the hearing aid is broken up into segments. The difference between channels and bands, however, is related to what is going on inside each of these segments. Bands are simply the number of segments the frequency response has been broken into. Channels, on the other hand, refer to the number of segments that are working independently of one another, usually the way that signal processing has been divided. Until you learn more about what goes on inside each channel, it is sufficient to say that we need to focus our attention on the number of channels within a hearing aid. With all this said, it's possible that a given hearing aid manufacturer might call channels bands, or bands channels. Usually, a band is a subdivision of a channel, for example; a hearing aid could have 8 channels and 16 bands (two bands in each channel).

To confuse the issue even more, hearing aid software also has "handles." Handles are used to "grab" a group of channels or bands to facilitate programming. A 20-channel hearing aid might have five handles, with each handle controlling four channels. Remember that bands and channels involve gain and processing; handles are a programming interface and only indirectly involve signal processing. Because the number of bands, channels, and handles varies across manufacturers and even models for the same manufacturer, we recommend you get the lowdown from the rep of your favorite manufacturer.

Linear Versus Compression

These two contrasting pairs really describe how gain and output are being manipulated or calculated within each channel of the hearing aid. A linear hearing aid (or a linear channel within a hearing aid) applies equal amounts of gain to all inputs. In general terms, we would want to apply linear gain to a patient who has a linear loudness growth function. As you know from Chapter 4, most patients fitted with hearing aids have a cochlear hearing loss, and therefore they *do not* have a linear loudness growth function. For this reason, most of the hearing aids fitted today are *not* linear (although there may be certain channels, usually in the low frequencies that are programmed at or near linear gain). Therefore, we devote most of our discussion to the various key aspects of nonlinear gain, often referred to as compression.

We start with a comparison of compression to linear. Figure 8–6 shows the

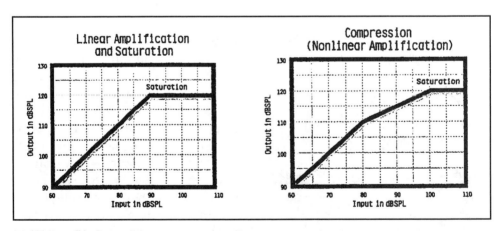

Figure 8–6. Input/output functions, along with saturation levels for a linear and compression hearing aid circuit. Notice on the graph on the right where the compression becomes activated 90 dB input). Most modern hearing aids begin compression for inputs around 40 dB SPL (80 dB input). Most modern hearing aids begin compression for inputs around 40 dB SPL.

difference between a linear and compression hearing aid. For the hearing aid providing linear amplification on the left, notice how the output grows in a linear manner as the input increases up to 90 dB SPL. In other words, the *gain* stays the same as the input increases Observe that a 70 dB input = 100 dB output (30 dB of gain) and likewise, an 80 dB input = 110 dB output (again, 30 dB of gain). When an input signal of 90 dB SPL is reached, the hearing aid goes into saturation (think of this as a ceiling), meaning that the output will not increase for higher inputs, which then indirectly reduces gain. As we mentioned earlier, it is important to remember that the saturation level (OSPL 90) varies with each hearing aid and must be set by the hearing aid fitter.

Let's now talk about compression. A hearing aid with compression varies the gain as the input changes, once the input is above the compression kneepoint. The graph on the right-hand side of Figure 8–6 shows this. Notice how now the output change is not a straight line. This is because as the input increases, the amount of gain applied to it varies, starting at inputs of 80 dB SPL. When the input level goes above 80 dB, there is no longer a 1 to 1 relationship between input and output, and the input/output function no longer progresses along a 45-degree angle. In the example shown in Figure 8–6, the hearing aid becomes "nonlinear" for a high input level of 80 dB SPL. Most of today's hearing aids actually become nonlinear at a much lower input level, say 40 to 45 dB SPL, although it could be as low as 25 dB or as high as 50 to 60 dB depending on the manufacturer and the channel(s) involved.

One way to think about *input* compression is to know that its most common use is to "repackage" sounds into the dynamic range of the end-user. If the patient's world of sound has an 80 dB range, but the patient only has a 40 dB range, we need to shrink the world. For now it's important to know that there are several types of compression, different types of compression within the same hearing aid, within the same channel, and changes are occurring several times per second for many listening situations.

The Basics of Compression

You've probably all driven a car. And, while reading this chapter you've been thinking about output limiting and different types of compression for hearing aids (at least you should have been). Well, here are some examples that might help you remember four possible choices:

The Scenario: Understanding Compression Really Is Like Driving a Car!

- You are driving down a city street going 35 miles per hour, no doubt listening to some good music.
- You see a stop sign one block away. Think of that stop sign as your patient's LDL (i.e., UCL, TD), and the speed of your car as the gain of the hearing aid. The LDL (stop sign) = 100 dB.

■ The stop sign is for a very busy highway: cars traveling 65 mph. You need to stop at the sign to avoid an accident. So, you're going to use your brakes.

■ Think of the point that you hit your brakes as the compression knee-point (one city block = 60 dB), and the pressure that you apply on the brakes as the compression ratio.

Choice #1: You continue driving 35 miles an hour until you are only 100 feet from the stop sign. At this point you slam on the brakes as hard as you can. There is a squealing of tires, your car slides sideways, you bump your head on the windshield, you chip your tooth on the steering wheel, but you do not slide out into traffic. This happened to a teenager in Ryder, ND about 45 years ago.

Type of circuitry? Output limiting using peak clipping (it's nasty, but it does get you stopped at the stop sign without serious injury).

Choice #2: You continue driving 35 miles an hour until you are only 100 feet from the stop sign. At this point you slam on the brakes as hard as you can. This time you do not slide sideways, your ABS works fantastic, no bumped head, no chipped tooth. You stop cleanly at the stop sign.

Type of circuitry? Output limiting using AGCo, kneepoint = 110 dB SPL, ratio = 10:1 (equivalent to slamming on the brakes). It's an unusual way to drive, but some-times it's necessary to go that fast until the very end. Other times, it simply happens due to a lack of attention or driving instruction.

Choice #3: Starting a block away, you put your foot on the brake at a constant pressure. The pressure is such that it allows you to come to a rolling stop at the stop sign.

Type of circuitry? AGCi (WDRC), linear compression, kneepoint = 40 dB SPL, ratio = 2:1. Works pretty well, but remember that the pres-sure on the brake is directly related to the point when you first start braking and the location of the stop sign. Had you stepped on the brake mid-way through the block (e.g., a kneepoint more like 60 dB SPL or so), you would have had to apply more pressure (e.g., a ratio around 3:1).

Choice #4: Starting a block away, you put your foot on the brake. This time, however, you start with a very light pressure, and then, the closer you get to the stop sign the more pressure you apply. Again, you come to a rolling stop at the stop sign.

Type of circuitry? AGCi (WDRC), curvilinear compression, kneepoint = 40 dB SPL, ratio = variable from 1.5:1 (soft inputs) to 6:1 (loud inputs), effective ratio = 2:1. Or, the same could be accomplished using two kneepoints between 40 and 80 dB SPL inputs. This is an alterna-tive method to linear compression for stopping at the same place— utility depends on the driver (dispenser), the vehicle (hearing aid), and road conditions (patient's loudness growth function).

Nearly every hearing aid today uses at least one type of compression, and many use at least two different types.

Understanding how the various types of compression work is essential for fitting and fine tuning all hearing aids. Compression is often referred to as automatic gain control (AGC) because the gain of the hearing aid changes automatically as the input intensity changes. Because there is no one simple way to describe compression in a modern hearing aid, it helps to contrast different types of compression to each other, and discuss how each type of compression is designed to contribute to a successful fitting. This section examines the very basics of hearing aid compression—enough to get you started fitting your first pair of hearing aids.

Input/Output Functions

To understand compression, the best way to introduce the concept is to obtain a good understanding of input/output functions. Once you understand input/output functions, your knowledge of compression will fall into place (we think). As you already know, input + gain = output. For the input/output function, we use a chart that has input on the "x-axis" and output for the "y-axis." The input/output function of a given hearing aid is then displayed by the diagonal line. At any point on this line gain can be determined by subtracting the input values from the output. The place on this line where it bends or changes angle (deviates from 45 degrees) is called the compression kneepoint (with a little imagination the entire function can be viewed as a very thin leg, with a bent knee, but missing a foot!). The "kneepoint" is where compression begins, and is also referred to as the compression threshold. You might see abbreviations such as CT for compression threshold, CK for compression kneepoint, or TK for threshold of kneepoint, all meaning the same thing.

Again, refer to Figure 8–6: observe that the gain is linear to the left of the kneepoint. This means that for any increase in input there is an equal increase in the output. On an input/output graph, linear gain is represented by a straight 45-degree diagonal line. With compression, the gain is nonlinear because the slope of this 45-degree diagonal line changes slope. Figure 8–7 shows a simple input/output function for a hearing aid. You also will notice on this input/output function the level in which the hearing aid goes into saturation. Saturation is the point where increases in input result in no further increases in output. Like a sponge that can no longer hold water, a saturated circuit can no make sounds any louder beyond a certain point. In most cases, this "saturation" point is not true saturation, but rather output limited, accomplished with output compression, which is what we talk about next.

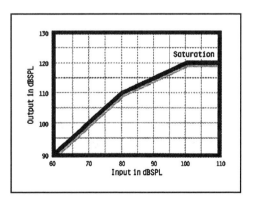

Figure 8–7. An input/output function with the saturation sound pressure level (SSPL) indicated.

Input Versus Output Compression

Compression can be classified into two major categories: input compression and output compression. One major difference between input (AGCi) and output (AGCo) compression is where the volume control is placed on the hearing aid circuit. In a traditional hearing aid with a manual volume control wheel, the patient is able to manipulate compression in very distinct ways, depending on whether the device has input or output compression. Even though many hearing aids today do not have manual volume control wheels, input and output compression is still an important consideration.

Figure 8–8 schematically shows the difference between AGCi and AGCo for three different volume control settings, respectively. For output compression hearing aids, the volume control placed ahead of the amplifier, whereas for the hearing aid using AGCi, the volume control is after the amplifier. This might seem like a relatively benign difference; however, this small variation in VC placement can result in dramatic differences in how the patient adjusts the hearing aids for their hearing loss, and how the hearing aids are programmed.

For the output compression function, which is the left side of Figure 8–8, changes in the volume control affects gain, but not MPO. In other words, as the user increases the volume control,

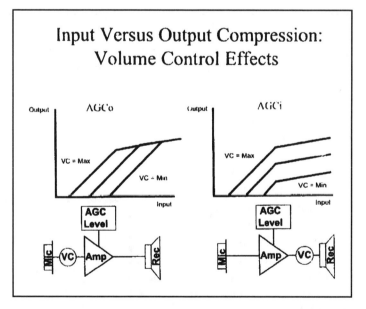

Figure 8–8. Input/output graphs along with circuit schematics for AGCi and AGCo compression. The position of the VC determines the effect of the gain and output as the volume control is manipulated by the user. From *Compression for Clinicians* by Ted Venema. Copyright © 1998 Singular Publishing, Inc. All rights reserved. Used with permission (p. 62).

gain increases, but there are no changes to maximum output. The effects of input compression are a lot different. When the VC is changed, using AGCi processing, both the gain and maximum output are affected. This is shown on the right side of Figure 8–8.

Figure 8–9 is an input/output graph, showing changes in output as gain changes. The effects of compression can also be examined by looking at changes in frequency response as a result in gain changes. Because hearing aid test boxes and specification sheets use this format, looking at changes in frequency response might be more helpful when learning about the differences between AGCi and AGCo. Figure 8–9 shows the effects of the VC on gain and MPO between for both input and output compression.

For the AGCo circuit on the left, as the VC changes, the MPO stays the same, while the gain for lower intensity inputs changes. Compare this to the ACGi in the right side of Figure 8–9. Here, both output and gain change as the input signal changes.

So far, our review of input and output compression might seem somewhat theoretical. In the real world there are important clinical uses for each type of compression, as input and output compression have different clinical application, but usually are found in the same hearing aid and both are applied and often adjusted for the same patient.

AGCo is used to limit the maximum output of loud sounds. Think of it as setting the ceiling for loud sounds— ensuring that those loud sounds fall

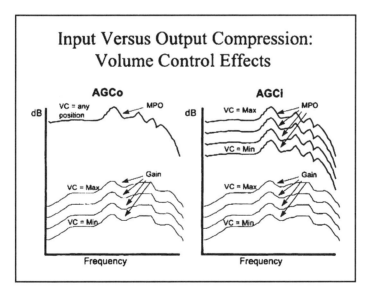

Figure 8–9. Frequency responses showing a comparison of the volume control effects of AGCo and AGCi. Notice how the AGCo adjusts the gain, but not the output, whereas the AGCi adjusts both the gain and output. From Venema, *Compression for Clinicians* by Ted Venema. Copyright © 1998 Singular Publishing, Inc. All rights reserved. Used with permission (p. 64).

below the patient's LDL. Input compression, on the other hand is commonly used for mild to moderate hearing losses to manage the incoming speech signal. That is, ACGi is used to restore loudness (or nearly restore loudness) for soft and average and loud inputs. Let's turn our attention to a specific type of AGCi, called wide dynamic range compression (WDRC) as it compares to AGCo.

Wide Dynamic Range Compression

The compression type utilized in nearly all hearing aids is AGCi, and when the AGCi kneepoint is relatively low (~55 dB SPL or below), this is referred to as wide dynamic range compression (WDRC). It is called this because a "wide" range of average speech is in compression. In order to understand how WDRC works, we compare it to the most common use of AGCo, called output-limiting compression. These two different compression types are usually found in the same hearing aid, but relate to different fitting goals.

WDRC

- This is a specific type of input compression that has several unique properties associated with it. It is associated with low-threshold kneepoints (less than 55 dB SPL; as low as ~25 to 30 dB SPL on some instruments)
- It has low compression ratios (less than 4 to 1, most commonly around 2 to 1).
- Because of the low kneepoints and relatively small ratios, compression takes place over a wide range of input levels, including nearly the

entire average speech signal; thus it receives the name WDRC. This characteristic of WDRC is shown on the right-hand side of Figure 8–10.

- WDRC processing provides a weak amount of compression over a wide range of inputs. The simple rule to remember is that as input goes up, gain goes down.
- Recall from Chapter 3 that most people with mild-moderate cochlear pathology have LDLs similar to people with normal hearing. An advantage then, of WDRC is that little or no gain can be applied for loud inputs, but significant gain can be applied to soft inputs, making them audible.
- Our final point: The fitting result of WDRC is that soft sounds become louder, but WDRC itself doesn't make soft sounds louder—it makes average sounds softer. If average sounds are softer, you (via programming) or the patient (via the VC) will turn up gain. When you turn up gain—soft sounds become louder.

ACGo Compression

- Output limiting compression (shutting things down on the top end) typically is associated with output compression (AGCo).
- Remember that "limiting compression" is a fitting method; "output compression" (AGCo) is a hearing aid circuit.
- Output limiting compression is associated with high compression kneepoints and high compression ratios. A high kneepoint means that the hearing aid begins to compress at relatively high input levels. Below the high kneepoint, the hearing aid

would linear gain if there were no companion AGCi circuit.

■ The kneepoints used for output limiting usually are around 100 to 115 dB (re: 2-cc coupler). Why? Because this corresponds to the LDL of the average hearing impaired patient (when converted to 2-cc values).

■ The compression ratio of an output limiting compressor is usually around 10 to 1, which means that there is only a 1 dB corresponding increase to the 10 dB change in output. This is shown on the left-hand side of Figure 8–10. Although that might sound like a lot of compression, it occurs at a high kneepoint, and that point—you need to stop things fast (think back to the car example).

■ Our final point: Consider that output limiting compression is used as a partner with WDRC. WDRC takes care of the soft to loud speech sounds; output limiting takes care of the very loud sounds. On postfitting visits, it's important to know which is which when you start making "mouse clicks."

Clinical Applications of Output Limiting Compression and WDRC

We've already discussed many of the clinical applications, but here is a review. WDRC does most of its work for soft and average level sounds by providing appropriate gain to maximize listener comfort with loudness, and provide audibility for soft sounds. It's not the purpose of WDRC to control maximum output (although it will do this if you program it that way). Output limiting compression only is called into action when the amplifier output exceeds the

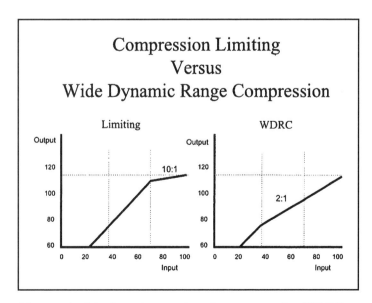

Figure 8–10. Input/output functions comparing WDRC to compression limiting. From *Compression for Clinicians* by Ted Venema. Copyright © 1998 Singular Publishing, Inc. All rights reserved. Used with permission. (p. 69).

AGCo kneepoint, which should be set according to the patient's LDL. Remember, it is common for both types of compression to be implemented in the same hearing aid.

For higher level inputs, the high compression kneepoints and aggressive ratios of output compression limiting are well suited for protecting the user from uncomfortably loud sound. WDRC and output compression limiting have unique applications for mild to moderate-severe hearing losses. When the loss is severe, however, it might be necessary to forego making soft sounds audible. If making soft sounds audible is not a fitting goal, then WDRC applications may not be needed. You might want to raise the kneepoint to 60 to 65 dB or so. Remember that with WDRC, maximum gain will always occur at the level of the kneepoint setting. So if average speech is your main focus, a higher kneepoint might work better.

TAKE FIVE: Does All This Make Sense?

- Output limiting can be AGCi, but usually is AGCo.
- WDRC always is AGCi
- AGCi usually is WDRC, but can be output limiting
- AGCo is always output limiting

You may have noticed that we have referenced some of the figures in this chapter from Ted Venema's book, "Compression for Clinicians." Ted has published a second edition of his excellent book in 2006. Either edition is an essential reference for learning more about the ins and outs of hearing aid compression.

More on the Parameters of Compression (Table 8–1)

Just like high-performance sports cars are defined by their performance standards, such as how fast it goes from 0 to 60 miles per hour, and the G force it products when you round a corner going 90 mph, compression systems are defined by their parameters. These parameters are compression threshold or kneepoint, compression ratio, and their time constants: attack and release time. Although the terms we use to describe the parameters of compression are not quite as sexy as G forces and mph, it will go a long way toward your success if you understand them.

Compression Kneepoint

We've discussed this to some extent already, but in our experience, you can just never get too much on this topic. The compression threshold or kneepoint is the lowest input level needed to provide a reduction in gain relative to linear amplification. This is best understood by looking at a simple input/output function. For a hearing aid employing linear amplification, increases in the input level result in equal changes in the output level. For example, in Figure 8–11, where the dark diagonal line represents the change in output, the angle change is considered the compression kneepoint. This change in the input/output function signifies a reduction in gain relative to the increase in input.

Compression Ratio

The compression ratio determines the amount of compression, or in simple terms, the "squash effect." It is the amount of change in input relative to

Table 8–1. A General Overview of Basic Parameters of Compression, with Typical Range of Settings for Each

Output Compression Limiting	Wide Dynamic Range Compression
High Kneepoint (>85 dB SPL)	Low Kneepoint (35 to 45 dB SPL)
High Ratio (10:1)	Low Ratio (1.2:1 to 4:1)
Fast Time Constants (20 to 30 msec)	Fast or Slow Time Constants (20 msec to >3 seconds)

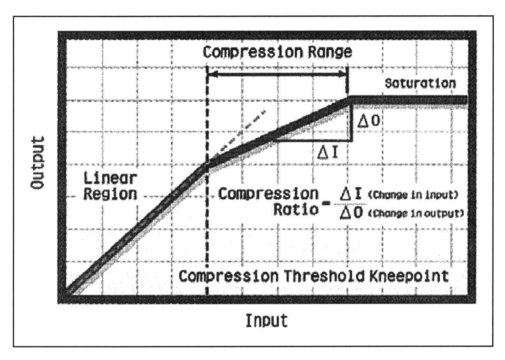

Figure 8–11. Various compression parameters are illustrated.

the resulting change in output. For example, if an input signal change of 10 dB results in an output change in the input of 10 dB, the ratio is 1:1, or linear. If the change in input of 10 dB results in an output change of 5 dB, the ratio would be 2:1. Compression ratio can be calculated by dividing the change in input by the change in output. Input/output functions for various compression ratios are illustrated in Figure 8–12.

When thinking about the amount of compression that is appropriate, we must also think about overall gain. In some instruments, it is possible to adjust kneepoints, ratios, and overall gain to obtain the appropriate loudness perceptions for the patient. To accomplish this effectively, it is important to think of these perceptions for three areas: soft, average and loud inputs. If a patient only has problems with loud inputs,

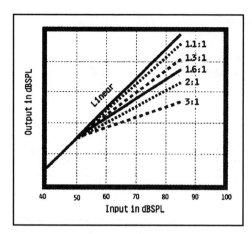

Figure 8–12. Input/Output functions for various compression ratios. Notice that a higher compression ratio (e.g., 3:1) reduces the most amount of output as input increases.

your adjustment will be much different than if he has problems with soft, average, *and* loud inputs. In Chapter 10, we provide you with a "cheat sheet" for adjusting soft, average and loud sounds based on the patient's complaints.

Behind The Scenes: Do You Care?

To further confuse things, different manufacturers handle compression adjustment differently in their software. You usually will have the option of clicking on a term that describes what you want to do, rather than specifically changing a kneepoint from 45 dB to 55 dB, or making a ratio 2.3:1 when it was 2.7:1. However, you still (sort of) need to know what is happening behind the scenes. Let's say you have a patient who needs more gain for loud inputs. In some software, you would increase gain for loud inputs by increasing overall gain, in other software you would raise the WDRC kneepoint, in other

software, you'd make the WDRC ratio smaller, and in yet other software you'd raise the AGCo kneepoint. Which one of these four actions does your favorite manufacturer use? Do you care? So much to think about, so little time!

Attack and Release Times

The attack and release time tell us how long it takes the hearing aid circuitry to respond to changes in input. With many WDRC products, a very low kneepoint is used, and therefore the hearing aid is nearly always in compression. In this case, you would not think about the hearing aid going in and out of compression, but rather, how long it takes to readjust gain while it is in compression.

As the name suggests, "attack time" is the time it takes to adjust to new input levels. If you are sitting in a quiet room, and someone starts talking at 65 dB SPL, how long will it take for the hearing aid to adjust to the prescribed gain for a 65-dB-SPL input? Usually, you want this to happen quickly. The release time, on the other hand, is the length of time it takes for the hearing aid to come out of compression and restore gain to a new setting. Again, for hearing aids that are always in compression, the release time isn't when the hearing aid goes *out of compression*, but simply how long it takes to *establish a new gain setting* based on the current input. If a person was in speech that was fluctuating greatly, you wouldn't want a long release time, as the hearing aid would not be appropriately adjusting to the different fluctuating inputs.

Figure 8–13 shows schematically how attack and release time work with a sudden intensity increase. The upper

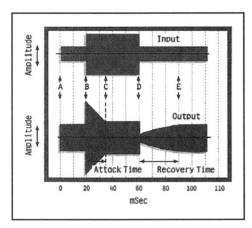

Figure 8–13. A schematic showing how attack and release (recovery) times adapt to changes in hearing aid gain.

takes a few milliseconds for the signal to become compressed. The distance between Time B and Time C is the attack time of the instrument. It is preferable for the attack time to be short (2 to 12 milliseconds).

The intensity of the input signal in Figure 8–13 decreases to nearly its initial intensity level at Time D. The loud signal is no longer present, so the hearing aid needs to return gain back to the pre-compression levels. The time it takes to do this is shown as the distance from Time D to Time E. This is the recovery time or release time.

Although it's preferable to have a short attack time, this is not always the case with release times. Current products have release times as fast as 20 to 30 milliseconds, and as long as 3 to 5 seconds. If the release time is too fast, the hearing aid may have an audible pumping sound. If the release time is too slow, the hearing aid gain may not be restored quickly enough, resulting in "dead spots." Not all patients, however,

part of Figure 8–13 shows the signal prior to entering the hearing aid, and the bottom part shows the signal being amplified by a compression hearing aid. Time A to Time B shows the signal amplified before compression. The intensity increase that occurs at Time triggers the onset of compression. This

TAKE FIVE: Attack, Release, and a "Woof"

A patient has hearing loss of around 50 dB HL, and has LDL around 100 dB HL. The hearing aid has a compression kneepoint of 40 dB SPL, and you have programmed it to deliver 25 dB of gain for a 50 dB SPL input (soft sounds) and 10 dB of gain for an 80 dB SPL input (loud sounds). The patient is sitting listening to his wife talk softly around 50 dB SPL, and his dog barks—an 80 dB SPL "woof." Would the hearing aid deliver 25 or 10 dB of gain for the woof? This depends on the attack time. If the attack time is fast (as it usually

is), the hearing aid will quickly readjust compression, and only deliver 10 dB of gain. The patient's wife continues talking in her soft voice following the woof. Will her voice how receive 25 or 10 dB of gain? Well, this depends on the compression release time. If the release time is long, 5 seconds or so, her voice would not receive the full amount of programmed gain until this time has passed. If the release time is very short (<100 msec), the full amount of gain would be restored very quickly.

may be able to take advantage of the theoretical advantages of a fast release time. It's not a simple matter.

Just like the compression kneepoints and ratios, with some products, release times can be adjusted by the hearing aid fitter. Unlike kneepoints and ratios, however, we don't recommend changing or adjusting them until you gain some experience. There really isn't a clinical test that is sensitive enough to give you the answer regarding which is best. And not only is it difficult to know what release time is best, what is best for one listening situation, may not be best for another. Currently, there are products available with very quick release times, and other products with quite long release times—both products are enjoying commercial success and patients are reporting benefit and satisfaction. It appears that as long as

---

TIPS AND TRICKS: "Compression Tidbits"

These are a few compression terms that are used from time to time. They are good to know about, and you might just get asked about them during one of your fittings.

BILL and TILL: When hearing aids were only two channels, these two terms were coined to describe variations of compression applications. Bass Increase for Low Levels (BILL) was used to describe hearing aids that had more compression in the lows then in the highs (a better term might be Bass Decrease for High Levels, BDHL, but this is a much less attractive acronym). When more compression was applied in the high frequencies, which nearly always is the case today, this was referred to as Treble Increase for Low Levels, or TILL. That is, the frequency response tends to "flatten out" for high inputs, but provides significant gain for the highs (much more so than the lows) for the soft inputs.

Syllabic Compression: A term used to describe a relatively short release time (e.g., <150 milliseconds). The origin of this term is the notion that if a patient is using a hearing aid with a release time this quick, he would not miss more than one syllable before the hearing aid restored gain to the new input level (e.g., syllables are around 75 to 150 msec, which all relates to modulation based noise reduction. See Chapter 9.

Adaptive (Dual) Compression: This is a circuit that tries to capture the best aspects of short and long release times. In this case, the release time is related to the duration of the input signal. For most inputs, a long release is in effect, but if a short duration signal occurs (e.g., door slam), the short release time will be activated and temporarily will replace the long release.

Automatic Volume Control (AVC): AVC has a relatively long attack and release time, which can vary between 150 ms and several seconds. AVC doesn't respond to rapid fluctuations in sound inputs, but does respond well to general overall changes in sound intensity. Therefore, in theory, it reduces the need for a manually adjusted volume control, and in theory, would work best for people with larger residual dynamic ranges.

you keep your release times within a "reasonable range," you probably won't get into much trouble.

Multiple Channels

As we mentioned earlier, today's products have multiple channels. Recall that within a channel, it is not only possible to have independent control of gain, but also compression (both kneepoint and ratios). Imagine a patient who has a downward sloping hearing loss (most do) going from 30 dB HL at 500 Hz to 70 dB HL at 4000 Hz. His LDLs range from 100 dB HL to 110 dB HL, and therefore his dynamic range varies from 70 dB (lows) to 40 dB (highs). At this stage of your reading (and hopefully clinical practice), it should be clear that if your goal is to "repackage the world" into his dynamic range, you will need more aggressive compression in the high frequencies then in the lows. This clearly is the advantage of multiple channels. In a case like this, your prescriptive fitting approach will provide you with suggested compression ratios, and the manufacturer's fitting software will program the hearing aid accordingly: in a 20-channel instrument, you might have 20 different settings of compression. This is a huge advantage over the single channels devices used as recent as the 1990s.

If you keep the kneepoint relatively low for all frequencies (to maintain the benefits of WDRC), you probably will end up with compression ratios of ~1.4 to 1.7 in the low-frequency channels, 1.8 to 2.4 for the mid-frequency channels, and 2.5 to 3.0 for the high-frequency channels. The goal of course is to maximize audibility of soft sounds, without

making loud sounds too loud, and to accomplish this across the entire amplified spectrum of sound.

Multichannel for AGCo

It's not just for WDRC anymore! We've always known that multichannel processing would be helpful in programming AGCo, and it now is available in many instruments. Just as we don't want the same *gain* for all frequencies, we also don't want the same *maximum output* for all frequency regions. Multichannel AGCo allows us to set the kneepoints in different channels to correspond to the patient's LDL for that frequency range. For example, if you see that the MPO exceeds the patient's LDL at 2000 Hz by 5 dB, in the "old days" of single channel AGCo (only five years ago), you would have to turn down the kneepoint by 5 dB for ALL outputs, just to tackle that 2000 Hz problem. Today, all you have to do is go to the corresponding channel for 2000 Hz, turn down that kneepoint 5 dB, and all the other outputs more or less stay the same. Headroom is not unnecessarily reduced.

The key is to get the AGCo kneepoint set pretty close to correct during your pre-fitting programming. Don't expect the automated programming to do this for you; you'll have to make a few mouse clicks on your own for this one. But you know the math; if not, go back to Chapter 6 and review.

Expansion

Another feature that is often combined with WDRC compression is audio expansion. Expansion compresses signals *below the kneepoint* and is used to minimize annoyance from amplified microphone noise and low-level environmental sounds. Expansion often allows the patient to use the gain necessary to make soft speech audible without the negative side effects of excessive amplification of ambient noise.

You can think of expansion as compression in reverse: when sound is *below* the kneepoint, it is squashed. It has no effect whenever the signal is *above* the kneepoint. If you want to make soft sounds softer, you *raise* the kneepoint

(more sounds in compression). It will squash any sound below the kneepoint, including speech (so don't put the kneepoint too high). The kneepoint usually is placed around the SPL level of soft speech, which also tends to be around the WDRC kneepoint for most fittings.

It is probably easiest to understand expansion if you think of an input/gain function, rather than an input/output function (See Figure 8–14 below: look at the lower line). Notice, that as the input increases *below* the expansion kneepoint, gain is EXPANDING.

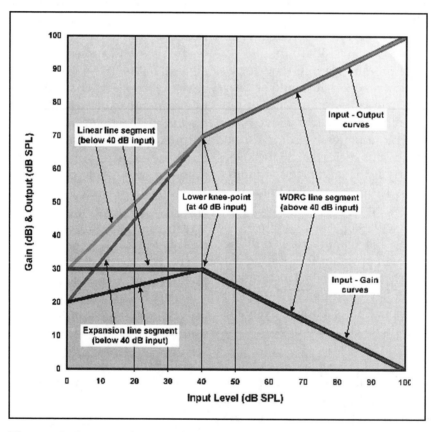

Figure 8–14. Input/output and input/gain curves for compression and expansion. The top two curves are input/output curves, and the bottom set are input/gain curves. Note the compression kneepoint (CK) is 40 dB. The lower line on the chart illustrates the effects of expansion for inputs below the 40 dB SPL kneepoint.

TAKE FIVE: Controlling Expansion (Maybe)

When expansion was first introduced for use with hearing aids, there was considerable programming of the features available (e.g., kneepoints and ratios). The problem, however, was that dispensers tended to confuse expansion with compression, and move a kneepoint up, when it should have been moved down. A somewhat bad fitting just became worse. Manufacturers then started to use general terms like "strong" (high kneepoint) and "weak" (low kneepoint) for programming, to avoid some of the confusion. Today, many manufacturers have totally eliminated your ability to program expansion, and many "fitters" don't even know it's there. In fact, in some software, you can't turn it off if you wanted to!

One of the main patient benefits is to reduce microphone noise: in fact, some manufacturers label the feature "microphone noise reduction," some manufacturers call it "soft squelch, and "others call it "low level noise reduction." [As half the world is on a diet, the term "expansion" often is avoided!]

In Closing

Knowing when the hearing aid is processing sound in a linear or nonlinear manner takes some thought. We close this chapter by trying to put it all together on one graph (as you have figured out by now compression is best expressed graphically). Figure 8–14 shows both input/output and input-gain curves. Notice that the compression kneepoint is 40 dB SPL. In order to intuitively understand how expansion and compression work, take a careful look at the *input/gain* curves. As inputs below the kneepoint get louder, gain is expanding and as inputs above the kneepoint become louder gain is being compressed.

You can think of this chapter as a cross-country Route 66 tour of compression with a few pit stops thrown in along the way. We've stopped at a few old familiar drive-ins, but also saw some new changes too. Taken alone, this journey is not enough to get you started, but there is no better time to start the process of becoming wise about the basics of hearing aids than reading and understanding this chapter. It is enough to get you ready for the next chapters on advanced hearing aid features and hearing aid selection. Before you leave this chapter, and move on to another roadside attraction, take the time to really understand the concepts gain, output, and compression. And buy a soft-top sports car the next time you're out! Life is too short not to own one.

9

Advanced Hearing Aid Features

Today's features versus the hearing aids of the past —a lot like the differences between major league and minor league baseball!

To the untrained observer, both major league and minor league baseball would appear to be the same. The rules are the same, the critical field dimensions are the same, and the players look about the same. However, as you gain a better understanding of some of the nuances of the game, you begin to see some of the differences in both quality and performance between the two leagues. As we go through the features of today's "major league hearing aids" you'll see how these advances can enhance patient benefit, and how they are different from their "minor league" cousins.

Thinking Digital

If this book had been written a decade or so ago, about this point in time we would have introduced you to those magic words, *DIGITAL PROCESSING*. We then would have had an entire section on bits and bytes, aliasing and antialiasing, Nyquest frequencies and perhaps even something about Nyquil! But, things have changed. Although this detailed explanation was a big deal in the late 1990s, digital hearing aids have rapidly become the "standard" fitting; it's nearly impossible to find a hearing aid that is *NOT* digital. There even are "disposable" digital hearing aids. So, today, simply being digital is no big deal!

Given that a "digital instrument" can be anything from a $49 disposable to a single-channel linear peak clipper to a "gazillion-channel-super-duper-directional-noise-blocker," it's not so important that you think about *HOW* a hearing aid does something, but rather, think about *WHAT* it does. Think about the features that your patient needs. It could be that after you select the features needed, you will only find all of these features in a high-end digital, but perhaps not. Most "entry level" products today have four or more channels, WDRC, AGCo, digital noise reduction, and directional technology. Not bad! That may be enough for many people!

How Does It Really Work?

Neither the major league player or the minor league really understands the physics behind the pitch called the "slider." What exactly makes it look like a fastball, and then make it drop and curve as it nears the plate? The difference, however, is that a good major league batter will hit it about twice as often as the average minor league player.

Like the baseball analogy above, we believe that it's not really necessary that you know how *digital processing* works. What is important to know, is how *digital hearing aids work*! The aim of this chapter is to get you started with this understanding process by providing some practical information on advanced hearing aid features.

To fully understand the superior performance of modern hearing aids, we turn back the clock 20 or so years and examine the performance of hearing aids in 1990. For you sports fans, comparing today's hearing aids to those of another generation is like watching ESPN Classic. The uniform styles look a little outdated, the players' hair is longer, a few more mustaches, but the game is still essentially the same. If you were fitting hearing aids back then, you were still fitting a device that was proven to be effective, you just had a little less to think about and a few more compromises to make.

Fundamental Acoustic Standards

What you had to "get right" 20 years ago is a good starting point for fitting a hearing aid with today's advanced features. You can think of this starting point as the "Classics." The following characteristics never go out of style no matter how advanced the technology gets. If you get these things right, the chances are very good that your patient will be satisfied no matter what level of technology you fit him with. We believe that 80% or more of a successful fitting hinges on these factors. Think of these basic requirements as the starting point for our entry into a discussion of advanced hearing aid features.

Smooth and Undistorted Frequency Response

This characteristic refers to the quality and shape of the frequency response of the instrument. Any audio device has a frequency response. Probably the best example of how frequency response affects sound quality and intelligibility is the old transistor radio (you even may have been using a similar one back in 1990 to listen to that ball game the first time). Often, the frequency response of these small radios was not smooth, and the bandwidth was limited, resulting in very poor sound quality. Hearing aids are the same way; if the frequency response is in a very limited narrow band, or distorted, it will result in very poor sound quality for anyone who uses it. We know that good sound quality is highly correlated with hearing aid success.

<table>
<tr><td>

TAKE FIVE:
Brewtowns and K-Amps

In 1982 the St. Louis Cardinals defeated the Milwaukee Brewers in seven games to take the "brewtown" World Series. It was also the year Mead Killion and Tom Tillman published fidelity ratings on a variety of sound systems. Using the "golden ear" of Julian Hirsch of *Stereo Review* magazine, Killion and Tillman determined that an "experimental K-Amp" hearing aid had comparable fidelity ratings to expensive stereo equipment.

</td></tr>
</table>

Loudness Comfort and Audibility

To state the obvious, all hearing aid users require sounds to be heard. We refer to this concept as audibility, and we discuss this important attribute in detail in Chapter 10. However, there is always a balance between making sounds audible and making them comfortable. This balance was especially critical with previous generations of hearing aids. For example, in a single-channel hearing aid it is possible to make virtually all soft speech sounds audible by turning up the volume control to full on (or the point just below where the hearing aid starts to feedback). All would be well for the patient for hearing soft sounds, that is, until a sound of average or loud intensity comes along, forcing the patient to turn the volume control wheel down, thus, making many soft speech sounds inaudible. Ensuring that the soft and medium intensity sounds of speech can

be heard, while loud sounds are not too loud, is an essential requirement of all hearing aids (we talked about this in Chapter 8 when we addressed WDRC). If you were fitting single-channel hearing aids in the early 1990s, striking a balance between audibility and comfort was a constant challenge. Only about 20% of products had WDRC. Today's hearing aids routinely utilize WDRC and expansion to maximize audibility and comfort of soft and average inputs, whereas output compression (AGCo) is used to keep loud sounds from becoming too loud, all accomplished over several independent channels.

These are the basic components of amplification that make up a large share of patient benefit and satisfaction, things we talk about in Chapter 10. But there are many other features available that can move that "okay" hearing aid fitting, with "okay" patient satisfaction, to an excellent fitting, and one hopes, above average satisfaction.

Advanced Features— The Building Blocks

At most minor league baseball parks they serve only the basic food items we've come to appreciate when attending a sporting event: hot dogs, peanuts, soda pop, and beer. On the other hand, if you've been to a major league ball game recently, you know you can get everything from sushi to Pad Thai to liver pâté. And wash it all down with a glass of high-priced Chardonnay! Advanced features are to hearing aids what gourmet food is to attending a major league game at a brand new ballpark. Of course, you can get all the traditional fare at the game, but if you want to splurge, typically pay a little extra, there is an abundance of other high quality dishes available. And you know, many more customers are highly satisfied because of this. Before you get too hungry, let's start by reviewing some of what's on the menu of a hearing aid with advanced features.

When we think of high-end digital products and what these products can do that the entry-level products cannot, it is useful to break down all the individual features of these products. Here are the advanced features that we discuss in this chapter:

- Multiple channels
- Multiple memories
- Signal classification
- Noise reduction
- Directional microphone technology
- Frequency lowering (compression)
- Adaptive feedback control
- Data logging
- Data learning (trainable gain, compression, microphone strategy, etc.)
- Wireless connectivity
- In situ testing

Granted, some of the entry level products on the market have a version of these advanced features, but often the high-end product has an "enhanced" version. For example, an entry level product may have one type of noise reduction, the high-end product from the same manufacturer may have three different types of noise reduction all working independently within the same hearing aid.

One way to gain a deeper understanding of how advanced features interact with the hearing aid selection and fitting process is to view this technology through the lens of the patient. In other words, how does each advanced feature contribute to the overall success of the fitting? And does the additional cost of the feature equate to enhanced benefit? This is also an effective way to learn how many of the advanced features found in a modern hearing aid contribute to solving many of the problems associated with hearing loss. Let's look at several advanced hearing aid features found in modern hearing aids and relate them to the needs of the patient with hearing loss by unveiling the basic building blocks of hearing aids.

When high school baseball players are drafted by a major league team, they begin their professional career in the minor leagues. In case you were wondering, the minor league baseball system has four classes or layers. This means that for a ball player to make it to the major leagues they have to pass through these four minor league layers, called Rookie, A, AA, and AAA. To move up to the next level a player has to prove he is worthy of a promotion by playing at a high level. Moving from one layer—getting it right at one level before moving to the next—also applies to selecting and fitting advanced features.

When fitting hearing aids to people with sensorineural hearing loss, there are some things we generally have to "get right" to maximize the benefits and performance for the patient. We have listed these roughly in order of importance. That is, each feature builds on the next, a type of layering of features. Advanced features found in most modern hearing aids allow you to improve four different patient needs effectively (Figure 9–1):

- Audibility, intelligibility, and loudness comfort in quiet listening situations
- Listening comfort in background noise

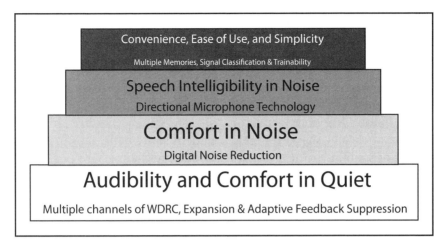

Figure 9–1. The "building blocks" of hearing aid features. For each of the four blocks, several key advanced features are listed that are designed to address it.

- Speech intelligibility in background noise
- Added convenience and ease of use

We've taken the 10 special features that we listed previously, and placed them within these four general categories (although some could fit in more than one). They're not in the same order as listed originally, but don't let that bother you.

Building Block #1: Audibility, Intelligibility, and Loudness Comfort in Quiet Listening Situations

Although most patients will probably enter your office with complaints related to speech understanding in background noise, it is probable that they also are having problems in quiet listening situations too. Moreover, nearly everyone spends far more time communicating with others in relatively quiet situations. That's why our first building block is ensuring that we make speech audible (especially soft speech), which should lead to improved intelligibility. The amplified signal also needs to be "acceptable," which means we need to give the patient appropriate loudness for the entire frequency range. What features help us do this?

Multichannel Processing

Today's high-end digital products have several channels of AGCi (WDRC), 10, 20, 30, or more. It seems like every year we hear of a new product that has even more channels. Many audiologists believe that "more is better" when it comes to channels, so manufacturers keep adding more whether they are necessary or not. In general, hearing aids with more channels are more expensive, and more, in fact, usually is better, although there may be a point where "X-amount" is enough. We're not too sure what that number is. We do know, however, that multiple channels of WDRC is the amplification strategy that allows the hearing aid (with your programming help) to repackage sound into the user's residual dynamic range (refer to Chapter 10 for details).

With more channels it is possible to apply different compression characteristics to different frequency-specific inputs to more closely shape the gain and output according to the patient's residual dynamic range and loudness growth pattern, and improve audibility. How many channels are enough? The latest research says between 5 and 8, although if the audiogram is relatively flat (e.g., fairly equal hearing loss between 500 to 4000 Hz), you can do a pretty good job using only 2 to 4 channels.

If you model the compression correctly, you provide audibility for a wider range of inputs. In most cases, improved *audibility* usually equals improved *intelligibility*. How many channels are enough for this? Current research says between 8 and 16 channels (after four channels, the added improvement is reduced considerably).

TIPS and TRICKS: How Many Channels?

There is at least one study suggesting that seven channels are needed to match a prescriptive fitting target with better than 90% accuracy. This may vary from manufacturer to manufacturer, depending on how the channels overlap and many other factors. We discuss matching prescriptive targets in Chapter 10, but for now keep in mind it's a good thing to have enough channels to match a target with precision. This is especially important for those steeply sloping audiograms, as seen in Chapter 5.

Recall from our earlier discussions that expansion can be helpful in reducing the output of low-level noises that might be annoying to the hearing aid user. Indirectly, expansion often allows us to provide greater audibility for soft speech, which should lead to greater patient benefit and satisfaction. Again, with more channels it's possible to program more effectively the expansion kneepoints so that they correspond with the speech spectrum and the patient's hearing loss.

Think back to our discussion of the speech spectrum (Chapter 2 and you'll recall that soft speech is considerably more intense in the lower frequencies than in the 3000- to 4000-Hz range (a difference of 10 to 15 dB). Hence, we need multiple channels for expansion so that we can use different expansion kneepoints for different frequency regions. In most hearing aids, expansion *cannot* be adjusted by the fitter, except maybe to turn it on or off. It is preprogrammed by the manufacturer and it's working behind the scenes (and we hope your patient will thank you for it, indirectly of course).

Multiple channels of AGCo also are important. This not only assists in optimizing comfort with loud sounds, but also is helpful for maximizing speech intelligibility. With multiple channels it is possible to shape the output of the hearing aid to mimic the patient's LDLs across frequencies. This will maximize the residual dynamic range, allowing for the dynamics of speech, but yet not allow the peaks of speech (or environmental sounds) to become uncomfortable.

Finally, multichannel processing is also useful for digital noise reduction and directional technology (more on that when we get to those categories).

Frequency Lowering

A special feature that is somewhat new to hearing aids is frequency lowering. This can be accomplished through frequency transposition, or using frequency compression. Current algorithms are designed to move or compress high frequencies (e.g., around 3000 to 4000 Hz and higher) to lower frequencies.

The underling theory behind frequency lowering goes back to our discussion of audibility and its importance. Although audibility usually is a good thing, there are three cases when we might *not* want high-frequency audibility when we are fitting hearing aids:

- The hearing aid is not able to deliver the desired high-frequency gain without continued feedback problems.
- The hearing loss is so severe that it is not practical to attempt to provide audibility.
- The patient has cochlear dead regions (which often is consistent with Reason #2, but dead regions also can be present in milder cochlear hearing losses (e.g., 60 to 70 dB HL).

When one or more of the above situations exist in a downward sloping hearing loss, it might be appropriate to consider using frequency lowering. The fundamental notion is that it's better to make high-frequency speech signals (e.g., "s" and "sh") audible at a *different* lower frequency, than not make them audible at all. This could be especially helpful for young children developing speech and language.

Research using frequency lowering techniques with adults is just emerging, and it's difficult to determine what impact this technology has for improving speech intelligibility in quiet listening conditions. It could be that there is an acclimatization period, which can be accelerated with auditory training. Like many features, verification of course is critical when using this feature. It is important to know if indeed the desired signals have been made audible when frequency lowering has been activated; your probe-mic measures are an excellent way, and one of the only ways, to make this determination.

Adaptive Feedback Suppression (Figure 9–2)

We now move on to the third special feature that has a significant impact on improving audibility, and improving

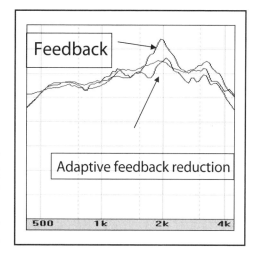

Figure 9–2. An example of acoustic feedback (large peak in sound energy at 2 kHz) and adaptive feedback reduction that have been activated on the hearing aid. Note the reduction in the energy peak at 2 kHz when the adaptive feedback reduction algorithm is activated.

speech intelligibility in quiet (and in noise too, but we leave that discussion for a later category). The benefit of this feature is often overlooked, as it's not as "sexy" as Bluetooth, digital noise reduction, or directional technology. Moreover, hearing aids are not supposed to have acoustic feedback, so when you tell your patients that their new ultra-expensive hearing aids won't whistle, the typical response is " . . . huh?"

The benefit of advanced feedback cancellation algorithms, however, is significant, especially with OC fittings. A good feedback suppression system can provide 15 dB or more of added stable gain (ASG)—the difference in gain with the feature turned "on" versus "off." This can make a huge difference in the audibility of speech (especially soft speech), and subsequently improve speech understanding. The degree of ASG available does vary considerably from manufacturer to manufacturer, so it's something you'll need to check out in your office before you start with fittings.

TIPS and TRICKS: Ear Canal Geography Matters

Another factor to consider with adaptive feedback suppression algorithms is the size and shape of the patient's ear canal. One good performing adaptive feedback suppression system might yield an average ASG of 15 dB, but on a specific individual with unusual ear canal geometry you might find the ASG to be only half that number. The important point is remember every patient is different and averages can be misleading.

Note that in our heading we used the word "adaptive." This is an important distinction. Many of the earlier digital products had "feedback control systems." In many cases, however, all this contributed was a reduction of gain—we were doing that back in the 1950s with body aids. Adaptive feedback control is a much more intelligent system. The hearing aid can detect the presence of feedback, and then apply an algorithm to reduce it. This can be done in two ways:

Narrowband notch filters: Once the feedback frequency is detected, a narrowband notch filter is applied at this frequency to eliminate the feedback. In theory, once the notch filter has been activated, the resulting real-ear output is relatively unchanged from what is was before the feedback occurred. You don't see this approach as the primary feedback stopper much any more, as phase cancellation (our next category) is more effective. It is possible (even probable), however, that some type of filtering or "gain-locking" approaches are still used in many high-end products as a *supplement* to phase cancellation.

Phase cancellation: Once the feedback frequency is detected, the hearing aid introduces a signal that is 180 degrees out of phase from the feedback signal, which then serves to eliminate the feedback. In some cases, the frequency also is slightly shifted, which makes the process more effective. In theory, once the phase cancellation has been activated, the resulting real-ear output is relatively unchanged from what it was before the feedback occurred.

It's important to note that adaptive feedback control does not make up for a bad fitting (e.g., a bad ear impression resulting in an unusually "leaky" fitting). Its primary purpose is for transient feedback that might occur when the patient's hand is placed close to the ear (when adjusting the VC or changing programs), or when an object like a telephone receiver is placed near the ear. An exception to this is OC fittings, which we discuss shortly.

TIPS and TRICKS: What Does "Stable Gain" Mean?

When thinking about acoustic feedback, we often use the term "maximum stable gain." In this sense, by *stable gain* we mean that the person can talk, move around, and the hearing aid will not go into feedback, and there is no distortion present due to oscillations. When we activate an adaptive feedback system then, it is possible to measure *added stable gain*. This is the amount of gain that is available to the user with the feedback cancellation system turned on, compared to when it is turned off. Some clinicians use this measure to judge the "goodness" of various products. One downside of this approach, however, is that if the hearing aid does not have a lot of gain, you will have a ceiling effect (max gain is reached) which could *underestimate* the effectiveness of the feedback canceller. Also, this measure tends to penalize hearing aids that are very stable *without* the feedback suppression algorithm; there is not as much room for improvement.

From a clinical standpoint, what we really are the most interested in is, "What amount of gain can be obtained with the feedback suppression algorithm activated?"

OC Fittings

As mentioned in previous chapters, OC fittings are very popular, reportedly accounting for 75% of the fittings in some offices. We dare say that if it were not for the adaptive feedback algorithms that are now available, this product would be far less popular. With OC fittings, there is nearly always a substantial amount of sound leaking out of the ear canal, as that is the acoustic design of this style instrument. With OC instruments, a good feedback system usually allows us to achieve as much as 10 to 15 dB more stable gain than we could obtained if this feature were not available (it does vary greatly from product to product).

Given that patients seem to prefer OC fittings, more gain leads to more audibility, and audibility usually leads to intelligibility, adaptive feedback reduction probably is the best feature to date for digital products!

Any Downsides?

There are not many downsides to a good feedback reduction algorithm, except increased battery drain if it is running continuously or most of the time. There can be some "chirping" with some systems, but that's a minor thing compared to a continuous whistle at 110 dB SPL.

One possible, but minor, side effect of adaptive feedback reduction algorithms is that they sometime confuse tonal sounds, such as a musical passage, as the whistling associated with feedback. Because the adaptive feedback system "thinks" the tonal sound is acoustic feedback from the hearing aid, it tries to reduce the gain of the incoming tonal sound. This particular side effect causes the hearing aids to produce a warbling like sound called entrainment. Often, you can address this side effect by going into the fitting software and making some adjustments to how the adaptive feedback settings; however, on some occasions you may have to change the form factor or vent size to fix the problem. In recent years, manufacturers have mostly solved this problem by having the hearing aid "remember" the feedback frequency.

Building Block #2: Listening Comfort in Background Noise

After reading the chapters on sensorineural hearing loss and basic hearing aid components, it probably wasn't too surprising to just read that many of the common problems associated with sensorineural hearing loss can be alleviated by making sounds audible and comfortable. Some communication needs, however, like listening in noisy environments, are not addressed by just making sounds comfortable and audible. Fortunately, digital electronics has given hearing aids the ability to separate certain noises from speech, or at least reduce the output of the noise, which should help your patients have a more relaxed listening experience in background noise. Notice that we do not say that digital noise reduction will provide "improved understanding in noise," but it's possible that that also could happen indirectly. Although we discussed three different hearing aid special features in the previous section, we only discuss one now: digital noise reduction.

Processed-based noise reduction, more commonly known as digital noise reduction (DNR), can be defined as any type of scheme in which a mathematical calculation is employed by the hearing aid's signal classification system to separate a desired signal (usually speech) from an undesirable signal (usually background noise). Or, in some cases, there is not separation, but rather and automatic reduction of gain in the channels where noise is dominant.

DNR algorithms are one of two types of noise-reduction strategies employed by modern hearing aids, with the other being spatially based noise reduction schemes. Spatially based noise reduction schemes use directional microphone technology to manage background noise. (We talk about that in the next category.)

Noise Reduction: A Little History

The notion of "noise reduction" certainly is not a new idea ushered in with the advent of digital hearing aids. In fact, attempts at analog noise reduction have a relatively long and storied history. Starting with body aids, there was a low-frequency reduction available that was advertized as "noise reduction." In the 1980s single-channel analog hearing aids were sometimes equipped with active low-cut tone controls as a way to manually reduce low-frequency types of ambient sound. Also in the 1980s, automatic signal processing (ASP; simply AGCi compression in the low frequencies) was introduced as a method for automatically reducing low-frequency sounds, a technology made famous when President Regan was fitted. Many remember the days when BILL (bass increase at low levels) and TILL (treble increase at low levels) processing were promoted as methods to improve speech understanding in background noise. In addition to manual low-cut switches, ASP and BILL/TILL schemes, two proprietary signal processing schemes, Adaptive Compression and the Zeta Noise Blocker, were introduced around this time with mixed results.

Although many of these analog noise reduction/speech enhancement schemes were popular throughout the 1980s to mid-1990s, research indicated that they were ineffective at improving speech intelligibility in noise and often contributed to poor sound quality. With the introduction of digital signal processing in commercially available hearing aids in the mid-1990s, a processed-based solution to reducing background noise once again was a possibility. Since the introduction of digital hearing aids in the mid-1990s, processed-based noise reduction strategies have grown more complex.

In the late 1990s and early 2000s, Mark McGuire, Sammy Sosa, and Barry Bonds were shattering home-run records, all of them passing the home-run record for a single season, which was 62 set by North Dakotan Roger Maris in 1961. At the time, fans were suspicious that many major league stars, including these home-run hitters, were using performance-enhancing drugs. Fans wanted to know what each star was putting into their body to improve performance. Although by no means illegal, what goes on inside the DNR system of each hearing aid often remains shrouded in mystery. Yet, we often hope we hit a home run when we fit a pair of hearing aids with this technology to our patient.

DNR: How Does It Work?

Often, the interworking of noise-reduction algorithms are shrouded in mystery. When it comes to under-standing how various types of noise-reduction algorithms actually work, hearing aid manufacturers don't make it any easier for clinicians because they often use proprietary terms and jargon to describe how their products are different from the competition. Even though there are important differences across product lines, there are some commonalities that can help us demystify the black box.

TAKE FIVE: The Black Box

In many professions, the concept of a "Black Box" is popular. For example, in the field of finance there is "black box trading," which is the use of a special computer algorithm to automatically decide when to make a stock transaction for a client. The use of the term "black box" is more commonly associated with computers. As hearing aids have a lot in common with computers these days, there is a lot of mystery surrounding what's in the hearing aid's "black box." We'll try to help you understand what's inside the black box.

Modulation Based. Today, most hearing aids have more than one type of noise reduction scheme. Many schemes are *modulation based*, and these are the easiest to understand. The signal classification system on board the hearing aid analyses the signal, looking at the number and depth of modulations—as well as many other characteristics (e.g., speech usually has 4 to 6 modulations/second). Modulation-based noise reduction systems work under the premise that speech has fewer modulations

(Hz) with more depth (dB) than noise stimuli. Typically, modulation frequency and depth are analyzed independently in each channel of the instrument (Figure 9–3). If the input signal is classified as noise the intensity of the signal is reduced, and if it's classified as speech the intensity level may be increased, or more commonly, the signal in that channel remains at programmed gain. The important point to remember regarding modulation based noise reduction, is that when noise is found to be the dominant signal in a given channel, gain for *everything* is reduced: noise *and* speech. There is not

---

TIPS and TRICKS: It's All About the SNR

The way most modulation-based DNR systems work fits reasonably well with the patient's speech understanding ability. It's unlikely that someone with a hearing loss bad enough to be fitted with hearing aids, will be understanding speech in background noise at an SNR of +2 dB or worse. Usually, these patients require an SNR of +5 dB or better. While it might seem like a negative that modulation-based DNR turns down the gain for speech as well as noise, it probably doesn't matter much, as this feature is only reducing gain for a given channel when the DNR is such that the patient isn't understanding speech anyway.

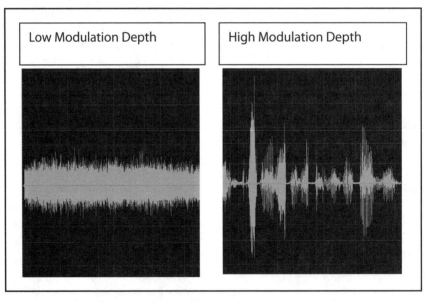

| Low Modulation Depth | High Modulation Depth |

Figure 9–3. A comparison of modulation depth. The left signal has a low modulation depth. The signal on the right has a high modulation depth. Modulation depth is one of many characteristics used by the hearing aid's on-board signal classification to identify nonspeech and speechlike signals.

an improvement in the signal to noise ratio within that channel and, hence, we would not expect an improvement in speech understanding.

Filtering and Subtraction. In addition to modulation-based noise-reduction strategies, most hearing aids employ some combination of filtering, spectral subtraction, or co-modulation detection. Each type of processed-based noise reduction strategy has its own operating principles and complexities that go well beyond the scope of this chapter. In general, these type of DNR systems are geared toward cleaning up the speech signal when speech is at least somewhat the dominant signal (e.g., SNRs of +2 to 5 dB or so). One method is to look for gaps between speech signals and reduce the "noise" for this short duration. The trick of course, is to pull out the noise without also pulling out some of the speech. Now if the talker would be willing to say the same word over and over a few hundred times, some averaging could occur, and the process would be much more effective. Unfortunately, in most conversations, the hearing aid only has one chance to get it right.

Impulse Noise. Impulse noise reduction (termed things like "sound smoothing," "sound relax," etc.) is not geared toward speech understanding, but simply designed to reduce annoyance. That is, the classification system looks for very sharp peaks in the onset of a signal. If found, it's assumed that this is noise (probably an irritating one) and is not speech. The initial peak of this signal is then reduced, giving the noise a duller sound.

TAKE FIVE: More on DNR

In almost all hearing aids dispensed today, there is more than one type of processed-based noise reduction scheme in operation. Often, there are three or more schemes working simultaneously. Kate's textbook, *Digital Hearing Aids*, reviews many of the technical differences of the various types of noise reduction algorithms. Although you need to have a basic understanding of how DNR algorithms work, it's more important for you to have a detailed knowledge of the advantages and limitations of DNR schemes in general, and how to effectively communicate this information to patients during the prefitting appointment. With a term like "noise reduction" it's very easy for the patient to develop unrealistic expectations.

Selecting DNR Parameters

It is important to keep in mind that digital noise reduction and boosting overall gain can be active simultaneously, and in theory could complement one another; one works best when noise is dominant, the other works best when speech is dominant. *Also*, this is happening independently in each channel. In some channels noise reduction could be reducing gain, whereas in other channels it might not have an effect because the dominant signal is speech.

When fine tuning the DNR feature on a hearing aid, there are some parameters that you need to consider. How each parameter is set—by either you or the manufacturer—can have a tremendous impact on the outcome of the fitting.

Gain Reduction. Once the hearing aid's signal classification system has determined that the input signal is noise for a given channel, how much does it reduce the noise signal? All products reduce gain in varying amounts across the frequency range, and might reduce it differently for different noises. With some products the "max" setting may result in a 4 to 6 dB reduction, while with other products, "max" could mean a 12 to 15 dB reduction for some noise inputs.

Gain Enhancement. Once a signal has been classified as speech, does the hearing aid boost the gain of the speech signal? The amount of gain enhancement varies across frequency as well. Some products have been known to even boost high-frequency gain when the SNR is adverse (it probably won't do any harm). We recommend using your probe-mic system with a real-speech input, and then measure the output for DNR-on versus DNR-off. This will help you understand what is happening when DNR is activated.

Activation Time (onset and offset time). Recall that with compression we call the time constants attack and release. It's a little different with noise reduction, so the common terms are "onset" and "offset." What you'll want to know is: once the input signal has been classified as noise, how long does it take to reduce the noise signal? To reduce it to its maximum? This could be as fast as a second or two, or as long as 5 to 10 seconds.

In addition to activation time, another consideration is speed of the gain recovery (offset time). In other words, when the input signal that was classified as noise is no longer present, or speech is present that is more intense than the noise, how long does it take for programmed gain to recover? Again, this is something very easy to observe in the real ear with your probe-mic testing.

Turn on a noise (make sure it's a real noise, e.g., white noise, speech noise, pink noise, etc. without modulations) with the hearing aid's DNR on max. Watch the output on the screen until the maximum reduction occurs. How long did it take? Now, with the noise still on, start talking above the noise. What happens and how long did it take?

SNR and Level Effects. Two other factors that can impact the DNR effects is the SNR of the signal, and the overall level of the noise. At what SNR is the noise reduction scheme activated, and how much is gain reduced at various signal-to-noise ratios? Is the noise reduction the same when speech is present? With some instruments, you can select noise reduction to occur for all signals, or only for speech-in-noise conditions.

You'll also want to know if the degree of gain reduction increases as a function of the overall noise level (*Hint:* it does for most instruments)? If a manufacturer advertizes 10 dB of noise reduction, is that for a 60 dB SPL noise or an 80 dB SPL noise? This of course is important to know when you're verifying the DNR feature with your probe-mic equipment. Using a noise input of 60 dB SPL might not be very impressive if the hearing aid wasn't designed to have much noise reduction at this input intensity.

TAKE FIVE:
Even More on DNR

There are significant differences across manufacturers for each of these DNR variables. Most of these differences can be observed both in a 2-cc coupler and in the actual ear using probe-microphone measures and a carefully controlled input signal (both speech and noise to answer different questions). Even though there are key differences across manufacturers, there is no published evidence suggesting one manufacturer's implementation of processed-based noise reduction is more beneficial than another. How slow, how fast, and how much for whom for what listening conditions are still research questions that need to

Assessing True Patient Benefit

Minor league baseball players are constantly being assessed relative to their major league potential. You might hear about a young guy in AA ball being a potential "five tool" player (hit for power, hit for average, good fielder, good throwing arm, and excellent speed). But just like special features with hearing aids, what is needed is "real-world evidence." For every highly hyped rookie who made it big (think Carlos Rodriquez of the Colorado Rockies), there has been one who was a flop (think David Clyde of the Texas Rangers). It's been over 10 years since DNR was introduced, and it certainly has not been a flop, but has it lived up to the hype?

A primary goal of any hearing aid fitting is to restore audibility of speech. In most cases simply restoring audibility for quiet sounds does not solve all of the communication problems associated with hearing loss. Professionals have to rely on advanced features, like noise-reduction algorithms to alleviate many of these existing communication problems. According to popular opinion, processed-based noise reduction schemes have the *potential* to improve several important dimensions of communication:

Improved Speech Intelligibility. It does seem reasonable that if noise is reduced, speech intelligibility should improve. Not surprisingly, marketing claims have sometimes touted the potential of noise reduction algorithms to improve speech understanding ability. To date, however, there is no research indicating that DNR significantly improves speech intelligibility in background noise. With modulation-based DNR, both speech and noise are reduced, and therefore the SNR doesn't really improve. With spectral subtraction and Wiener-filter-based approaches, the "cleaning" of the mixed speech and noise signal does not appear to be significant enough to improve speech recognition for standard clinical speech tests. There have been limited reports of "ease of listening" improvements, but more research in this area is needed.

Make Loud Sounds Less Annoying. One type of noise reduction algorithm is able to recognize impulse like sounds that usually are annoying to a hearing aid user. Although the primary function of AGCo is to keep the hearing aid's MPO below the discomfort level of the patient, noise-reduction schemes, which may be faster acting than the AGCo, have the potential to protect the patient from sudden, high-intensity transient sounds. These are sounds that may still be below the patient's LDL and the AGCo kneepoint, but are still certainly are annoying. Limited studies have shown that this type of DNR indeed does make transient sounds more tolerable. The general thought is that if the patient is not bothered as much by these noises (e.g., the clanging of dishes in a noisy restaurant) they will be better able to focus on the conversation, and there may be an indirect benefit in speech understanding.

Improve Listening Comfort in Noise. Overall listening comfort, sometimes referred as "more relaxed listening," is believed to be improved with the use of processed-based noise reduction. Traditionally, patients have had to reduce the gain on their hearing aids or remove them when bothered by background noise. Some studies have indicated that DNR does improve listening comfort and reduce the annoyance from noise. We know that long-duration noise can be fatiguing. If the patient is more alert

because of DNR, will their speech intelligibility improve? Perhaps.

Cognitive Issues

Noise can affect cognitive performance. One of the hardest thing to do in all of sports is to hit a 100 mph fastball. There is not so much crowd noise in the minors, but in the majors there certainly is. When is crowd noise the loudest? In the top of the 9th inning, with two outs, when the opposing batter is trying to hit a 100 mph fastball!

Perhaps an overlooked byproduct of DNR is that it has the potential to lighten the cognitive workload. In other words, when noise reduction is activated, the brain may be able to release attention-related resources to be used for other tasks occurring simultaneously. For example, let's say you are sitting in your family room trying to learn an important new skill by watching a DVD, while trying to ignore the din from the kitchen as your husband uses the blender or another noisy appliance for several minutes. What if the noise of the blender was softer? Would you be able to better concentrate on the task?

TAKE FIVE: Do No Harm

Although there is no evidence suggesting that processed-based noise reduction improves speech intelligibility, there is also no evidence suggesting that it degrades speech intelligibility either, at least to the point at which patients no longer prefer it turned off. One of the basic tenets of physician training is first, "do no harm" to patients they are evaluating and treating. The same probably holds true for dispensers

and one way to "do no harm" is to recommend processed-based noise reduction technology for all your patients. Even though virtually all hearing aids now have it, it's nice to know it shouldn't make things worse. And . . . it's certainly possible that things like relaxed listening, ease of listening, and brain resource allocation could indirectly make things better.

In theory, DNR has the potential to reduce cognitive workload by reducing the sounds of the blender and you are able to focus your attention on a more important task for a longer period of time. A few recent studies have suggested that indeed DNR has the potential to reduce cognitive effort.

Building Block #3: Speech Intelligibility in Noise

Many surveys of patients who have tried hearing aids indicate that an inability to understand speech in the presence of background noise is the major reason why hearing aids are rejected. The good news is that directional microphone technology can address many of the problems associated with understanding speech in noise. Because directional microphones have been implemented in hearing aids for many years, much research has been conducted with them. Therefore, we go into some details on how directional microphone hearing aids work as well as review many fitting considerations. Directional microphones happen to be the only one of our 10 special features that have been proven to improve speech recognition in background noise.

Directional Microphone Technology

Directional hearing aids have been around since the early 1970s, but really didn't have a large market penetration until the 1990s. Given their effectiveness, we have observed a surge in the number of hearing instruments dispensed with directional microphones over the last 10 years, and, today, the majority of hearing aids have directional technology (this technology is not available with CIC instruments due to space limitations).

Directional microphone systems depend on noise to be spatially separated from speech, or other sounds the listener wants to hear. It might seem obvious, but it is worth noting that this spatial separation is not done by the directional microphone system directly. Rather, it is up to the end users to place the sounds they want to hear directly in front of them and the noise off to the side or behind them. When the end user is properly situated in a listening environment, directional microphones are highly effective at improving the signal-to-noise ratio. As we discuss later, unfortunately, when the listening environment becomes more reverberant, there is less spatial separation of the speech and noise signals due to reflections, and consequently the SNR improvement is diminished.

Microphone Methods to Achieve Directionality. Traditionally, there have been two ways directionality has been achieved in a hearing aid. The first method, which was employed in the early directional hearing aids, was to use a single *directional* microphone with two inlet ports. The rear port employs an "acoustic" delay (using a physicial damping material) which is tuned to equal the external delay of the same sound traveling from the rear port to the front port. The effect is that signals from the back are out of phase at the microphone and cancel, providing the desired directivity. This is referred to as the acoustical delay method or "single microphone" approach. As it is a directional *microphone*, the *hearing* aid is always directional. This approach is seldom used with today's hearing aids.

The second method, and by far the most common, uses two omnidirectional microphones with *electronic* delay. When both types of directional microphone systems are properly working, they provide about the same signal-to-noise ratio improvement, however, the two-microphone system provides much more flexibility, as tuning can be automatic and adaptive during use. Given the overwhelming popularity of the two-mic electronic delay system, we focus on this design.

When two omnidirectional microphones are placed into a hearing instrument a dual microphone system is created. Figure 9–4A is a schematic of a directional microphone system using electronic delay. Subtracting the output

of the rear microphone from the output of the front microphone and adding an electronic time delay to the output of the rear microphone provides an improved signal-to-noise ratio. The distance between the two microphones determines the amount of delay to the signal from the rear microphone. For example, due to their size, traditional BTEs allow a maximum distance between the two microphone ports of 12 to 16 mm, whereas smaller custom hearing instruments only allow for 4 to 10 mm of maximum distance. This means, the wider the spacing between the two microphone ports the better the directivity. If the ports are too close together, there will be little or no directional effect. This is one reason why we don't have directional microphone technology with CIC instruments.

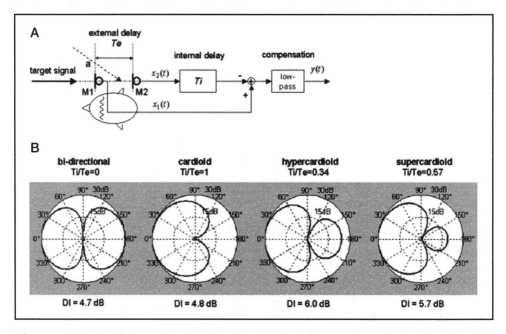

Figure 9–4. A. Schematic of a directional microphone using electronic delay. M1 and M2 denote the two microphone arrangement in proximity to the right ear. **B.** Four common polar plots found in directional microphones. Note the patterns are aligned to correspond with the head at the top of the figure. Typically, the 0° azimuth is positioned at "12 o'clock" (see Figure 9–5).

One important consideration in the design of a hearing aid with two omni-directional microphones is called "matching." The use of dual microphones as described above, assumes that the two microphones have equal sensitivity at all frequencies. Hearing aid component manufacturers generally take several measures to ensure that the sensitivities of the two microphones are sufficient and supply them to hearing aid manufacturers in matched pairs.

It also is possible for the signal processing within the hearing aid to monitor the relative sensitivities of the two microphones and adjust the electrical gain to compensate the differences in microphone sensitivity. Many digital hearing aids now employ dynamic matching that constantly compares the relative sensitivity of the two microphones. Any differences in level or response can be corrected by changing the gain or frequency response of the microphone.

TIPS and TRICKS: Clean Ports Are Critical

Because the directivity of a hearing aid depends on phase and timing differences of the sounds entering the two different ports, it is important to keep these ports clean. A port plugged with "gunk" can render an excellent directional instrument into an omnidirectional one. Directional microphone ports can be cleaned in the clinic using a vacuum pump and suctioning equipment. If you conduct a key word search at Google on "hearing aid repair equipment" you are likely to find such a system. A handy tool to have!

One concern related to microphone matching is called electronic drift, which refers to when the two microphone system is out of electronic alignment (although many hearing aids can "re-calibrate" the system). However, what is more likely to cause the microphones to be mismatched is dirt and debris that has collected in the ports. This can alter the timing of the sound reaching the microphone, which then alters directivity. This is why it is important to check the directivity of your patient's hearing aids follow-up visits, to ensure that all is working properly.

Frequency Response Equalization. Directional microphones inherently reduce low frequency output. This is referred to as an unequalized frequency response. That is, if you have gain programmed to NAL-NL2 targets in the low frequencies for the omnidirectional mode, and you then switch to the directional mode, the output will no longer match NAL-NL2 targets unless amplifier gain is altered simultaneously. The exact amount of low-frequency gain reduction varies, but typically there is a 6 dB per octave roll-off of low-frequency energy beginning around 1000 Hz. When the low-frequency response is increased to be the same (or close to) the omnidirectional response, this is referred to as an "equalized frequency response." To equalize, it is necessary to increase low-frequency amplifier gain, which can make the hearing aid sound "noisy" (only in quiet; it will not sound noisy in background noise, the situation when directional amplification would be used, as the background would be considerably louder than the amplifier noise). As we discuss later, equalization must be taken into consideration when fitting directional microphone instruments—the directionality will be less effective if audibility of the low-frequency target speech is missing.

Polar Plots (patterns).

When evaluating a minor league pitcher to determine if he has major league potential, one important question is "how fast is his fast ball?" While you can go by your own visual inspection, or the "crack" you hear when the ball hits the catcher's mitt, it's something that also needs to be measured objectively. This is accomplished using a radar gun. Directional hearing aids need to be assessed objectively too.

There are several ways to measure the directionality of hearing aids: some are conducted in the laboratory and some you conduct in the clinic. The most common laboratory method is to plot the output intensity for a 360-degree pattern for sound arriving at the microphone. These are referred to as polar plots or polar patterns. A polar plot is constructed by measuring the output of the hearing aid at several points within an imaginary sphere around the hearing aid microphone. These results are plotted relative to the output at a 0-degrees azimuth in both the horizontal and vertical planes.

Polar plots can be expressed in two ways. One way is to show polar plots for several key frequencies (.5, 1, 2, and 4 kHz), because the directivity and gain is not equal for each of them. Figure 9–5 shows a frequency-specific polar plot. Notice how each polar plot is slightly different. Another way is to average the four key frequencies together and express the polar plot as a single line. This looks similar to Figure 9–5, except the fine

separate lines on the polar plot have been averaged and plotted as a single line.

Polar patterns can be measured with the hearing aid positioned in the sound-field (e.g., attached to a microphone stand), or with the hearing aid placed in or on the ear of the KEMAR (an electronic manikin used for acoustic research). As you would predict, the field measures *without* the KEMAR are the "prettiest," as there is no shadowing or deflections, resulting in smoother curves. These are the curves often used in specification sheets (Figure 9–6A) The KEMAR curves, are somewhat more "real world" as they show how the directionality actually works on the head, which also includes the directional effects of head reflections and head shadow (Figure 9–6B). It's common for a custom instrument to be "more directional" with the KEMAR measure, as concha effects can enhance the directivity in the higher frequencies.

In general, polar patterns represent the theoretical limits of the four two-input directional microphone configurations. Look back at Figure 9–4B, which illustrates the polar patterns for four conventional directional microphone designs:

- Cardioid (upside-down heart appearance)
- Hypercardioid (more reduction from back, but not at 180 degrees)
- Supercardioid (more reduction from back, but not at 180 degrees)
- Bidirectional (figure-8 pattern).

In actual use, these patterns will be much different due to head and pinna contributions. Moreover, with most products these patterns are continually

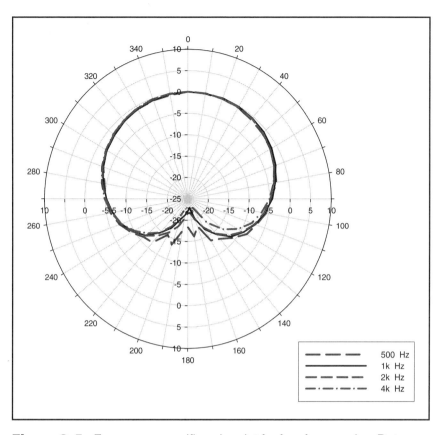

Figure 9–5. Frequency-specific polar plot for four frequencies. Data provided by Y. Wu, University of Iowa.

morphing, and at any given time the pattern may not resemble any of the patterns shown here. Consider also, that polar patterns are easily influenced by reverberation—the published ones that you are used to seeing often are obtained in an anechoic chamber.

In recent years, there have been some modification to the standard polar patterns, in an attempt to enhance overall performance with directional products.

■ Focused hypercardiod: In this pattern, in additional to the atten-

uation of sounds from the back, attenuation also is applied to sounds from the sides for the *frontal* hemisphere. This results in a narrower frontal region where sound receives maximum output centering on 0-degree azimuth.

■ Anti-cardioid pattern: In this case, the hearing aid automatically switches to an anti-cardioid (reverse cardioid) pattern when speech is from the back, background noise is present, and the overall background noise level is relative high.

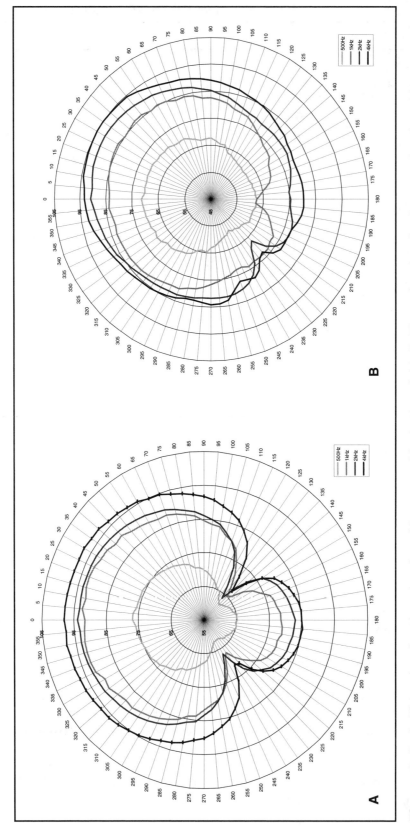

Figure 9–6. **A.** The polar plots for a hearing aid measured in the free field. **B.** The polar plots for the same hearing aid measured on the KEMAR.

TAKE FIVE:
Unique Polar Patterns

Focused hypercardiod and anti-cardioid patterns are relatively recent advances in directional microphone technology. Considering that most sounds of interest come from in front of the listener, you might wonder where a patient would benefit from the use of these newer patterns. Can you think of some common listening situations where an anti-cardioid might be beneficial?

The Directivity Index. The polar pattern can be used to calculate the hearing aid's directivity index (DI). The DI is a ratio that compares the output of the signal at 0-degree azimuth to the output of the average of all other azimuths. It will vary by frequency and usually is conducted for individual key frequencies, and then averaged to obtain a single DI value for a product. For example, a given product at 2000 Hz, with a cardioid polar pattern, might have an output of 90 dB SPL at 0-degree azimuth and 70 dB SPL at 180-degree azimuth: a front-to-back difference of 20 dB. However, if we average the output from all the measured azimuths between 0 and 360 degrees, we might find that the *average* is 85 dB SPL—the DI therefore would be 5.0 dB (90 dB minus 85 dB). The average DI when the hearing aid is placed on the KEMAR might be quite different due to microphone placement, pinna, and head shadow and head diffraction effects.

Common Directional Hearing Aid Features. There are different types of direc-

tional microphone technologies, but nearly all of today's high-end digital employ two omnidirectional microphones to accomplish the directional effect. Two features that most digital directional products have:

Automatic Switching: As mentioned earlier, the digital hearing aid, through its signal classification system, is capable of detecting the overall input level, spectrum (e.g., speech? noise? music?) and the azimuth (front? back? side?) of the sounds in the patient's listening environment. This internal digital knowledge can be used to "steer" the hearing aid toward the most suitable microphone mode.

With many directional products, the hearing aid will automatically switch to directional when the user is in a noisy situation, and will automatically switch to omnidirectional when the user is in a quiet listening environment. This feature is especially useful for those people who don't like to take the time to switch, forget to switch, or are unable to easily switch due to dexterity problems. The automatic switching algorithms vary from manufacturer to manufacturer, but usually the overall input signal needs to be ~60 dB SPL, and the signal detection system must detect noise as part of the input (e.g., there would be no reason to switch to directional if the patient was simply listening to loud speech).

Adaptive Polar Pattern: Directional hearing aids with dual microphones easily can be adjusted to different polar patterns, depending on the electronic delay that is introduced. Different patterns have polar nulls at different azimuths. With an *adaptive directional* product, the hearing aid automatically (and rapidly) samples all possible polar patterns and determines if there is one specific pattern that results in a significant lower output. If so, the system then locks on that specific algorithm and makes the necessary adjustments to the polar pattern so that maximum attenuation is given to sounds from that direction. It also can track a moving noise source (within the rear hemisphere), moving the null of the polar plot to be consistent with the location of the noise source.

As you might guess, the observed patient benefit with adaptive directional is most effective when there is only a single noise source, and there is minimal reverberation; listening to car noise on a busy street, or an air conditioner in a quiet room, for example. If there is not one specific source of noise, or the room is reverberant and the noise is bouncing around the room, the hearing aid will classify the listening situation "diffuse field" and will default to the best algorithm for that condition (usually hypercardiod).

TAKE FIVE: A Real Fish Story

Not all hearing aid patients are satisfied customers, but one of the most glowing letters from a patient that we've seen supporting adaptive directional technology came from a fellow who worked at the famous Pike Place Fish Market in Seattle. While meeting with the public in the open market area, there was a constant stream of forklifts traveling behind him unloading fresh fish. He was a long-time user of directional technology, but noticed a significant improvement in his ability to understand his customers when he switched to the new adaptive directional hearing aids. The reasons should be obvious: the customers were in front, the noise was from behind; the noise was loud enough to trigger directional processing, the noise was a true broadband noise (not other speech signals), the adaptive could track the noise, and there was little reverberation.

TIPS and TRICKS: Directional Mics and Happy Hour

Some hearing aids with directional technology have the capability to create different polar patterns for different frequency ranges, sometimes termed "multifrequency directionality." For example, if there was a low frequency noise, such as a vacuum cleaner, originating from the back of the patient, the algorithm would establish a cardiod pattern for this frequency range. If, at the same time there was a mid-frequency noise, such as a kitchen blender coming more from the side of the patient, the algorithms would establish a hypercardiod pattern for this frequency range. The actual real-world benefit of this type of processing has yet to be determined, but if you have a patient whose husband insists on vacuuming while she is blending her margaritas, this could be the product for her (although we'd recommend counseling)!

Relation Between DI and Speech Understanding. As the DI calculations are based on intensity differences between sounds arriving from the front and sounds arriving from all other directions, it seems likely that these DI measures should provide a reasonable prediction of speech understanding in noisy situations. That is, if the DI is 5 dB for one directional instrument, and 2 dB for another directional instrument, it's tempting to think that the first instrument would be 3 dB better in improving the SNR for the patient.

Although the DI is similar to an SNR improvement, it is not quite the same. The DI is a relatively good predictor of speech understanding in noisy indoor environments in which the level of the competing noise stimuli is more azimuth dependent than in outdoor environments. For mild to moderate-severe losses, and when the patient is more or less surrounded by noise, an approximate 7 to 10% improvement in speech understanding can be expected for every 1 dB improvement in the DI. For severe to profound losses a 3.5% improvement can be expected for every 1 dB of improvement. If we then look at a hearing aid that could be set in either the directional (DI = 4 dB) or the omnidirectional (DI = –2 dB), it's possible that a 42% improvement in speech understanding could occur (i.e., 6 dB improvement in DI). Importantly however, these improvement values only apply if the patient is in the ~25% to 75% portion of his speech intelligibility function.

Factors Affecting Directional Microphone Performance.

There are many factors that could prevent even the most talented athlete from reaching the major leagues. One of the proverbial stories of the "can't miss" prospect who didn't pan out is the guy who does everything—he can run, throw, and slug home runs—but he can't hit a curveball to save his life. He has all the tools, but one small flaw is exploited by competitors as he

TAKE FIVE: What Is the AI-DI?

It has been suggested that the preciseness of the DI can be enhanced by using a weighting system based on the frequency-specific importance function of speech. One method suggested is the Count-The-Dots audiogram that we discussed in Chapter 6. As you might recall, the density of the dots (frequency importance for understanding speech) is much greater in the 2000-Hz range, than at lower frequencies such as 500 Hz. It's possible then, to use a weighting system so that the DI for 2000 Hz counts more heavily toward the "average" DI than the DI for 500 Hz. This is referred to as the AI-DI. Using this method, a hearing aid with a DI of 5.0 dB at 2000 Hz and 2.0 dB at 500 Hz would have a larger average DI than a hearing aid with 2.0 dB at 2000 Hz and 5.0 dB at 500 Hz. For most hearing aids, however, the difference between the average AI-DI and the average DI are small (because most products have a similar DI at all frequencies). Most manufacturers and researchers today simply use the average DI.

TIPS and TRICKS: Can You Have a Negative DI?

It's tempting to think that omnidirectional hearing aids have a DI of 0 dB. That is, it seems logical that the absence of directivity would be "0." Unfortunately, this isn't true. The average DI typically is worse than 0 dB, except for deep fitted CIC or ITC products (which can still utilize pinna effects for directionality). BTEs, in the *omnidirectional mode*, typically have an average DI around −2 dB. This is because of the poor microphone placement (no pinna effects) and because the greatest output results from signals coming from around 45 degrees, not directly from the front. So, if a directional product only had a DI of 2.0 (which could be true of a mini-BTE OC product) it may still be 4.0 dB better than the same hearing aid in the omnidirectional mode.

---

reaches the major leagues. The same holds true for directional technology. You can have the most sophisticated directional system on the planet, but if the microphones aren't properly aligned or the vent size is not properly accounted for, the performance is significantly compromised. Maybe you can't hit the curveball either, but at least you can account for the following factors that can compromise performance of directional systems.

Venting Effects: Venting negatively affects the directivity of the hearing aid fittings. If a vent is present, low frequency sounds (<500 to 1000 Hz), such as background noise, pass through the hearing aid or earmold without being amplified. Moreover, there will be little gain in the low frequencies; it's not possible to take away gain when there is no gain!

Studies have shown that directivity is significantly reduced with increasing vent size. Consequently, maximum directivity is achieved with no vent. For obvious reasons, "no vent" is not a viable option for the majority of patients. Research has shown that vents 1 mm or less do not significantly compromise directivity for sounds below 1000 Hz.

When there is not directionality in the low frequency, the overall effects of directionality are not as obvious to the patient, and they may not have that desired "ah-ha" response when they switch to directional in your office. However, hearing aids with large vents and open-canal fittings still maintain good directionality in the higher frequencies (when there is significant gain). Behavioral research has shown that indeed this high-frequency directionality does result in improved speech recognition in noise, although not as great as if there also was a significant directional effect in the lows.

Microphone Port Alignment Effects: The impact of microphone alignment on directionality is the primary reason manufacturers request an ear impression with the horizontal plane marked when a directional microphone is ordered on a custom hearing aid. Clinical studies have demonstrated that directivity is negatively impacted with as little as a 10- to 15-degree deviation between the microphone port alignment and the horizontal plane.

Depending on the stature and posture of a hearing aid user, the horizontal plane can vary significantly for different individuals. Finding the horizontal plane for an individual with correct posture is relatively straightforward and there is little deviation from individual to individual.

However, many of our patients have affected posture due to osteoporosis and other spinal abnormalities. If this is the case for a hearing aid user, then the horizontal plane is atypical. When marking an impression you will want to be aware of typical head position for a particular user.

The lengths of earmold tubing for directional BTE hearing aids can also affect microphone alignment, thus negatively affect directionality. When fitting a directional BTE, it is important to keep the microphone ports horizontally aligned above the ear. As little as 20 degrees out of alignment can reduce the directional benefit by 0.5 dB.

Microphone port alignment can be a particular problem with the mini-BTE instruments that have become popular in recent years. One of the attractions of these products is that they are comfortable to wear and barely visible. Optimizing comfort and reducing visibility, however, can result in a placement on the ear that negatively impacts the directional effect. As with many things in the fitting of hearing aids, it's often necessary to reach a reasonable compromise.

Effects of Distance and Reverberation on Directionality: A common finding in hearing aid research is that it is difficult to predict real-world hearing aid benefit and satisfaction on an individual basis using speech intelligibility test results obtained in the clinic. Among the many factors that impact on this outcome, the acoustics of the patient's everyday listening environments is one that contributes significantly. Room acoustics relates to the way sound is propagated and perceived within an enclosed space. Room acoustics can be influenced by resonant modes, diffraction, and diffusion.

Reverberation time is the parameter commonly used to describe room acoustics, although background noise and distance from talker also are important factors in determining if communication is successful. The best possible directional microphone/digital noise-reduction hearing aids may provide little or no additional benefit in some environments. It's important, therefore, to understand the relationship among common speech signals, different listening environments, and hearing aids.

Understanding the potential benefits and limitations of directional hearing aids across a variety of listening environments is essential when counseling persons with these types of devices. It is important to advise patients that the effectiveness of directional microphones

---

TIPS and TRICKS: Alignment

Before a patient walks out the door with their new hearing aids, check to make sure the microphone ports are aligned within 15 degrees of the horizontal plane. In some cases, it might be possible to adjust the hearing aids to maximize alignment, and not reduce comfort. If the mics are not aligned, performance will be compromised. This is pretty easy to check by using real-ear measures of front-to-back performance.

will be degraded as room reverberation and speaker distance increases. Armed with this information patients can develop more realistic expectations for their instruments' performance in noise.

As a speaker moves farther from the hearing aid user, speech intelligibility in noise decreases. Also, as room reverberation increases directional benefit decreases, thus decreasing speech intelligibility in noise. For directional technology to be effective, the direct desired sound (termed "near field") reaching the microphones (e.g., the speaker's voice) must have greater amplitude that same sound which has been reflected and is reaching the same ports (termed "far field"). It's common for patients to expect that directional technology will improve their speech understanding in a place of worship, where in nearly all cases, the reflected sound is greater than the direct sound, making directional processing no better than omnidirectional.

Low-Frequency Gain. Earlier, we discussed the effects of equalizing the frequency response, Studies have shown that the equalization of the frequency response to be the most effective for hearing aid wearers with low-frequency thresholds that were poorer than 40 dB HL. Individuals with low-frequency hearing thresholds better than 40 dB HL do not tend to show an improvement in speech understanding from equalizing the frequency response—probably because in many cases their hearing is good enough to hear the low frequency speech sounds without amplification. The rule of thumb for all losses greater than 40 dB HL at 500 Hz is to always equalize (increase the gain) the frequency response in the directional mode (Figure 9–7).

Compression Effects on Directivity. The short answer is that compression has no negative effect on directionality,

---

TIPS and TRICKS:
Speech Understanding and Reverberation

The early components of reverberation combine with the direct speech signal to increase the effective signal level, but the late components of reverberation combine with background noise to increase the effective noise level. For full audibility, the average level of the effective signal needs to be 15 dB above the average level of the effective noise in the frequency range 750 to 3000 Hz. However, if the hearing aid user has less than full audibility because of noise and reverberation, the only option is to move closer to the talker, perhaps within 2 feet or less. This is sometimes a little impractical, but full audibility of the useful information is not always necessary. Speech is a highly redundant signal, meaning that there often are multiple cues for the same piece of language information. As a result, we usually can maintain intelligibility despite a significant loss of acoustic cues.

The simple message, however, is that if a hearing aid user is having difficulty because of noise or reverberation, moving closer to the talker is an obvious way of reducing those difficulties, as it will nearly always improve the signal-to-noise ratio.

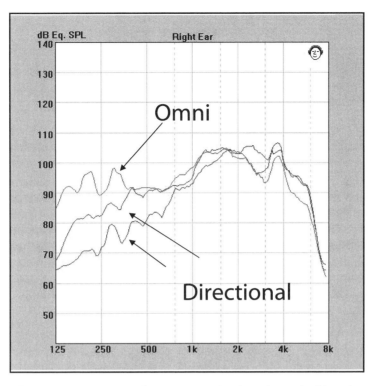

Figure 9–7. The low-frequency reduction of a typical hearing aid in the directional microphone mode (lower curve). The middle curve is the result of applying additional low-frequency gain.

but we continue anyway. If you assess directivity in your clinic or office, compression can make it appear that the hearing aid has less directionality than it really does.

An interaction between compression with low kneepoints (40 to 45 dB SPL) and directivity is possible due to the way in which directional microphones work. WDRC hearing aids provide more gain for sounds arriving from azimuths for which amplitude is reduced by the directional microphone than for those sounds arriving from azimuths for which there is little or no gain reduction. That is, the directional microphone reduced the input, but WDRC boosts it back up to some degree because it provides more gain for soft sounds. This interaction results in a reduction in the magnitude of directivity on hearing aids with low kneepoints compared to hearing aids with higher kneepoints. This simply is because in clinical testing the signals from different azimuths are not presented at the same time, as they occur in the real world. The good news is that studies have shown that compression does not affect directivity (better or worse) when it is measured in real-world listening environments in which noise is arriving at the microphone from multiple sources at the same time.

TIPS and TRICKS: Exceptions

Although directional hearing aids clearly have been shown to improve the SNR, and subsequently speech understanding when the primary talker is in front, and noise is surrounding or from behind, there are conditions when traditional directional technology may not be beneficial. One such case is when speech is not from the front, but is coming from the side or from behind, and noise is present (if noise is not present, the hearing aid would of course remain in the omnidirectional mode). Although typically, for this condition, the hearing user would simply turn his or her head, and directional technology would still be okay, there are some listening situations where turning one's head is not easily possible, or not recommended. Everyday use cases for this would be driving a car, walking side-by-side with someone in a hallway or down a street, or sitting next to someone at a conference table. In recent years, manufacturers have added some unique algorithms to assist with these types of listening situations:

Manufacturer A: As part of the hearing aids signal classification system, using modulation detection (in this case sometimes referred to as "voice activity detection") the azimuth of a speech signal is detected. If this speech signal is detected in the rear hemisphere, *and* the classification system detects that noise also is present, *and* the overall SPL meets the algorithm trigger (e.g., ~52 dB SPL), the hearing aid will automatically switch to an adaptive reverse cardioid pattern.

Manufacturer B: When the on-board signal classifier detects speech is present in one hearing aid and not the other it attempts to preserve the differences in signal-to-noise ratio between the two ears. In theory, this helps maintain important intensity and timing differences between the two ears and may enhance binaural hearing.

Manufacturer C: For a bilateral fitting, one hearing aid has a fairly "narrow beam" directionality, and the other hearing aid stays in omnidirectional.

The bottom line is that manufacturers have unique ways in which they implement automatic signal processing in their devices. It's always a good idea to ask the manufacturer representative to explain how they signal processing algorithms operate and for data from well-designed studies to support their claims.

Real-World Benefit of Directional Hearing Aids. Although laboratory studies consistently have shown significant improvement in speech understanding in background noise for hearing aids with directional microphones, less consistent benefit has been obtained in real-world use. Field trial studies suggest that the performance of directional microphones in everyday listening is highly dependent on the characteristics of the listening environment. Location of the talker, the talker's distance from the user, amount of noise, and reverberation are among the conditions that can affect directional microphone performance. These same field studies suggest that the omnidirectional mode is preferred in quiet listening environments and in the presence of background noise when the talker was not located directly in front of listener and/or when the talker was more than 10 to 12 feet from the user. The directional mode appears to be preferred when background noise was present and the talker was located in front of and/or 10 feet or closer to the hearing aid user.

One of the limitations of switchable directional microphones is that the user must manually set the microphone mode. Studies have shown that this is a problem for many patients. In one study, nearly one-third of owners of switchable products did not know how to make the manual switch between the omni and directional modes, or they knew, but simply didn't do it—a strong vote for automatic switching. In well-controlled studies, where the subjects used different types of directional technology, and also omnidirectional, but they were blinded to what technology they were using, the results favoring directional in background noise, have not been as strong as you might think. They are many variables, which we've already discussed, that can account for this.

TIPS and TRICKS: When 3 dB Matters

In addition to reverberation, and distance-from-speaker, another important factor is the relationship between the patient's performance-intensity function in noise, and the SNR of their common listening conditions. In a diffuse sound field we might expect a directional hearing aid to provide a 3 dB SNR advantage. Let's take a patient who has a performance-intensity function that is 10% at an SNR of +3 dB, is 50% at an SNR of 6 dB, and then reaches a plateau of 80% at an SNR of 9 dB. When he is sitting in Ryder at Nick's Café, where the SNR is 6 dB, he will like the 3 dB directional improvement, as it will improve his SNR by 30%. But that isn't his most important listening situation. He wants to understand all the good jokes at the K-Bar in Makoti when he plays in the Wednesday night pool league. The SNR during joke telling at the K-Bar is usually 0 dB. His directional technology will improve the SNR to +3 dB, but he still will only understand 10%! His conclusion? His hearing aids only work part of the time: they work at Nick's Café, but not at the K-Bar. The teaching point here is that directional technology only works when a 3 dB improvement matters for a given individual.

TIPS and TRICKS: A Dozen Things Your Patients Need to Know About Directional Microphone Products

This section outlines key findings, supported by peer-reviewed clinical evidence, about directional microphone technology. We've provided some strategies on how to communicate this information in a practical manner to your patients. Weaving these facts into your conversations with patients, will help you build credibility and trust.

1. When working properly, directional microphones are the only clinically proven strategy for improving the signal to noise ratio of the listening environment. For the vast majority of patients, directional microphones are an important advanced hearing aid feature.

2. Hearing aids with directional microphones have the highest overall satisfaction rating of any "high-end" feature, according to MarkeTrak survey data.

3. Both fixed and adaptive directional microphones perform equally in everyday listening situations. In other words, there is not an inherent performance advantage for the adaptive directional technology.

4. Based on the fact that at least one-third of patients either forget or do not understand how to operate the switch, automatic directional technology is easier to use and more convenient. This may translate into improved patient benefit and satisfaction.

5. Performance quality of directional microphone technology is related directly to vent size, port alignment, and low-frequency gain. These factors must be accounted for whenever possible by the diligent professional during the fitting process.

6. For every 1 dB improvement in signal-to-noise ratio, the patient can expect approximately 7 to 10% improvement in speech intelligibility for listening situations where they are performing in the 25 to 75% intelligibility range. For severe losses, 1 dB of improvement results in less improvement in speech intelligibility.

7. The patient's success with directional microphone technology is highly dependent on their ability to learn how to use the devices effectively and to situate themselves in a room in such a way that they optimize use. It is up to the dispensing professional to teach the patient how to use the directional instruments. Additionally, it is up to the dispensing professional to teach the patient to recognize listening situations in which directional technology will work well, and situations where it might fall short of expectations.

8. Because microphone ports can easily become clogged with debris, thus affecting directivity, patients are urged to return to the office at least two times per year to have the instruments tested (for directionality) and cleaned.

9. Approximately 80 to 90% of adults with aidable hearing loss will benefit to some degree from directional microphone technology, compared to conventional omnidirectional. The advantages and

limitations of adding directional mics to hearing aids will depend on the patient's hearing loss and the SNR of their common listening situations, which needs to be discussed individually with each patient.

10. The expected directional benefit will not occur when the listening situation is either too easy or too hard. This may be difficult to predict on an individual basis, as the performance intensity function for listening in noise for a given patient is difficult to predict (the results of the QuickSIN will provide a good estimate).

11. In some cases, especially those with severe SNR loss, or people with concominent cognitive problems, directional mics will not meet the signal-to-noise ratio improvement needs of the patients. In these events, personal assistive listening device technology should be discussed and demonstrated for the patient.

12. The DIs of directional products vary greatly among manufacturers, and within manufacturers for different models. Clinical evaluation of directivity is necessary.

Building Block #4: Added Convenience and Ease of Use

When a minor league player makes to it the majors, they're often asked what's the biggest difference. A common answer is: "I'm glad those long bus rides are over." Convenience is a good thing in baseball . . . and with hearing aids too!

One of the biggest challenges associated with fitting hearing aids is getting patients to actually use them. As we mentioned before, as many as 15% of people who *own* hearing aids, never use them. Over the past few years, there has been an increase in the number of features added to hearing aids that are intended to make them easier to use or more automatic. These features do not directly contribute to hearing aid benefit, but in many cases, could provide the extra "user comfort" that increases satisfaction and results in more daily use (which indirectly will lead to increased benefit).

Signal Classification

A unique feature of digital instruments is the ability to analyze the input signal, and then make decisions regarding the intensity level and spectrum of the signal. That is, within some boundaries, different signals are classified. Although this analysis varies somewhat from product to product, factors that are used to make this classification usually include:

- Overall SPL
- Frequency-specific SPL
- Modulation rate
- Modulation amplitude
- Modulation depth
- Rise and decay times

As mentioned, the sound classification system, to some extent, eliminates the need for several memories. We have already talked about several "features" (e.g., DNR, directional, etc), but in many cases, these features only work effectively if there is appropriate steering conducted by the classification system. Here are some common examples (all of which can take place without ever changing memories):

- The classification system determines that you are in a relatively noisy area, and that speech is also present: the directional microphone feature is activated.
- The classification system determines that you are in relatively loud background noise, and the dominant signal is noise (not speech): the directional microphone system is activated and the modulation-based noise reduction is turned on.
- The classification system detects that you are outside and it is windy (determined by the time it takes to travel from one inlet port to another): features to reduce wind noise can be implemented.
- The classification system detects that you are listening to music: certain parameters automatically will be adjusted.
- The classification system determines that you are in speech-in-noise, it is a trainable hearing aid, and you increase gain: the hearing aid will "remember" that you like more

gain for speech-in-noise for that input level.

The classification systems of hearing aids continue to improve each year, and in many current models, these features appear to work quite successfully. Research has shown that for many signals, like speech-in-quiet, the classification system is correct over 90% of the time. The classification systems also are quite good at detection broad spectrum noises (e.g., vacuum cleaner, air conditioner, etc).

Obviously, the hardest thing is to classify is when background *speech* becomes *"noise."* Are two talkers who are talking at the same time considered noise? Three talkers? Four talkers? And which one of the four talkers is the one you want to hear, versus the other three who are "noise"? Nothing comes close to doing this as well as the brain (well, at least most brains). This is why Mead Killion coined the term "ABONSO"— the Automatic Brain-Operated Noise Suppression Option.

Multiple Memories

It is common for most high-end digital products to have multiple memories. Nothing much different here than with

---

TAKE FIVE: Not Quite as Good as the Brain

You can think of the signal classification system as the brain of the hearing aid. Even though it's pretty smart, it's not as sharp as the human brain. For example if the signal classification system "thinks" you're listening to music and you're not, the sound of the hearing aid may abruptly change when you don't want it to. This unexpected change in the sound can be annoying to patients and can cause them to complain about their hearing aid making "funny noises" This is something to keep in mind when troubleshooting these types of complaints.

the analog products of the past, except that typically it's now considered a "standard" feature, and switching from memory to memory happens automatically with some products. With small CICs, if the memories are not accessed via remote control, the manufacturer might not offer extra memories, as placing a button on the CIC faceplate can be difficult (the memories are of course are still on the chip, just not accessed by the fitting software). As mentioned in the previous section, if the signal classification is working properly, a lot of good things can happen within a single memory automatically. However, in many cases, it's still useful to have a dedicated memory for certain types of listening, so that the user can override the automatic functioning.

As most digital products also have directional microphone technology, some manufacturers reserve a memory for this feature. Other manufacturers have the hearing aid automatically switch to directional in the same memory. In these instruments, you might want a dedicated omnidirectional memory as a back-up.

Most products also have a telecoil option that can be programmed independently, a big advantage over hearing aids of a few years ago, when the telecoil program was influenced by what was programmed in the "acoustic" program. This is a good use of a memory for many people. Some of today's products automatically switch to the T-coil memory when the phone is brought to the ear.

An additional memory can be dedicated to a "music" program. We know that a person's LDL for music is usually higher than for annoying noises, or even speech. You might want to raise the AGCo kneepoint, therefore, in the music program. We also know that it is important to hear the dynamics of music. Commonly used WDRC, especially if it is fast acting, will reduce these dynamics. Usually, then, the music program has less compression than the program dedicated to listening to speech, or speech-in-noise.

TIPS and TRICKS: There Always Are Exceptions

As we mentioned a few pages back, most of today's hearing aids have an automatic/adaptive directional microphone system. If the noise is loud enough, the hearing aid automatically switches to directional, and if the noise if from a given location, the polar pattern adaptively will lock on this noise and reduce the output. We recently heard of a patient who complained about his new hearing aids not working as well as his old ones. He found that when he went for his morning walk to get the news-paper on a country road, he could not hear the approaching cars very well—he could with his old hearing aids. The problem? The car noise was loud enough to trigger directional processing. The adaptive directional feature then locked on the noise, tracked it, and made if softer (perhaps enough to be inaudible). The hearing aids were doing exactly what they were designed to do—but the patient didn't like it. A perfect example of when a dedicated omnidirectional program is the solution.

As signal classification systems become more sophisticated, and hearing aids become more automatic, the need for memories will be less. For example, the hearing aid could automatically detect that music was present, and then automatically turn off directional technology, DNR, adjust gain, input and output compression, and so forth, all within the same memory.

Data Logging

At one time, the major league batting potential of a minor league player was mostly evaluated by looking at his batting average, runs scored, runs batted in, and home runs. Today, much is logged, so that we further examine these categories related to day games versus night games, grass versus turf, righties versus lefties, home versus away, and so on. We can do a lot of logging with hearing aids too, which we hope will help us to bring all our patients to the majors.

Recall our previous discussion of the hearing aid's signal classification system. It is constantly monitoring the input signal in an attempt to measure overall intensity of the signal, and classify the signal type. It certainly is possible for the hearing aid to store all this information, and it does. The hearing aid also can store all actions that take place: VC changes, on-off changes, use of DNR, use of directional, changes of programs, and so forth. When all this information is stored, it's called "data logging."

Like other features we have mentioned, data logging can provide an indirect benefit for the patient. Data logging can be used at different times and for various purposes throughout the fitting process. The four most common general uses appear to be: coun-

seling at the time of the fitting, routine counseling during the postfitting visits, troubleshooting patient complaints, and using data logging results to change the programming of the hearing aids (often related to hearing aid "training").

Day of the Fitting. Some dispensers include a discussion of the data logging feature as part of the hearing aid orientation on the day of the fitting. It makes sense that this would help show the patient that the two of you must work together during the adjustment period, and that the hearing aid will be recording information that will facilitate this. It alerts patients that it's important for them to take an active role in the hearing aid adjustment process. Moreover, it reminds them that these are intelligent products, which should give them some sense of security during the sometimes trying initial-use period.

Follow-Up Counseling. Many dispensers rely heavily on the data logging findings during the first postfitting visit. The logged information certainly can add an important *third* set of data for counseling when it is coupled with the objective probe-mic findings and the patient report of benefit using a self-assessment scale such as the COSI (Client Oriented Scale of Improvement). For example, how about this scenario? The post-fitting COSI tells us that the patient still can't hear his granddaughter's soft voice. Do the probe-mic findings show that we made soft speech audible? If so, does the data logging show he's using both hearing aids (or even one hearing aid)? The correct programs? The prescribed gain or VC setting? You see how it all works.

One of the first things that most dispensers look at during the post-fitting visit is the hearing aid use data. Here are examples of findings that may need explanation:

- Minimal hearing aid use: What's the problem? Poor performance? Unrealistic expectations? A change in lifestyle? Illness?
- Minimal use for only one hearing aid: Poorer performance with two versus one? Has the patient given two hearing aids a fair shot? A cosmetics issue? Uncomfortable fit?
- Much *less* use than verbally reported: Why the discrepancy? Trying to please dispenser or family members? Using a dead battery?
- Much *more* use than verbally reported: Neglecting to turn off hearing aids at night, or when not using them?
- Minimal use of additional programs: How does this compare with environment logging? Understand the purpose of the different programs? How to switch? Are all the additional programs really necessary?

Data logging also can be useful for comparing the use of different programs versus the results of environmental classification. For example, you might observe that a patient uses the "noise/directional" program 80% of the time, yet the classification results show he is in quiet 85% of the time. Why is this? Is he confused about which program to use? Does he even know which program he is using? Or is there something about the "noise" program that makes this fitting better for listening in quiet.

You'll probably be able to find the answer with a little discussion, but the topic might never have come up if data logging had been ignored. Of course, much of this assumes that the environment classification systems are correct, a topic we addressed earlier.

In some cases, using data logging is helpful in reinstructing a patient regarding some of the hearing aid features. For example, if you're fitting directional products with automatic switching between the omnidirectional and directional programs, it allows for a visual representation of what has been happening with the hearing instrument, thereby assuring the patient that the hearing aid is indeed switching to reduce background noise in response to environmental changes. Speaking of changes, it's also helpful to observe if the patient is using a VC setting that is close to the default fitting. In particular, if he is maxing out the VC range, then maybe he wasn't fitted with the right instrument, or doesn't have the best earmold plumbing.

Troubleshooting. In addition to routine counseling issues, often on the return clinic visit or during unscheduled visits, the patient has a specific problem he wants solved. Sometimes, it relates to the programming of the hearing aids, other times it concerns use and operation. The savvy dispenser eventually will solve most of these problems, but data logging often can speed things up and add new insights. This is especially true when the patient does not have all the details quite right. Patients with poor finger dexterity and/or sensitivity often believe that they are making changes when they are not, and may then infer that the hearing aid isn't working correctly. This can sometimes lead to an unpleasant confrontation during counseling. Datalogging can provide an unbiased answer.

Data logging also can help obtain a gain setting that is acceptable to the patient. Although some clinicians are pretty rigid about having their patients stay close to the gain prescribed by a validated prescriptive method, others believe that patients should choose what they like, which, for the most part, they can do with a VC. Today, however, because of the popularity of the mini-BTE OC fittings, and mini-CICs, many hearing aids are being fitted without a VC, and most patients don't want to be bothered with a remote. So, if you're a fan of "let-the-patient-decide fitting approach," how do you get the gain right? It's a common complaint on return visits.

One option is to lend the patient a remote and then use the VC data logging findings for the fixed setting. Or, if the products that were purchased didn't have data logging, you could lend the patient OC products that did, and then use the resulting logged data as a guide to program his instruments. Some instruments even allow for storing the settings for a given listening situation.

Data logging also helps you add some "evidence" to your fitting practice. It is common, for example, to fit to a given prescriptive response. This could be something like the NAL-NL2, or maybe the proprietary fitting from your favorite manufacturer. Data logging will provide real-world evidence regarding if your "first fit" is reasonably acceptable to your patients.

Changing the Fitting. Changing the fitting is a little different from routine post-fitting counseling, as we are refer-

ring to an adjustment based on information from the data logging. This could be as straightforward as adding or deleting a program, or it could involve more detailed programming changes such as altering gain, frequency response, or even compression parameters.

In several products, the software interprets the results of the data logging and gives the dispenser suggestions for possible fitting changes. The dispenser and the patient can then team up to optimize the fitting and decide what, if any, changes are needed. The key term here is "team up," as when the patient and the dispenser look at a specific graph together, and then make a decision to make a change, this has a greater impact than when it is more or less arbitrarily done by the dispenser.

Data Logging for Data Training. Data logging of course is an essential feature of trainable hearing aids, which we discuss in detail later. This could mean that a new "trained" fitting is sitting in the software, waiting for the dispenser to accept or reject it. Or, it could mean that the dispenser lets the hearing aid and the patient loose on their own, and the programming changes automatically. Although some would say we already have theoretical prescriptive methods that provide us with desired gain and output for each patient, others would contend that this is just a starting point that applies only to the "average" patient using "average" technology, and that each individual patient needs to refine the fitting in his or her own environment.

Today, data logging can record the users preferences for different listening environments (based on signal classification), for all input levels, including gain preferences for loudness and frequency response for each environment being logged. The hearing aid can then be trained to automatically reprogram to these desired setting, when the situation is detected. In other words, ongoing gain, frequency, and compression training, automatically switching to different settings for speech-in-quiet, noise, music, and so forth, all in the same hearing aid program. This certainly will be much closer to a "tailored fitting," and it seems logical that all this will increase patient satisfaction. But will it be a better fitting? Check out our section on trainable hearing aids for more on this topic.

In general, data logging seems to be a feature that most dispensers find very helpful for counseling. As audiologist Bill Heob describes it:

Data logging is a blank slate that comes to life after patients are given examples of what the graphs, charts, and percentages on the computer screen might imply. After patients understand the basic parameters from their data logs, they often view the data in a much more personal way. The data generate tangible information that allows patients to see how their personal auditory environment can be interpreted by their audiologist and how it can be incorporated into the unique programming of their sophisticated, powerful new hearing instruments.

Trainable Hearing Aids

All baseball players go to spring training in late February for six weeks of fine tuning. Today, nearly all hearing aids also have the ability to be trained. Baseball players benefit from the extra training, and in theory, your fittings benefit from it as well. Think of it this way, during the off season, one baseball player spends all his time hunting, fishing, and hanging out at cool bars in Hawaii. The second fellow spends his time working out, watching videos of his previous at bats, and in the batting cage. Who do you think will have a more successful season? Of course, the guy who actually did the training will have a better year (although Babe Ruth and Mickey Mantle may have been exceptions to this rule). Patients that appropriately train their hearing aids are likely to be more successful, and most probably more satisfied with the fitting.

As briefly mentioned in the preceding section, what has developed in the past few years is hearing aids that can "learn" regarding the information that has been gathered with data learning. That is, let's say that you fit a patient

---

TAKE FIVE: The Female Perspective

Although data logging sounds like a pretty good thing, a recent survey revealed that about 30% of dispensers don't use it. The same study, by looking at demographic data, examined why it seems to be embraced by some, and shunned by others. Although many aspects of the dispensers profile were examined (e.g., audiologist vs. dispenser, years experience, education, age, etc.) only one factor was significant: gender. Females tend to use data logging more than males do. Noted Pittsburgh audiologist Catherine Palmer provided an explanation of this at a recent meeting: "Women like to tell you what to do, and then check up on you to see if you are really doing it."

with gain consistent with NAL-NL2 targets. BUT, we know that the standard deviations for the "average person" are around ±5 dB (that is, target is really a "range" not a precise number). Your patient is one of those who just happens to like 4 dB below target. So what happens when he uses his hearing aids is that he, on average, turns gain down 4 dB. If you prefer, you can have the hearing aid "learn" this and *automatically* reset the start-up gain to be 4 dB lower.

The first generation of products only had learning for overall gain, but now we have products that also can learn frequency response, microphone strategy, and compression; that is, going back to our previous example, if the patient only turned down gain 4 dB for loud, but not soft, the hearing aid wouldn't change overall gain, but a bigger ratio would be learned. The end result then would be the same gain for soft and average, but less gain for loud.

Trainable hearing aids can be either time based or event based, and both types are available among manufactures. With time based, the hearing aid takes a "snapshot" every minute or so, and stores the gain setting, the listening environment and the SPL. This is then averaged over many days. With event based, learning only occurs when a change is made, and again everything is stored at the time of that event. There are some advantages and disadvantages of each of these training models; in most cases similar results are obtained.

Another aspect of trainable hearing aids that potentially could lead to direct patient benefit is specific learning for different listening environments. That is, within the same program, gain changes, and frequency response changes are paired with the level of the input signal, and the classification of the input signal. This is how it would work. Let's say that you fit your patient to NAL-NL2 targets for Program #1. He goes out and uses his hearing aids and finds that he needs soft speech about 3 dB louder (average and loud speech inputs are okay), and he also needs another 3 dB for the frequencies above 2000 Hz. Any time noise is louder than about 75 dB SPL, he turns down gain 5 dB (on average; gain is okay for noise inputs less than this). He likes his music pretty loud, and he always turns the gain up about 5 dB for music. Within a short period of time, whenever one of these environments is detected, the hearing aids automatically will adjust to his preferred settings. And this all happens within the same program.

This all sounds pretty impressive, but will this always result in a better fitting? How do you define "better"? Should the training of the hearing aid be limited to ensure some minimal level of benefit? Some say this training will help with acclimatization. But, to state the obvious, the brain can't acclimatize to sounds that aren't audible. Consider this example. You've just fitted hearing aids on a 70-year-old man with a high-frequency loss of 50 to 60 dB in the range of 2000 to 4000 Hz. He's a new user. You know he needs audibility for soft sounds, so you give him 30 dB or so of gain for soft inputs in the 2000 to 4000-Hz range. His hearing aids are trainable, and can be trained independently for different input levels and different frequency regions. To no one's surprise, he doesn't like hearing these new high-frequency sounds, and he soon trains his hearing aids to provide little or no gain in this frequency region.

What's left is an ear canal output that more or less mimics his real-ear unaided response. Again, to no one's surprise, he thinks this sounds "normal." He returns to your office after two weeks and is "happy as a clam." You're happy because he's happy. The manufacturer is happy because you're happy. It's a happy world. Well, sort of.

Research has shown that the starting point of the training can influence the ending point. In one study, when patients were started 6 dB over NAL targets, their ending point was 2 dB above target. When the same patients were started 6 dB below target, they remained 6 dB below. An 8 dB difference for preferred gain, *for the same patients*!

In another study, patients who were experienced users, and on average had been using gain 10 dB below target for soft speech, were all fitted to NAL targets. They were using instruments with compression training, so they clearly could have trained gain to resemble their old fitting. They did not: their trained gain was nearly identical to NAL targets for soft inputs. These studies clearly show that training can be influenced by the starting point, and therefore it is important to use a reasonable starting point for all training. Moreover, the training should be monitored so that a patient would not unknowingly significantly reduce speech understanding while trying to maximize listening comfort.

Automatic Acclimatization. Another feature that more or less fits under the "trainable" umbrella is what is called "automatic acclimatization." We've addressed acclimatization several times in preceding chapters. The general notion is that many new hearing aid users need some time listening to the signals

their brain had forgotten about, before the brain can use these signal most effectively. Providing the user these signal on Day #1 may be a bit too much, however, and lead to hearing aid rejection. Some dispensers have the patient come back at periodic intervals and gradually increase gain. On the other hand, if the patient returns happy, do you really want to bump up gain and make him unhappy? A compromise is automatic acclimatization.

As the name indicates, the hearing aid can be programmed so that the gain of the instrument can increase at a prescribed amount over a prescribed time frame. For example, you could fit a patient 5 dB below the NAL-NL2 target and then have the acclimatization feature increase 1 to 2 dB per week until the desired gain setting was obtained. This option is relative new, so we're not too sure how it will interact with the training of the hearing aid. Who knows . . . the one feature might raise gain the desired 5 dB whereas the other feature will train it back down where it was in the beginning.

Wireless Connectivity

The history of "wireless" transmissions dates back to the 19th century. One of the most notable experiments was conducted by Nicola Tesla, who is credited with developing alternating current and radio transmission technology. Tesla demonstrated "the transmission of electrical energy without wires" that depends upon electrical conductivity as early as 1891. The Tesla effect (named in his honor) is a term for an application of this type of electrical conduction. Tesla orchestrated the most impressive display of wireless technology in the late

1800s at Colorado Springs, Colorado. Using what he called "terrestrial stationary waves," he lighted 200 lamps without wires from a distance of 25 miles.

In general, today we usually think of "wireless" as a radio frequency or electromagnetic signals that carry some type of communication signal over a desired pathway. In recent years, wireless communication has become common place for both commercial and home use, ranging from garage door openers to computer peripherals, from global positioning systems (GPS) to satellite television transmission, and, of course, the wireless device most of us are the most familiar with, the cellular telephone. Although the total grows significantly daily, it recently was estimated that there are over four billion cell phones in use in the world.

A wireless technology, introduced in 1998, that is rapidly growing in use is the Bluetooth protocol. Bluetooth is radio technology for exchanging data over short distances and developing personal area networks. It is commonly used to connect and exchange information between devices such as GPS receivers, computers, cameras, video games, stereo headsets, MP3 players, and, of course, mobile telephones (Figure 9–8). Bluetooth technology allows for wireless, streaming use of cellular phones, making them more practical, convenient, and safer. Nearly all cell phones sold have Bluetooth, and it's estimated that the majority of new cars sold will have Bluetooth as a standard or optional feature.

It is not surprising that over the years, wireless technology also found its way into the hearing aid industry. Recall that we discussed the telecoil and other induction loop systems in

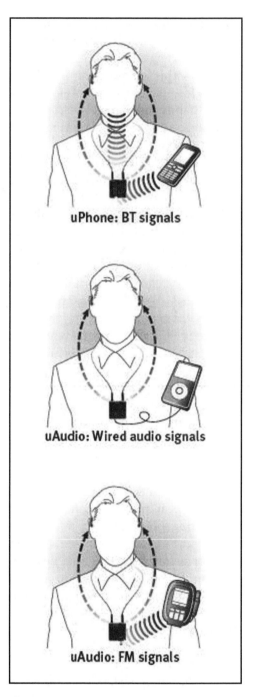

Figure 9–8. An example of a wireless gateway device using Bluetooth transmission with a cell phone, MP3 player, and remote control. Reprinted with permission from Unitron, all rights reserved.

Chapter 8. Another common use of wireless technology with hearing aids for the past 30 years has been FM transmission, a wireless application often used with hearing-impaired children. This is an effective method of overcoming the negative effects of background noise and talker distance, resulting in an improvement in the signal-to-noise ratio at the listener's ear. In this chapter, we discuss two new areas of wireless connectivity that commonly are being implemented in today's technology.

Hearing Aid to Hearing Aid Communication. In 2004, wireless transmission was introduced which used magnetic transmission to communicate between the two hearing instruments, and also between hearing instruments and an optional remote control accessory. This wireless connection enables the right and left hearing instruments to work together in a harmonized system. The input obtained from both instruments is shared so that important decisions concerning signal processing are based on this combined intelligence, which allows for symmetric steering of important functions such as digital noise reduction and directional technology. The notion is that with the analysis from both hearing aids, the signal classification system will be more effective. This communication is also important for receiving Bluetooth transmissions (which we discuss shortly), as a single signal can be delivered bilaterally to the user.

User commands regarding VC adjustment and program selection are also transmitted wirelessly between hearing aids, maintaining symmetric function and optimizing day-to-day user efficiency. This is especially help-ful when smaller hearing aids, such as mini-CICs, are used. For example, using only a single button on the hearing aid, a person could have a VC bottom on the right hearing aid, and a program button on the left hearing aid; pressing either button would change the volume or the program in both hearing aids simultaneously. The connectivity is also helpful for people who only have good dexterity with one hand. They can operate both hearing aids using only one control.

TAKE FIVE: Ear to Ear

Wireless communication between hearing aids uses near field magnetic induction (NFMI). Similar to a telecoil, NFMI has a limited transmission range, so it works well for ear-to-ear communication between hearing aids, but not for other applications.

Bluetooth Applications. Working together with, and complementing the hearing aid to hearing aid wireless function is the recent introduction of Bluetooth technology in hearing aids. This can be used with a wide range of hearing instruments and has been designed to connect hearing-impaired listeners to the world of modern communication technology.

Using Bluetooth as a streaming device, the hearing aid user can connect to his cell phone, television, stereo system, MP3 player, or other audio products. The end result of using Bluetooth transmission is that the signal-to-noise ratio of the listening situation has been improved. In other words, the microphone is placed closer to the sound source and Bluetooth is used to transmit the signal directly to the amplifier and receiver in the hearing aid. Figure 9–8 shows some examples of how Bluetooth transmission works with various consumer electronics paired with hearing aids. Notice in Figure 9–8 that the patient has to wear the device around his neck, although this is not necessary for many systems. The streamer or gateway device allows the consumer electronic device to "connect" with the hearing aid using Bluetooth as the transmission signal.

TIPS and TRICKS: Transmission Signals

Recently, some manufacturers have introduced wireless features that do not use a streamer or gateway device. When a 2.4-GHz or 900-MHz band is used a streamer is not needed, and the signal can be transmitted directly to the hearing aid. This can be a nice advantage as you don't need to wear or carry an extra device. There are some disadvantages associated with the wireless devices using a 2.4-GHz or 900-MHz transmissions signal. As the world of wireless connectivity in hearing aids is rapidly evolving, we will let you sort of the pros and cons of the various transmission signals with your manufacturer's representative.

In Situ Testing

Okay—we made it to our last feature! First, let us say that we not too fond of

this term, as some people call probemic measurements in situ testing (in situ means something like "in place" or "in place of"—our Latin isn't too good). But it's the best term we have, and is commonly used, so we use it. What we are referring to is the use of the hearing aid to deliver signals to the ear, which then requires a response from the patient. To some extent, the hearing aid is being used in place of an audiometer, although most would recommend it as a supplemental measure, as all standards and guidelines require a hearing test conducted by a calibrated audiometer. This technique currently is used to estimate thresholds, loudness levels, or LDLs, but also could be used to present speech material, or conduct special tests such as gap detection or the TEN test. The reason we have this feature listed in this category is that it could indirectly lead to improved patient benefit.

We talked about this in Chapter 7, but one of the problems of fitting hearing aids is that we continually are required to go back and forth between dB HL, dB SPL (re: the real ear) and dB SPL (re: the coupler). The advantage of using the hearing aid as the tone generator is that we have eliminated one of the variables—the residual volume of the ear canal. The problem of course is that the stimulus is a digital signal, we don't have an audiometer dial in HL. How would you like to tell your patient, your hearing threshold changed from "1001 to 1110" to "1001 to 1110"! So manufacturers need alogrithms that can take these digital measures and relate it to their fitting software. Some have done this, others haven't, but nearly all digital products have the capabilities of doing the testing.

In general, in situ testing seems like a good idea; however, it has been around now for several years, and hasn't really caught on as many people thought it would. Recently, advancements in this area have been hearing aids that are coupled to a probe in the ear, so a direct reading can then be taken from the signal delivered by the hearing aid. The fitting algorithm can then compare this to "average" or to what would be obtained in a 2-cc coupler, and make changes to the fitting. The question, of course, is, does all this really lead to a better fitting? To date, there has not been independent research to answer this question.

In Closing

So, there you have it: Ten or more special hearing aids features, added to the basic ones we discussed in Chapter 8. A lot to think about. Notice that some of these features are specifically designed to improve speech understanding and/or reduce background noise. Other features are geared more toward improving the overall "hearing aid experience" by making hearing aids more "hands free," flexible, and easier to use. Yet, some other features are there to help us do a better job in the fitting and counseling process.

When dispensing hearing aids, it is common to use many of these features to categorize hearing aids products from "Entry-Level" to "Mid-Level" to "Premier" (or whatever three terms you prefer to use). Obviously, if a pair of Premier hearing aids cost $1000 more than Mid-Level products, then you owe it to the patient to explain what they obtained (relative to benefit) for the extra $1000. If there is no logical explanation, then perhaps the Mid-Level products are okay for that specific patient.

Fitting a hearing aid with advanced features rather than one without them is a little like the difference between hearing the "crack" of a wood bat compared to the "ping" of an aluminum bat. In order to save money, in college they use aluminum rather than wood bats. If you're a baseball fan, you'd agree that the "ping" just doesn't sound like baseball. Advanced features are the same way. They may cost more, but it's probable they will result in a more authentic experience for your patient.

10

Hearing Aid Fitting Procedures

> *The selection and fitting of hearing aids is a lot like taking an airline trip. This one is headed to a fun place, and we'll be taking off before you know it! Sit back and get ready for the ride.*

In this chapter we review the necessary steps to actually *fit and dispense* a pair of hearing aids. This appointment, which is commonly referred to as the hearing aid delivery or fitting, takes about one-hour (maybe longer when you are getting started) of face-to-face time with the patient. There are a few tasks, however, that you need to do well in advance to ensure that this appointment goes smoothly.

Because we are fitting digitally programmable hearing aids, we often can take a "one-size-fits-all" approach. This means that any single hearing aid can fit a wide range of different audiogram configurations. All you need to do is fine tune or adjust the acoustic parameters (gain, output, compression) with computer software. This might sound easy, but it isn't. You need to know when and how to make these adjustments,

keeping your patient involved in the adjustment process.

To really understand how to program a hearing aid we need to start with some underlying philosophy. Once you know the starting point you will have a better chance of making the correct adjustments to the gain, output, or compression of any modern hearing aid. Typically, we use a starting point that is data driven; this often is referred to as a "prescriptive fitting approach." Once you've determine *what* you want, then it's necessary to determine if it's being delivered in the patients ear canal. This is where verification comes in. There are many different ways to *verify* hearing aid performance but, clearly, probe-microphone measures are the most valid and reliable. And, then, once the fitting is verified, a comprehensive orientation is needed. Finally, you'll need to be prepared to deal with troubleshooting some fitting problems that might come up, and provide the adjustments or fitting changes that offer solutions.

But, before all this fitting, verification, and troubleshooting occurs, the first step is to ensure that the hearing aids are working properly. This happens *before* the patient arrives, and involves 2-cc coupler testing.

Quality Control: 2-cc Coupler Measures

Ever try to board an overseas flight, or even cross the border between the United States and Canada without a valid passport? Just like you have to "get things in order" prior to your flight, you also have to prepare for your hearing aid fitting by ensuring that the hearing aid is working according to manufacturer's specifications.

Hearing aids are measured in a coupler long before they are placed on an actual ear. The 2-cc coupler has been used for over 60 years to measure hearing aid performance, and this device is the industry standard. It's important to point out again that the residual volume of the ear canal (when a hearing or earmold is in place) is *not* really 2-cc, and the impedance characteristics of the ear canal is not really the same as the steel coupler. Therefore, we would not expect that coupler gain and output will be the same as what is obtained in the real ear, and that is not the intended purpose. However, because the coupler is convenient and standardized, it is the ideal way to ensure that hearing aids are performing at a certain standard, and in the manner intended by the manufacturers. It is always possible that some-

thing was damaged during shipping, or that a given hearing aid somehow slipped through the manufacturer's quality control process. Moreover, as we discuss in a later section, coupler measurements are an excellent way to determine if the hearing aid is working as intended on follow-up visits—you will need a baseline for comparison.

Test Equipment for Coupler Testing

The following section regarding 2-cc coupler measures was partially adapted from the Audioscan Verifit User's Guide Version 3.4 and the Fonix 8000 Operator's Manual 2.0. These, of course, are only two of the seven or eight manufacturers of this type of equipment. Most of the instrumentation and measures we discuss, however, apply to all 2-cc coupler testing, regardless of manufacturer. It's important that you obtain a copy of the user's guide for the equipment that you are using to clarify specific details.

As shown in Figure 10–1, 2-cc coupler testing is conducted in a sound enclosure, commonly referred to simply as a "test box." These test boxes come in slightly different sizes and shapes, but all must meet the standards of ANSI S3.22. Within the test box, a loudspeaker presents the desired calibrated signal to the hearing aid; there is a regulating microphone to ensure the signal is presented at the desired level. Different types of input signals can be used, although for most measures, swept pure tones are utilized. The hearing aid is connected to a coupler, which in turn is connected to a measurement microphone to assess the hearing aid

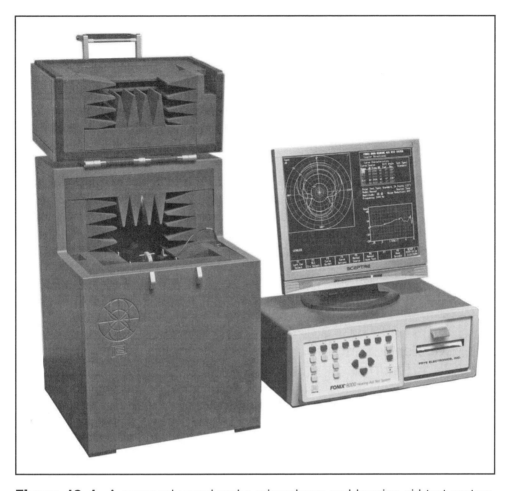

Figure 10–1. A commonly used probe microphone and hearing aid test system. The test box is on the left. Photo reprinted with the permission of Frye Electronics, Inc., Tigard, OR.

output. Standard couplers are shown in Figure 10–2.

■ **HA-1 2-cc Coupler:** Dimensions per ANSI S3.7 for testing in-the-ear aids, canal aids, and aids fitted with earmolds.

■ **HA-2, 2-cc Coupler:** Dimensions per ANSI S3.7 for testing behind-the-ear aids, eyeglass aids, and body aids.

■ **Ear-Level Adapter (BTE):** Snaps into the 1/4″ (6.35 mm) diameter cavity of the HA-2 coupler.

Equipped with a 0.6″ (15 mm) length of 0.076″ (1.93 mm) ID tubing, the adapter allows ANSI S3.22 specified connection of an ear-level aid to the coupler.

■ **Open Coupler:** Used for testing open canal (OC) instruments; however it is not a standard 2-cc coupler and should not be used to compare to manufacturing specifications

■ **CIC Coupler:** Used for testing CIC instruments. Like the OC coupler, it

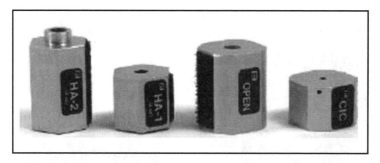

Figure 10–2. The most commonly used 2-cc couplers used clinically. Photo reprinted with the permission of Frye Electronics, Inc., Tigard, OR.

should not be used to compare manufacturing specifications.

TIPS and TRICKS: Coupler/Hearing Aid Pairings

In general, you will test certain style hearing aids with certain couplers—the BTE with the HA-2, for example. This is important so that you can compare your results to manufacturer's specs. However, don't feel bound by these rules when you are troubleshooting problems. For example, if you have concerns that the tubing may be pinched inside of the earmold, don't hesitate to run the BTE instrument (with its earmold connected) using the HA-1 coupler—as you would a custom instrument.

It's important to associate a given coupler with the hearing aid style. In general, you will conduct coupler testing for four different types of hearing aids. Listed below are the four types, and the coupler pairings that you normally will use:

- **BTE** instruments are coupled to the HA-2 coupler by means of a 10-mm (3/8th ") length of heavy wall #13 earmold tubing. The only purpose of this tubing is to seal the tip of the earhook to the coupler inlet. All of the tubing required by ANSI S3.22 is machined into the metal stem of the HA-2 coupler. The #13 tubing should be inspected regularly for cracks that will cause feedback. If you specifically want to see the effects of the earmold plumbing, it is possible to couple the BTE-with-earmold to an HA-1 coupler.

- **Custom** instruments are sealed to the HA-1 coupler with putty so that the end of the eartip is flush with the inside of the coupler opening. Putty should not extend into the coupler cavity or block the sound outlet of the instrument. *Vents should be sealed at the face plate end.* It is very important that the instrument be well sealed to the coupler.

- **Open Fit** instruments with thin tubing and dome plumbing must use the coupler and coupling system specified by the manufacturer. This may involve a hook that replaces the open fit slim tubing or an adapter tube that may be sealed to the opening of the HA-1 coupler with putty. The OC coupler can also be used.

■ **RIC (Receiver-in-the-canal)** instruments are coupled to the HA-1 coupler using putty to seal the receiver module or soft tip to the coupler opening. The OC coupler can also be used.

When conducting testing, you also will use battery substitution pills. They are used to power hearing aids, measure battery drain, and estimate battery life. The standard sizes are 675/76, 13, 312, and 10A/230. The *thin connecting strip* of each battery pill is *fragile*. When inserting pills into the hearing instrument battery compartment, take care that this strip is not pinched or bent severely as the battery door is closed. The general procedure is:

1. Select a battery pill that is appropriately sized for the hearing instrument that you are testing.
2. Insert the pill into the hearing instrument, carefully closing the battery door over the thin connecting strip.
3. Plug the pill's cable into the battery pill jack.
4. Turn the hearing instrument on.

Coupler Measures And The Real Ear

Manufacturers rely on 2-cc coupler measures during the quality control process because they are standardized. Every hearing aid made can be tested using the same cavity and test protocol.

As mentioned earlier, there can be some large differences, however, between the hearing aid response in a 2-cc coupler and an actual human ear. Using average data, we can make some reasonable predictions about the differences between the gain obtained in 2-cc coupler and in real ears. This is referred to as the COupler Response for Flat Insertion Gain (CORFIG). This term, coined by Mead Killion, can be thought of as a "correction factor" used to calculate the difference between the coupler and real-ear gain. The correction is not the same for all styles of hearing aids (due primarily to the microphone location), and there are no "standard" CORFIGs. You don't need to be an expert on all this, but here are the three components of the CORFIG, and a brief explanation of why they are important for determining the overall correction factor:

■ Unaided ear effects, termed real-ear unaided gain (REUG): A person usually losses their natural ear canal resonance and pinna effects when a hearing aid or earmold is placed in the ear. The coupler does not (the hearing aid does not go *inside* the coupler). This has the biggest impact in the 2000 to 4000-Hz range. **Advantage Coupler**.

■ Residual volume effects: When a hearing aid or earmold is placed in the ear, the residual volume is reduced well below 2-cc, which results in an increase in ear canal SPL (check out Boyles law from Chapter 2). The coupler, of course remains at 2-cc (hence the name!). This has an effect across all frequencies, but slightly larger for the higher frequencies. **Advantage Real Ear**.

■ Microphone location effects: When the microphone of a hearing aid is placed in the concha, or at the entrance of the ear canal, there is a boost in output because of pinna/concha effects. For coupler measures, the microphone always is placed in the same calibrated position. **Advantage Real Ear**.

So, to summarize the CORFIG, if the advantage for microphone location (most prominent in the high frequencies) and reduced residual volume exceeds the loss of the REUG, gain in the real ear will be greater than gain in the coupler. If the microphone location does not take advantage of pinna effects (a BTE fitting), and the residual volume is not significantly reduced, then coupler gain will be greater than real-ear gain. Keep in mind that we are talking about differences in gain. If you're interested in differences in output, that's a different correction (more on that a little later). But never fear, if you always measure real-ear gain and output with your probe-mic equipment, you really don't have to worry about this! It is good, however, to have a general idea of what probably will happen in the real ear when you see a coupler response curve.

The Hearing Aid Specification Sheet

So, you're taking a trip? Fortunately, the data about your trip are stored. Best to print out your itinerary so that you have all the times correct. You may need to refer to it often. We also need to know some facts about hearing aids: it's called the "spec sheet."

Now that we've covered some of the descriptors of coupler measures, let's turn our attention to the hearing aid specification sheet, or simply, "the spec sheet." No matter what type or style of hearing aid being fitted, a spec sheet is required to be sent with the hearing aid by the manufacturer.

The American National Standards Institute (ANSI) determines the data that must be reported on the spec sheet. The ANSI S3.22 1996 standards are currently used. (There is another similar standard in Europe called IEC.) The 1996 standard has been revised, now the S3.22-2003, which can be used as an option. The differences between the two standards are not too significant regarding the basic measures and a summary of the differences are shown in Figure 10–3.

ANSI S3.22-2003 has been designated a recognized standard by the FDA but is not yet mandatory. Manufacturers may use either version for reporting test data. The most significant change from the 1996 version is the requirement for the hearing aid to be set in its most linear mode for the setting of the gain control to Reference Test Setting (changed from Reference Test Position) and for all tests except attack and release and input-output (I/O) curves. These two tests are to be conducted with the AGC function set for maximum effect. The AGC test sequence will pause to allow AGC to be set prior to measuring attack and release time. Full-on gain is determined with 50 dB input SPL (60 dB was formerly an option) and frequency response curves are run at 60 dB SPL for Linear and AGC aids. The ANSI S3.22 2009 standard also has been released, but is not in common use at this time.

| Tests defined in the standard | Differences in Standards | |
	1996	2003
Full on gain (HFA FOG)	run at 50 or 60 dB SPL	run at 50 dB SPL
Maximum output (HFA OSPL90)	AGC set by mfg suggestion	AGC set to min effect
Frequency response	at 50 or 60 dB SPL	at 60 dB SPL
Equivalent input noise	gain at 60 dB SPL	gain at 50 dB SPL
Harmonic distortion	AGC set by mfg suggestion	AGC set to min effect
Battery drain	AGC set by mfg suggestion	AGC set to min effect
Telephone coil sensitivity	AGC set by mfg suggestion	AGC set to min effect
AGC input/output	AGC set by mfg suggestion	AGC set to max effect
AGC attack and release time	AGC set by mfg suggestion	AGC set to max effect

Figure 10–3. A hearing aid data sheet. It is provides an example of the ANSI S3.22 1996 standard governing the specifications of hearing aid characteristics. These measures are calculated by the hearing aid manufacturer and reported on each hearing aid spec sheet. On the left-hand side of the figure, nine separate hearing aid characteristics are listed.

The following are the measures that you will be the most concerned with:

1. OSPL90—This is a measure of maximum power output. It is reported as both a peak measure and high frequency average measure (HFA) by taking the average output at 1000, 1600, and 2500 Hz.
2. Gain—There are three separate measures of gain reported on the ANSI '96 spec sheet. Both the peak and HFA gain for a 70 dB SPL input are reported. In addition, reference test gain for an input of 60 dB is reported.
3. Total Harmonic Distortion (THD) —This is measured by putting a pure tone signal into the hearing aid and analyzing the resulting amplified sound wave. An artifact resulting from the amplification of this signal would be classified as distortion. On the spec sheet THD is measured with three different pure tones (500 Hz with a 70 dB input, 800 Hz with a 70 dB input, and 1600 Hz with a 60 dB input). THD is expressed as a percentage. A percentage score of 1% or less is acceptable.
4. Automatic Gain Control (AGC)— Both the attack time (when input signals become compressed) and the release time (when the input signal is no longer being compressed) are recorded.
5. T-coil—Two measures of telecoil performance are recorded. Simulated telephone sensitivity (STS) and sound pressure level of the inductive telephone simulator (HFA SPLITS). STS describes how much the user has to increase the volume control so that the volume with the telecoil is the same as the volume through the microphone. The first term (STS) applies to

telephone use, and the second to looped room use. In the example in Figure 10–4, telecoil performance is depicted in the bottom family of curves, labeled Induction Coil Sensitivity.

6. Equivalent Input Noise (EIN)— As microphones and receivers generate internal noise, this needs to be quantified and reported. The EIN captures this noise by measuring the magnitude of the noise

	Next 16 Slim Tube (optional)	Next 16	Next 16 P (power)	Next 16 HP (high power)	
ANSI S3.22-1996 /IEC 118-7 2CC COUPLER TECHNICAL DATA					
Reference Test Frequency ANSI IEC 118-7	HFA 2.5 kHz	HFA 1.6 kHz	HFA 1.6 kHz	HFA 1.6 kHz	
OSPL90 Maximum HFA at RTF	124 dB 108 dB 109 dB	125 dB 122 dB 121 dB	130 dB 125 dB 123 dB	135 dB 128 dB 125 dB	
Full on Gain (input 50 dB) Maximum HFA at RTF	53 dB 37 dB 37 dB	60 dB 52 dB 51 dB	70 dB 60 dB 57 dB	75 dB 65 dB 61 dB	
Basic Frequency Response Frequency Range (Hz) Reference Test Gain (ANSI 1996)	100-6300 30 dB	100-5900 45 dB	100-5600 48 dB	100-5600 51 dB	
Induction Coil Sensitivity (ANSI 1996, 31.6 mA/m) HFA SPLITS STS	89 dB -1 dB	104 dB -1 dB	108 dB 0 dB	111 dB 0 dB	
Current Drain at RTG	1.1 mA	1.2 mA	1.7 mA	2.2 mA	
Typical Battery Life	265 h	245 h	170 h	132 h	
Equivalent Input Noise at RTG	28 dB	20 dB	20 dB	20 dB	
Total Harmonic Distortion at 500 Hz at 800 Hz at 1600 Hz	1% 1% 1%	4% 2% 1%	1% 1% 1%	2% 2% 1%	

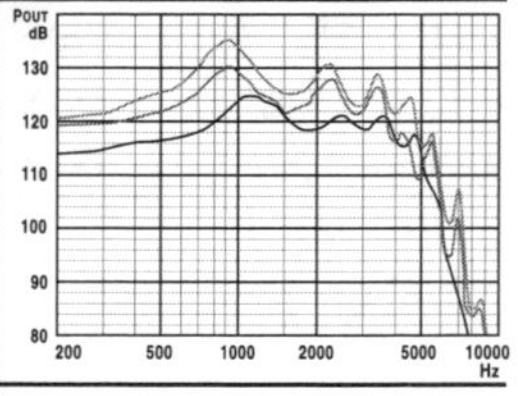

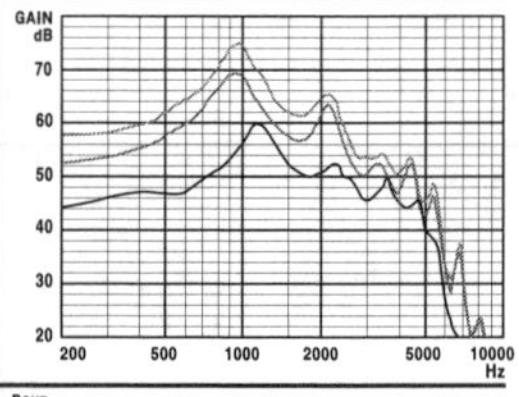

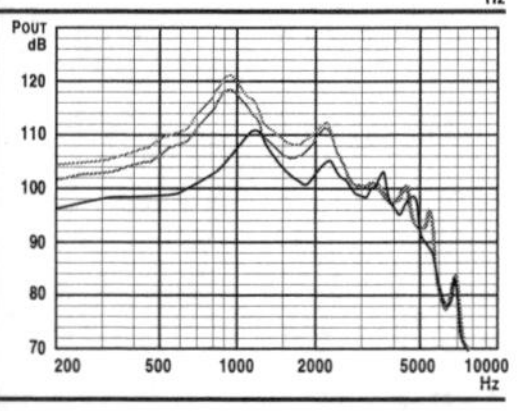

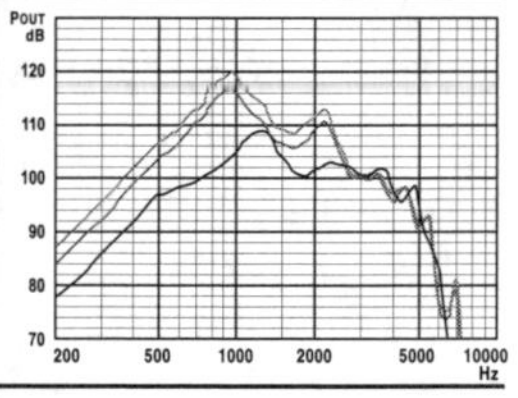

Figure 10–4. An example of a hearing aid specification sheet, using ANSI S3.22 1996 test results. Reprinted with the permission from Unitron, all rights reserved.

at the output of the hearing aid and then subtracting the gain of the hearing aid. In this example, there are two types of EIN reported, as one measure is completed with a 50 dB input and the other with a 60 dB input. There are many factors that determine the EIN result, as a rule of thumb this measure should be lower than 30 dB.

7. Drain—This is a measure of battery drain and it measured by using a battery pill. The single number measure, expressed in milliamps, reflects how much current is being drawn from the battery into the hearing aid.

8. Frequency Range—This is the range of frequencies between the lowest and highest frequencies where gain is 20 dB below the HFA gain.

Figure 10–4 shows how all these measures are displayed by the hearing aid manufacturer on the "spec sheet."

Figure 10–4 shows several 2-cc coupler curves for four models of a BTE hearing aid from a single manufacturer. All of the curves, with the exception of the bottom family of curves are measured using a 2-cc coupler and a pure-tone signal. The top family of curves represents the output for a 90-dB SPL input. The family of curves that are second from the top represent full-on gain measures for a 50 dB SPL input signal. Also shown are a family of curves, labeled Basic Frequency Response, which is the usable frequency of the instrument. Finally, there is another family of curves, labeled Induction Coil Sensitivity, which show the specifications for the telecoil on the instrument. As you can see, there is a lot of information on the spec sheet, and you actually could use your hearing aid test box to verify all of them. However, we advise you to pick out a couple of measures, perhaps full-on gain and OSPL90, and routinely measure them prior to the fitting. When you measure them, be sure to use the same intensity level for the input signal as shown on the spec sheet.

So far, we mostly have talked about using 2-cc coupler measures to ensure

---

TIPS and TRICKS: More On the "Spec Sheet"

As we've mentioned, there is a lot of useful 2-cc coupler information contained on the spec sheet that you will find shipped with each hearing aid. For custom products, the sheet shows the 2-cc coupler results for the very aid that you have in your possession. It is different for BTE products, however. What you usually will obtain is the "standard" specs for that particular model, but not necessarily that particular hearing aid. We assume that the aid was tested, and met the ANSI ± tolerances, and therefore, what you will measure should be very similar to the standard specs. In the case of an RIC or thin-tube product, it's possible that the standards specs were run using a tone hook and tubing, which of course would be different from what you would obtain running the product in an HA-1 coupler.

TAKE FIVE:
Okay, Are You Ready to Conduct Some Measurements?

Here's your assignment:

- Take a new hearing aid out of the box and locate its spec sheet. As it's a requirement for manufacturers to enclose it with all new orders, you should have no trouble finding it.
- Get familiar with the hearing aid test box and all the associated equipment. Print out the online manual, as there will be several good illustrations.
- Put in the battery pill.
- Attach the hearing aid to the appropriate coupler, and position it correctly in the test box.
- Ensure that the vent is sealed off at the canal tip with fun-tack (putty).
- Set the hearing aid to the full-on volume position. To do this, you have to attach the hearing aid to the programming computer using a Hi-Pro box and/or a NOAHLink.

- All adjustments are set in the neutral position (no reduction of response). All fitting software has a "test mode" that shuts off all automatic features.
- Conduct the following tests and then carefully observe if your measurements are the same at the ones from the manufacturer:
  - Gain for a 50 dB SPL input
  - Output for an 80 dB SPL input
  - Distortion
- The purpose of conducting HAT box testing in your clinic is to ensure that the hearing aid is meeting a specific quality control standard before you fit it to a patient. Remember, that because of the differences in results between 2-cc coupler testing and probe-microphone ear canal measures, the HAT box analysis is not a replacement for the latter during the actual fitting appointment.

that your hearing aids are meeting the quality standard set by the manufacturer. You don't want any surprises (like a dead hearing aid) on the day that the patient shows up for the fitting (Important fitting note: The probability of experiencing a dead hearing aid out of the box is directly correlated to patient's travel time to the fitting appointment). But in addition to the basic ANSI measures, there are many other things about the hearing aid that you can learn with 2-cc coupler measures. Here is a summary of some:

- Noise reduction: Turn the hearing aid to a typical "use gain setting,"

and deliver a signal of 70 dB SPL or so. Use an input signal that indeed is noise (not speech, a pure tone, or modulated noise), and measure the output. Turn on noise reduction, and observe the output for the same signal: it should be noticeably less. This procedure can be used to examine the effects of different DNR software settings (e.g., min, med, and max), or to determine the effects of DNR for different noise levels by conducting comparative testing at 50, 60, 70, and 80 dB SPL inputs.

- Directional technology: Some of today's test box manufacturers provide the option of testing directionality. The printout will show the directional effects for different input signals. This procedure also can be used to test the effectiveness of adaptive or automatic directional, by altering the input signal and changing the orientation of the hearing aid. Follow the guidelines from the equipment's manual.

■ Feedback suppression: Most of today's hearing aids have automatic feedback suppression. It's possible to test the effectiveness of algorithm in the test box. First, turn off the feedback suppression circuit, and force the hearing aid into feedback (one manufacturer recommends putting the monitoring earphones around the hearing aid to accomplish this). Then turn on the feedback suppression circuit and observe the effects.

■ Phase: There are some reports that hearing aids that are not "in phase" will not provide optimum *bilateral benefit* when worn. With some 2-cc coupler equipment, it's possible to assess the phase of the instruments.

■ Group delay: Digital processing takes time, and this processing time (input to output) is referred to as "group delay." As channels and features are increased, so is the delay. When the delay becomes excessive (e.g., >10 msec or so) it can become annoying to the patient. This is especially problematic for open-canal fittings. Some 2-cc coupler systems allow for assessing group delay.

■ Telecoil performance: There are several methods to check the functioning of the telecoil. One approach is to use a "wand" to produce the desired signal.

TAKE FIVE: Learn More

To learn more about 2-cc testing, and all the fun things that you can test, go to either the Audioscan or the Frye Electronics Web sites. Both sites have great training documents available to download.

Programming the Hearing Aids: Hardware and Software

Once you have conducted 2-cc coupler measures to ensure that the hearing aids are working according to specifications; it's time to do the initial programming of the hearing aids. This is also something you can do before the patient arrives (e.g., enter his audiogram and LDLs), although in busy clinics, it often happens while the patient is sitting in front of your probe-mic system. Regardless of *when* you do it, there is one basic rule to remember: the manufacturer will provide you the software to conduct "first fit"; you will use your knowledge and skills to provide "last fit."

If you are working in an office that's been programming hearing aids for a while, it's almost guaranteed that there's a little white box somewhere on a desk that's used to program hearing aids. With the proper programming cables, this box is used to program or "first fit" new hearing aids. Just about every hearing aid fitted today needs to be programmed by a computer (prior to about 1990 or so, all you really needed was a tiny screwdriver to make changes on a hearing aid). "Programming" a hearing aid means that we are plugging a cable or battery pill into the hearing aid, and connecting it to a special device that "communicates" with a computer.

There is an organization called the Hearing Instrument Manufacturer's Association (HIMSA), which has more than 100 member companies. These companies are involved in all aspects of hearing health care, including all hearing aid manufacturers. HIMSA produces a special software platform, called NOAH (not an acronym, just NOAH) that you can install on your office computer prior to installing manufacturer's fitting software. NOAH allows all hearing aid manufacturers to have a common framework to save and retrieve patient data. Currently, most offices are using NOAH 3 and an updated version (NOAH 4) was released in March 2011. You can program hearing aids by simply using a manufacturer's "stand alone" software, but since most offices fit hearing aids from several different manufacturers, it is more efficient to use the NOAH umbrella.

In addition to the NOAH platform, professionals have a couple of different hardware options to connect a hearing aid to the NOAH platform on their office computer. One way is to use what's called a Hi-Pro box that plugs into your computer with a cable—that's the white box we were talking about earlier. The other way is to use a more portable system using Bluetooth transmission, called NOAHLink. Both systems require programming cables, which are supplied by the hearing aid manufacturer (you can obtain these cables and the fitting software from the manufacturer, usually at no charge). The NOAHLink system, which was released by HIMSA in 2003, is probably the more popular of the two devices. As you can see in Figure 10–5, you are able to place the transmitter box around the patient's neck and the programming cables are

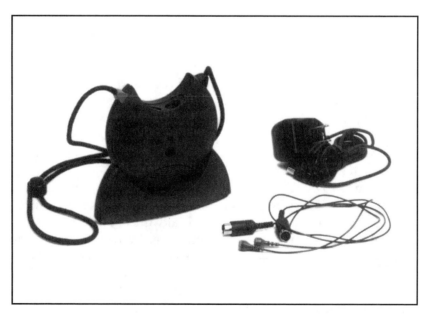

Figure 10–5. The NOAHLink programming system. Reprinted with permission of HIMSA.

connected directly to the hearing aids. This arrangement allows the patient to move around: to go from your test booth to your probe-mic room, for example, during the fitting and fine-tuning appointments.

Before any new hearing aid comes to market, HIMSA provides certification testing on all programming software to ensure that it works properly. Although HIMSA maintains a staff and has a Web site (http://www.himsa.com), field professionals always direct their NOAH, NOAHLink and Hi-Pro questions directly to a hearing aid manufacturer. In fact, you can purchase all of this programming hardware and software directly from one of your manufacturing partners.

TAKE FIVE:
Always Check First

When you buy a new computer for your office to program and fit hearing aids, it is always a good idea to check with a couple of your hearing aid manufacturing partners to make sure you are buying one that works well with NOAH. These programs can "eat up" a lot of space, so think big!

Recently, some hearing aid manufacturers have introduced their own wireless programming systems that don't use any programming cables. One example of this is the iCube system from Phonak. The upside to iCube is that it is completely wireless (hearing aid fitters typically have one desk drawer filled with dozens of programming cables), but the downside is you can only program Phonak hearing aids, so you still need cables for the other companies.

Using "First-Fit"

A few words about the preprogramming of hearing aid features. First, for features such as WDRC, the automated programming to a "first-fit" setting is invaluable. Given that some hearing aids have a "gazillion" channels (or more) we certainly do not want to go channel-by-channel and make decisions regarding what is the best kneepoint, compression ratio and release time. For other features (e.g., AGCo, DNR, directional, feedback suppression, etc.) there will be a "default" setting. You may or may not agree with this setting, but if you're just getting started (and you probably are or you wouldn't be reading this book), these default settings are probably better than what you could think through on your own. As you gain experience, and are armed with more information about the patient, you might want to override some of these settings.

As mentioned, if you use the "first fit" and default settings, you will have a fitting that probably is an "okay" starting point. In general, first fit settings are conservative: the notion is to make the initial amplification experience a pleasant one for the new user (e.g., gain is somewhat reduced, AGCo kneepoints might be set a little lower than necessary, etc.).

Regarding the selection of gain and output for different inputs, the manufacturers' software will allow you to select a validated prescriptive method such as the NAL-NL2 or the DSL 5.0, and the instrument will be programmed to these parameters (although sometimes with minor modifications). Simply selecting a prescriptive method in the fitting software of course, does not mean the output will meet that prescription in the real ear—that's what verification is all about. All major manufacturers also have a "recommended" (default) fitting algorithm, which they might call Siemens-Fit, Unitron-Fit, Oticon-Fit, and so forth. In most cases these fitting algorithms call for less gain and output than the well-known validated methods. The general notion is that the new user needs a fitting that provides "initial acceptance." You will have to decide during the verification process if you want to send the patient out the door with this fitting (and perhaps use training, automatic acclimatization, or repeat visits to increase gain), or if you will want to verify and adjust the output according to the standard fitting algorithms.

TAKE FIVE: Things to Remember About the "First-Fit" of Gain and Output

■ The manufacturer's software will do the "first fit," it's your responsibility to do "last fit."

■ Just because you select a given validated prescription (e.g., NAL-NL2) in the fitting software, this does not ensure that you will meet this target in the real ear (in fact, research suggests that often you will not even be within 10 dB of target at all frequencies).

■ Just because a given algorithm appears to meet targets in the simulated fitting screen, this does not mean that you will meet these targets in the real ear.

■ Most manufacturers' proprietary fitting algorithms are geared toward "initial acceptance;" this is different from the validated prescriptive methods which tend to be geared more toward speech intelligibility and preferred loudness levels.

To review, here are a few terms related to the initial programming of the hearing aids:

■ HIMSA: Hearing Instrument Manufacturers Association, which oversees deliver and quality control of manufacturer's fitting software

■ NOAH: Software platform produced by HIMSA

■ Hi-Pro box: A device used to program hearing aids. It requires a wired connection between the hearing aids and the Hi-Pro and the Hi-Pro box and the computer

■ NOAHLink: The more portable cousin of the HIPro box, NOAHLink eliminates some of the wires of the Hi-Pro box by using a Bluetooth transmission signal.

■ Programming cables: A connection from the Hi-Pro to the hearing aid. Hearing aids can be connected to cables with a programming pill, programming strip or direct connection into the hearing aids via a special port

■ Programming strip: Used with some products and attaches to the programming cable; makes connection with hearing aid by sliding into narrow opening at battery door.

■ Programming pill: Used with some products and attaches to programming cable; fits into battery compartment same as a battery.

- Stand-alone software: Software from a given manufacturer that can be used to program their hearing aids and is not run under the NOAH module.
- First Fit: The settings that the manufacturer believes are a good starting point for the fitting, not only for gain and output, but for special features.
- Default setting: To expedite the fitting process, the manufacturers have many "built-in" (default) settings that relate to First Fit. For example, the noise reduction might be set to "medium," the compression might be set to "fast release," and so on.
- Proprietary Fit: The manufacturer's algorithm that selects gain and output for different inputs for the First Fit. These algorithms are often termed "proprietary" as there typically are few published data describing how the various values were obtained.

The Verification Process

It's your lucky day. You just got upgraded to first class on your cross-country trip. Somewhere you have stored away a "formula" for how this will be different from sitting in coach. A more comfortable seat, better snacks, free drinks, and a friendlier flight attendant. But will all this happen? Only the verification process will tell you.

As mentioned at the beginning of this chapter, verification of the fitting is crit-ical. Is the hearing aid performing the way that you predicted, or the way that you desire it to perform? By "perform" we mean, while the patient is wearing it, not when it is attached to a coupler. We believe that the best verification approach is probe-microphone measures, and that is the focus of this section. There are alternative ways to verify the fitting, however. It's possible that these alternative approaches could be used *instead of* probe-mic measures, but we recommend that they be used to *complement* probe-mic testing. We summarize six different verification strategies that you possibly could use.

Probe-mic measures: Does the hearing aid gain and output meet the prescribed targets for different input levels in the real ear?

- Using probe-mic equipment, either the real-ear insertion gain (REIG) or the real-ear aided response (REAR), or both, is measured (calculated).
- These REIG or REAR values for different input levels are then compared to fitting targets from a predetermined prescriptive fitting protocol.
- The hearing aid parameters (e.g., channel-specific gain, WDRC, etc.) are adjusted until real-ear gain approximates the desired targets for each input level.

Functional gain: Does the hearing aid gain meet prescribed targets for soft input levels?

- Using frequency-specific signals, the patient's hearing thresholds are determined, both unaided and aided in the sound field; the difference of these thresholds is calculated, which is "functional gain."

■ These gain values are compared to prescribed targets for soft inputs from a predetermined prescriptive fitting method.

■ The hearing aid parameters (e.g., channel-specific gain, WDRC if very low kneepoints are employed) are adjusted until functional gain approximates the desired targets for soft input levels.

Audibility: Does the hearing aid gain provide appropriate audibility for soft sounds?

■ Using frequency-specific signals, the patient's aided hearing thresholds are determined in the sound field.

■ These aided thresholds are compared to desired threshold levels (while the general verification is to determine if soft speech is audible, desired levels may vary as the hearing loss becomes more severe). As general guidance, the count-the-dot audiogram from Chapter 7 can be used to determine aided audibility of the average speech signal.

■ The hearing aid parameters (e.g., channel-specific gain, WDRC if very low kneepoints are employed) are adjusted until aided thresholds approximate the desired levels.

Loudness ratings: Does the hearing aid gain and output result in appropriate loudness ratings (perceptions) for different input levels?

■ Using a range of loudness anchors, the patient performs loudness judgments for speech and/or narrow-bands of noise. The patient rates the loudness of different input levels (e.g., ~45 dB SPL should be judged as "soft"; ~65 dB SPL should be judged as "comfortable"; ~85 dB SPL should be judged as "loud but not uncomfortable.")

■ The hearing aid parameters (e.g., channel-specific gain, WDRC, AGCo) are adjusted until appropriate loudness judgments are obtained for all three input levels.

Speech intelligibility measures: Does the hearing aid gain optimize speech understanding?

■ While aided in the sound field (or mildly reverberant room), the patient is presented one or more standardized speech tests (in quiet and/or in noise), typically at a level ~50 dB HL; 65 dB SPL.

■ The patient's scores are compared to that of normal hearing individuals, or to expected levels of performance for someone with a similar degree of hearing loss.

■ The hearing aid parameters (e.g. channel-specific gain, WDRC) are adjusted until aided speech scores reach desired levels.

Speech intelligibility judgments: Does the hearing aid gain optimize the patient's ratings of speech understanding?

■ While aided in the sound field (or mildly reverberant room), the patient is presented a standardized speech test or different speech passages (in quiet and/or in noise), typically at a level ~65 dB SPL. Ratings could be obtained using bounded category scaling, or paired-comparisons if different stimuli are presented.

■ The patient's judgments of intelligibility (or ease of listening) are compared to expected levels of performance for someone with a similar degree of hearing loss.

■ The hearing aid parameters (e.g., channel-specific gain, WDRC) are adjusted until speech intelligibility is rated at the desired level.

Speech quality judgments: Does the hearing aid gain optimize the patient's ratings of speech quality?

■ While aided in the sound field (or mildly reverberant room), the patient is presented a standardized speech test or different speech passages (in quiet and/or in noise), typically at a level ~65 dB SPL. Ratings could be obtained using bounded category scaling, or paired-comparisons if different stimuli are presented.

■ The patient's judgments of quality are compared to expected levels of performance for someone with a similar degree of hearing loss, or in the case of paired-comparisons, the highest rated hearing aid adjustment.

■ The hearing aid parameters (e.g., channel-specific gain, WDRC) are adjusted until speech quality is rated at the desired level.

It's unlikely that you will use all six verification measures, although in one form or another, all six are used by some dispensers. Many also tend be used haphazardly—on a busy afternoon, the sound quality scaling procedure may turn into the simple question, "How does that sound?" or maybe even the statement, "Bet that sounds good doesn't it!"

Prescriptive Fitting Methods

Up to this point, you have spent your time gathering information about each patient's hearing loss and communication needs. You also have conducted some coupler measures, and you've conducted the initial programming of the instrument. Recall that we discussed the option of using a validated prescriptive fitting approach when we "first fit" the hearing instrument. We also discussed prescriptive fitting approaches when we examined how kneepoints and ratios were selected. Let's now take a closer look at prescriptive methods.

A prescriptive fitting method requires that we take the hearing thresholds we measured and put them into a formula. The formula subsequently generates a fitting target, actually multiple targets, as you will need different gain/output for different input levels. You can think of this prescriptive target as a starting point for the gain and frequency response of the hearing aid which typically is based on each individual's audiogram thresholds. Some fittings methods also use the patient's measured LDLs (more on that later).

Prescriptive fitting methods using auditory thresholds or loudness measures to generate a fitting target have been around for decades. An early approach (circa 1940s) that was easy to remember simply took half the amount of hearing loss to determine desired gain. Before prescriptive methods became the preferred way to select gain and output, professionals relied on something called the "comparative approach." Using the comparative approach, a number of different hearing aids with various gain and frequency response configurations were randomly placed on the patient and speech testing or quality judgments were conducted. Usually, the hearing aid that scored the highest on word-recognition testing was the device that the patient was fitted with (even if it was only a few percent better than the others). With the advent of programmable technology, comparative procedures have been all but completely abandoned in the United States, although they are still used in parts of Europe.

There are some components, however, from the comparative evaluation that are still with us. When, for example, you hear a colleague asking the patient during the initial fitting, "Does that sound better than your old hearing aids?" he is harkening back to the bygone comparative fitting era. Of course, there are times, mainly after the patient has been wearing his or her hearing aids for a while, when you can ask for subjective judgments, and the findings may be valid and reliable. But, true believers in a prescriptive fitting method assume that the gain, output, and frequency response derived from the prescriptive formula is probably the best starting point for any patient, even if it doesn't sound quite right. The probability of a patient picking the gain, output, and frequency response that is best for them during a single office visit (in an unnatural environment) is very unlikely, especially for new users. Refining the fitting in the real world is a different matter (see our section on trainable hearing aids in Chapter 9).

Equalization and Normalization

Over the years there have been dozens of prescriptive fitting formulas. If you look in some old books, you may find the methods of Lybarger, Libby, or Berger. There also was the IHAFF, POGO, and POGO II. In recent years, there really are only two underlying philosophies that we need to think about concerning prescriptive formulas: loudness normalization and loudness equalization. These two concepts might sound the same to you, but let us explain.

Prescriptive formulas based on loudness normalization attempt to give hearing-impaired patients the same amount of loudness that a person with normal hearing listening to the same sound would perceive. On the other hand, loudness equalization procedures attempt to take all the key frequencies of speech and make them the same loudness to the hearing-impaired patient. That is, enough gain is provided to place *average speech* at the patient's MCL for all key frequencies. In some cases, this results in fitting targets very similar to loudness equalization, but with a different philosophy.

In practical terms, loudness equalization procedures usually require less gain for soft sounds than loudness normalization procedures. In a steeply sloping loss, for example, the equalization method typically provides less audibility of soft speech for the high frequencies. There hasn't been a lot of definitive research on the topic but, in general, it's been found that true normalization provides too much gain, especially for the higher frequencies. Some researchers, such as Brian Moore of Cambridge University in the United Kingdom, have developed two parallel fitting methods, one for loudness restoration (CAMREST) and one for equalization (CAMEQ, now modified to CAMEQ2-HF).

DSL and NAL

Although there have been 20 or more hearing aid fitting methods that have been proposed in one form or another over the past 60 years, today, there really are only two prescriptive fitting methods for you need to remember. The first is the desired sensation level (DSL) method, which has been around since 1984, and has been modified several times. Most consider the DSL the "fitting of choice" for children. Its use with adults has been somewhat limited, but has increased significantly in recent years when a modification for adults was add-ed. In general, earlier versions seemed to prescribe a bit more gain than the average adult wanted (and maybe need-ed). The latest version of the DSL, Version 5.0, has specific targets for adults, considerably less than those prescribed for children.

TAKE FIVE: Children Versus Adults

Although there is not total consensus on this topic, many believe that prescriptive targets should be different for an infant or toddler, than for an adult. The reasoning behind this is that the young child needs to develop speech and language and, therefore, the audibility of speech is critical. This includes "incidental learning" (overhearing speech when not directly spoken to), so audibility for soft inputs also is important. With adults, who have already developed speech and language, audibility may not be as critical, as they can "fill in" many sounds based on their knowledge of the English language. Therefore, for methods such as the DSL 5.0 for example, the difference in prescribed gain can vary by as much as 10 to 15 dB for an infant versus an adult.

Historically, the fitting method which has been the most popular with adults is the one from the National Acoustic Laboratories (NAL) in Australia. There have been several revisions from the original NAL method of 1976, (originally called the Byrne and Tonnison method). These have been termed NAL-R (for revised), NAL-RP (for revised and profound), and the NAL-NL1 (for non-linear). The current NAL version is NAL-NL2, introduced in 2010. The NAL is a loudness equalization method that has been heavily researched and tweaked over the years. Here are a few things you might want to know about the NAL family of fitting targets:

- It's one of the only independently validated prescriptive fitting approaches in use today (the other is the DSL), and it is used in most all parts of the world.
- All versions of the NAL formula use a loudness equalization method. This means that the NAL formula strives to make all octave bands equally loud. Based on your knowledge after reading Chapter 2, you should know this means that less gain is applied to low-frequency energy compared to the high frequencies.
- Loudness equalization typically represents a reasonable compromise between restoring audibility and maintaining comfort of speech sounds.

■ Some version of the NAL formula has been used since 1976. It's been tweaked over the years to reflect changes in hearing aid technology and patient gain preferences

■ It's shown in systematic research reviews that the gain and output derived from the NAL formula is preferred as a starting point by about two-thirds of patients.

TAKE FIVE: More on Proprietary Algorithms

We talked a little about proprietary algorithms earlier when we addressed first fit, but here is a little more detail. Most hearing aid manufacturers have developed their own fitting method: these methods typically are referred to as "proprietary methods." In some cases, they might even take a common method, like the NAL-NL2, and then modify it, so that when you select NAL-NL2 you might not be using the same targets as you would see in the stand-alone software. These proprietary algorithms often are the default for the "first fit" of the patient's hearing aids. In general, on the day of the fitting, *underfitting* seems more acceptable to the patient than overfitting. Keeping the patient happy of course is important, and some people are willing to sacrifice audibility to accomplish this. Therefore, most proprietary algorithms prescribe less gain than the validated methods of the NAL and the DSL. If you verity to the NAL using your probe-mic system, then what you use for the "first-fit" doesn't matter much. If you don't verify, but simply use what shows up when you push the "magic button" then it does matter.

If you're just getting started using prescriptive fitting methods, here are a few things that these methods will do for you (there are some differences regarding what is provided by the NAL-NL2 versus the DSL).

■ Fitting targets in insertion gain for a wide range of inputs and different input signals.
■ Fitting targets in ear canal SPL output for a wide range of inputs and different input signals.
■ Desired settings for WDRC (kneepoint, ratio, etc.)
■ Targets for output limiting based on the LDLs that you enter or the algorithms predicted maximum output values.

■ Targets displayed for 2-cc coupler as well as ear canal gain and SPL.
■ Corrections based on the patient's age.
■ Corrections based on the number of hearing aid channels.
■ Corrections based on the method threshold data were collected
■ Corrections for hearing aid experience, gender, and listening in quiet versus noise.

The Need for Verification

It would be nice, and would save time, if we could just assume that prescriptive fitting methods, displayed as "simulated gain" on a fitting screen, translated into an accurate match of the prescriptive target in ear canal SPL. Unfortunately, as we've discussed, the results from the 2-cc coupler and what we see on our computer fitting screens usually is not what is actually happening in the real ear (refer back to our earlier discussion of the CORFIG). Probe-microphone measures are the gold standard when it comes to verifying that our prescriptive fitting method of choice is being met in the patient's ear canal. There really is no substitute method, and failure to assess the real-ear SPL when hearing aids are fitted is considered unethical practice by many. At the least, it goes against all published "Best Practice" guidelines.

Probe-microphone measures have been around for a number of decades; however, for reasons that are not clearly understood, not every clinician takes the time to do them. They are, however, absolutely necessary if you want to be sure your prescriptive fitting target is being matched. Any savvy consumer would expect that this procedure would be conducted, especially as the topic was addressed thoroughly in a 2009 *Consumer's Report*. After all, if one is purchasing a state-of-the-art electronic device for several thousand dollars, it would seem only logical that the programming is verified using a state-of-the- art device also. No matter what you might hear from others, there is no way to know if patients are getting the right amount of gain or output without conducting probe-microphone measures. In essence, they ensure that your patient is starting off with a reasonably good "first fit," and at the least, reasonable audibility.

TAKE FIVE:
Looking for the Truth

A recent survey of 309 audiologists and 111 Hearing Instrument Specialists indicated that only 45% of them routinely use probe-microphone measures in their practice. However, the survey included a "lie detector" question. The respondents were asked about a fabricated test, called the Binaural Summation Index. About 20% of them said they routinely did this test that doesn't really exist. What that means to us, is that there could be a 20% fudge factor, meaning that the 45% of routine probe microphone users could be closer to 25%.

Before we work through a simple step-by-step probe-microphone procedure, there are a couple of misconceptions that need to be addressed. Regardless of what you might hear, any hearing aid can be measured using a probe-microphone system. Probe-mic measures work just fine with digital instruments. They work just fine with open-canal instruments (using a slightly modified protocol). Probe-mic measures also are very reliable, perhaps the most reliable measure that you will make. Test-retest is around 2 dB. In addition, probe-microphone measures are a great way to show patients how those special features we discussed in Chapter 9 really *are* working. To get into the details concerning all of these test protocols is well beyond the scope of this book; however, there are some excellent sources for learning more. The major manufacturers of probe-microphone equipment, such as Audioscan, Frye Electronics, MedRx., and Otometrics, all have excellent Web sites with plenty of educational material available.

TAKE FIVE:
Added Convenience

We talked about Bluetooth hearing aid applications in Chapter 9. Bluetooth transmission is also available with some probe-microphone equipment. The big advantage is that the patient is not tethered to the equipment and you have a little more room to move around the patient and your equipment.

Probe-Microphone Equipment and Procedures

The basic probe-mic equipment often is part of your 2-cc coupler test system. Additional equipment you will need include:

■ An external loudspeaker to present the test signal
■ A regulating microphone at the ear to monitor the test signal
■ A probe tube in the ear canal, which is connected to the measurement microphone (see Figure 10–5).

The measures are plotted and analyzed much the same as when you conduct 2-cc coupler testing. The equipment will allow you to plot functions in gain or in ear canal SPL.

Three important things to remember when starting to conduct probe-mic measures is to:

☐ Get the patient in the right place.
☐ Get the reference (monitor) mic in the right place.
☐ Get the tip of the probe tube in the right place.

If you get these three things right, you have a good chance of obtaining a valid and reliable measure.

The Patient

Positioning the patient is important. Probably the biggest mistake dispensers make is allowing the patient to sit too far away from the loudspeaker. Two reasons why you want to have the patient sit reasonably close (around 1 meter) are:

■ It will improve the signal-to-noise ratio. Often, test rooms are noisy (more than one computer running, heating and air conditioning systems running, etc). If you want to test at soft levels like 50 dB SPL (and you should) then you will have to have the patient at a distance where 50 dB SPL is louder than the ambient noise reaching the monitor microphone; this allows for proper leveling/calibration.
■ It will present overdriving of the loudspeaker. The farther the person is away from the loudspeaker, the more output required to reach a given desired level. In some cases, with some equipment, you will overdrive the loudspeaker at the high input levels (the run will be aborted) if the person is seated too far away.

A commonly used method to ensure that the patient's head is located at the correct distance is to use a "calibrated string" measured to be one meter long. Tape one end of the string to the top of the loudspeaker, and then assure that the middle of the patient's head is at the other end of the string.

It also is important to have the person sit at the correct azimuth. Unless your equipment requires something different (e.g., Fonix 7000), we recommend a 0-degree vertical azimuth and a 0-degree horizontal azimuth.

The Reference Mic

For most systems, the reference microphone is part of the "probe assembly." The entire assembly is hung on the ear or fits next to the ear, which then places the reference mic just below the ear canal. This works fine. Ensure, however, that the mic doesn't twist, and you end of with the opening facing backward (the signal should be measured at a grazing angle).

It also is possible with some systems to place the reference mic at other locations, such as above the ear. This also works fine. Check with the manufacturer of your equipment to determine the recommended placement.

The Probe Tube

All systems use a probe tube, although the tubes are slightly different among manufacturers. Most systems require that you first "calibrate the tube" (follow the instructions in the manual). This procedure makes the probe tube acoustically invisible: it's as if the microphone itself is now located in the ear canal. At the time of testing, you will place this tube in the patient's ear canal. Poor placement of the probe tube easily can make the entire probe-microphone measure invalid. A few things to remember about placing the probe tube in the ear canal include:

- The tip of the tube needs to be relatively close to the TM. If the tip is within 5 mm, valid results should be obtained through 4000 Hz.
- The tip of the tube should be 3 to 5 mm beyond the tip of the hearing aid or earmold.
- The average adult ear canal is about 25 mm. The best reference for probe-tube placement is the intertragal notch. Although it varies from person to person, this notch usually is about 10 mm from the opening of the ear canal. The average distance, therefore, between the intertragal notch and the TM is about 35 mm.
- If the ring marker on the probe tube (or the black mark that you make using a Sharpie if no ring is present) is placed on the tube at 30 mm from the tip, and this mark is aligned with the intertragal notch, then the tip of the probe tube should be about 5 mm from the TM. This would satisfy both requirements of being close to the TM and extending beyond the tip of the hearing aid or earmold.
- As the tip of the probe is farther from the TM, the output in the high frequencies is reduced. If you are not aware of the poor probe placement, this inaccurate finding might prompt you to incorrectly add high frequency gain to match target when the hearing aid is programmed.
- Although it is tempting to slide the probe tube through the vent of the hearing aid, do not do this if the vent is 2 mm or smaller, as you

will alter the vent effects that you are attempting to measure.

Input Signal

The input signal that you typically will use will be real speech, modulated noise, or unmodulated noise, depending on what equipment you have, and what you are assessing. For checking the MPO of the hearing aid, you also will want to use a swept pure tone (i.e., a tone will drive the hearing aid to a higher output than a broad-band signal). You will present the test signals at different input levels; again, the actual levels will depend on what it is you are measuring. Common presentation levels are 50, 65, and 80 dB SPL for soft, average and loud, and a swept tone of 85 or 90 dB SPL for the MPO assessment.

As mentioned, there are different input signals available. These vary depending on the equipment that you are using, and the purpose of the test. Traditionally, we have used either pure tones or noise for probe-mic testing, and there still are some cases when you'll want to use these inputs:

- Swept pure-tones: Recommended to determine the MPO of the hearing aid, but a poor choice for other probe-mic measures. Using a pure-tone signal it is difficult to observe compression and channel interaction effects.
- Broadband noise: A commonly used noise for conducted REIG (e.g., pink noise, speech-shaped noise) but not recommended for REAR verification. Good signal for assessing the effects of DNR.

In addition to pure tones, and different types of noises, special speechlike signals have been developed in recent years for testing modern hearing aids. This is the signal we recommend for the majority of your probe-mic testing, including prescriptive target verification. Listed below is a summary of some of the more common ones used for probe-mic testing:

- ISTS: An acronym for the International Speech Test Signal. This signal was developed as part of the ISMADHA project (International Standards for Measuring Advanced Digital Hearing Aids) for the EHIMA (European Hearing Instrument Manufacturer's Association). The signal consists of concatenated speech (brief speech segments linked together) of six female speakers; six different languages.
- ICRA: ICRA is an acronym for International Collegium of Rehabilitative Audiology, the organization for which the signals were prepared by a working group dubbed Hearing Aid Clinical Test Environment Standardization (HACTES). There are different types of babble signals available (e.g., male, female, six-person) for different voice levels (normal, raised, loud), and these 11 noise signals have modulation characteristics similar to those of natural speech.
- Verifit Speech Test Signal: Male voice test signal developed by Bill Cole of Audioscan; it is filtered to provide the long-term average speech spectrum (LTASS) recommended for average vocal effort. Commonly referred to as the "carrot passage" as the speaker is talking about carrots.
- Fonix (Frye) Digital Speech: A modulated broadband signal; available in two varieties: ANSI and ICRA.

TIPS and TRICKS: Using *Live* Speech for Probe-Mic Measures

Our emphasis had been on using a calibrated speech or speechlike signal for probe-mic measures. This is good, because the ear canal SPL fitting targets need to be directly connected to the input signal. If you use the *wrong* signal, it could appear that you are not matching targets when in fact you are. Most of today's probe-mic systems also allow you to use *live speech*—this could be your voice, the patient's voice, a family member's voice, or Demi Moore's voice if she happens to be around. This approach can provide an impressive demonstration, and might be helpful for counseling and sales, as it has considerable face validity. We would *not* recommend using "live voice" for fitting the hearing aid, however.

Real-Ear Terminology

During your airline travels you've probably heard terms like an "open-jaw" flight reservation, sitting on the "tarmac," flying on a "code share," or taking a "red eye." You may even hear the "mile-high club" mentioned. Understanding terminology is important for getting you to and from a desired location, as well as talking to fellow travelers along the way. The same is true for probe-mic terminology.

Let's get familiar with real-ear measurement terminology. Remember all that talk earlier about ANSI standards, well ANSI S3.46 is the probe microphone standard that was established in 1998. Some of the terms used in the standard are slightly different from what has become common in clinical use and what was published in the now classic book by Mueller, Hawkins, and Northern, *Probe Microphone Measurements; Hearing Aid Selection and Assessment*—a book you really should have for your professional library, coffee table, or nightstand.

Two general rules regarding probe-mic terminology are as follows:

- If the measure refers to SPL in the ear canal, the acronym for the term will end in an "R."
- If the measure refers to a *difference measure*, generally because input has been subtracted from output, then the acronym for the term will end in a "G."

TAKE FIVE: Understanding "Response" Versus "Gain": A Lunchtime Conversation

Terminology can be confusing, and probe-mic terms certainly fall into this category. The following is a lunchtime conversation, recently recorded among seven audiologists. As all the ANSI probe-mic terms start with "RE," it's convenient to shorten the terms by only using the last two letters of the abbreviation. The key is to know the "G's" from the "R's."

Brad: You should have seen the patient I had this morning. His UR was 28 dB at 3K!

Casey: Brad, Brad. You mean his UG was 28 dB. If you used a 50 dB input, his UR would have been 78 dB, not 28.

Brad: Yeah, well, okay you're right. But anyway, when I put in the open tip for his OC fitting, the OR actually was –2 dB, so I guess the tip was more occluding than I thought.

Maureen: Very interesting Brad, but sounds like you're talking about his OG, not his OR. If you're using a 50 dB input, the OR would have been 48 dB.

Jay: Could someone pass the ketchup please?

Mike: I see an OG like that sometimes for my OC fittings too. How did your speech map results turn out?

Brad: I didn't do speech mapping, I did insertion gain, and my match to NAL-NL2 was pretty good.

Brian: You mean your match to the IR? I'd think with a UG that big, the IR would have a dip at 3K.

Gus: Brian, Brian. You're still using the old "IR" term? We dumped that 15 years ago. Gain is always gain, which is always a difference. The term is REIG, not REIR.

Jay: Anybody need another soda?

Brian: Okay, sorry, that REIR thing just sort of slipped out. I switched to speech mapping several years ago, so I use the AG for verification and don't think much about insertion gain anymore—oops, should I have said the AR rather than the AG?

Mike: Well Brian that was just a little "oops." We still use both the AG and AR terms, but usually when we do speech mapping, we indeed use the AR for verification.

Brad: So am I the only one who is still verifying hearing aids using the IG?

Gus: Well you are in the minority; our recent *Hearing Journal* survey showed that only about one-third of dispensers still use the REIG.

Maureen: I still do REIG calculations for some patients when the speech map results look really strange.

Casey: I can't remember the last time I used the IG. The beauty of speech mapping is that you don't have to worry about those nasty bumps and dips in the patient's UG.

Gus: When I do REIG calculations, I simply use the average UG, and then you don't have those problems.

Brian: What? You can do that? Isn't that cheating?

Mike: Hey folks, the party is over. Looks like our 1:00 patients are here.

Jay: Hey wait, doesn't anyone want to talk about the SAL test?

Probe Microphone Terms From ANSI

- **REUR**—real-ear unaided response—SPL as a function of frequency, at a specified measurement point in the ear canal, for a specified sound field, with the ear canal unoccluded. Commonly referred to as "ear canal resonance."
- **REUG**—real-ear unaided gain—*Difference* in decibels between the SPL as a function of frequency at a specified measurement point in the ear canal and the SPL at the field reference point, for a specified sound field with the ear canal unoccluded. This measurement serves as a baseline for calculating the hearing aid insertion gain. This also can serve as a correction factor for calculation of coupler gain for DSL and NAL fitting formulas. Some sample REUGs are shown in Figure 10–6.
- **REOR**—real-ear occluded response—SPL as a function of frequency, at a specified measurement point in the ear canal, for a specified sound field, with the hearing aid in place and turned *off*. Reveals how the earmold/custom hearing aid is attenuating sound. Used to examine the effect of a vent on the canal resonance, or how "open" an open fitting really is. It is not a direct measure of the occlusion effect, although if the REOR is similar to the REUR, there is a high probability that there is no occlusion effect.
- **REOG**—real-ear occluded gain—*Difference* in decibels, as a function of frequency, between the SPL at a specified measurement point in the ear canal and the SPL at the field reference point, for a specified sound field with the hearing aid in place and turned off. That is, if you use a 60 dB input signal, and the REOR at 3000 Hz is 58 dB, the REOG would be –2 dB.
- **REAR**—real-ear aided response—SPL as a function of frequency, at a specified measurement point in the ear canal, for a specified sound field, with the hearing aid in place and turned *on*. The overall configuration of the REAR should be somewhat similar to the output shown in the 2-cc coupler, with expected variations due primarily to microphone location effects.
- **REAG**—real-ear aided gain—*Difference* in decibels, as a function of frequency, between the SPL at a specified measurement point in the ear canal and the SPL at the field reference point, for a specified sound field, with the hearing aid in place and turned on. That is, if you use a 60 dB input signal, and the REAR at 3000 Hz is 90 dB SPL, the REAG would be 30 dB.
- **REIG**—real-ear insertion gain—Difference in decibels, as a function of frequency, between the REAR and the REUR, or the REAG and the REUG, taken with the measurement point and the same sound field conditions. Used to validate gain-based prescriptive targets. Because gain is always a difference value, and never an absolute value, there is no REIR, just REIG.
  - **REAG – REUG = REIG**
  - **REAR – REUR = REIG**

Other Commonly Used Terms

These next terms are not included in the ANSI standard; however, they are utilized in clinics, and might show up in various fitting software.

■ **RESR**—real-ear saturation response—SPL as a function of frequency, in the ear canal, with the hearing aid in place, turned on, with the VC adjusted to full-on (or just below feedback) with an 85 or 90 dB input signal (signal of an intensity to cause the hearing aid to reach it's MPO). This measurement is to determine if the maximum output of the hearing aid falls within the desired levels across frequencies based on the patient's LDLs. Also to determine if the maximum output of the hearing aid is at a "safe" level. You can predict the RESR from the coupler OSPL90 if you measure the patient's RECD.

■ **RECD**—real-ear coupler difference —Difference in decibels, as a func-

tion of frequency, between the output of the hearing aid in the real ear and in the 2-cc coupler, taken with the same input signal and hearing aid VC setting. Primarily used with infants and young children, where direct REAR measures or REIG calculations are difficult to obtain. The RECD can be used to predict the output of speech signals for different input levels, or to predict maximum output. The average RECDs for different age groups are shown in Table 10–1.

■ **REDD**—real-ear dial difference— *Difference* in decibels, as a function of frequency, between the output from an earphone (either insert or supra-aural) in the real ear and the audiometer dial setting. For example, if a patient's threshold was 60 dB HL, and the REDD was 12 dB, we would predict that the

Table 10–1. Average Values of the RECD Across Various Ages Reported by Dillon (2001) and Based on the Work of Scollie, Seewald, and Jenstad (1998)

Age (months)	250 Hz	500 Hz	1 KHz	2 KHz	3 kHz	4 KHz	6 KHz
1	5	12	18	21	19	21	22
3	5	11	15	17	15	16	16
6	5	10	14	15	13	13	13
12	4	9	13	14	10	11	10
24	4	8	11	12	9	9	8
36	3	7	11	11	8	8	7
48	2	7	10	10	7	7	6
60	2	6	10	10	6	6	5
adult	1	5	8	9	5	5	4

Source: Reprinted, by permission, from Dillon (2001) "Hearing Aids."

real-ear SPL threshold would be 72 dB (60 + 12 dB). The purpose is to convert the patient's HL results (e.g., audiogram, LDL's, etc.) into ear canal SPL values, sometimes referred to as an SPL-O-Gram. These values then can be displayed on the probe-mic equipment for verification purposes (e.g., the output is measured in ear canal SPL so the targets must be in ear canal SPL).

■ **RETSPL**—Reference equivalent threshold in SPL. *Difference* in decibels, as a function of frequency, between the output from an ear-phone (either insert or supra-aural) in the calibrations coupler (either 6-cc or 2-cc) and the audiometer dial setting. For example, if the hearing aid dial was set to 60 dB HL at 2000 Hz, and the output in the 2-cc coupler for the insert earphone was 62.5 dB, the RETSPL would be 2.5 dB. The RETSPL is not technically a *real-ear* term, but it is used for some corrections related to real-ear measures.

Making It Simple

The plastic-lined airsickness bag that you typically see today in the seat pocket in front of you was created by inventor Gilmore Schjeldahl for Northwest Orient Airlines in 1949. For many years these bags were labeled "For Motion Discomfort." Over the years, the airlines figured out that we all pretty much knew what these bags were for, so to keep things simple, they stopped the labeling.

Although all these probe-mic acronyms might have you thinking about those airline bags, we too have a way to make things a bit more simple:

■ **REUG**—The natural hearing aid the patient walked in the door with; the amplification his pinna and ear canal have been giving him all his life.
■ **REOG**—What the hearing aid or earmold does to the patient (acoustically) *before* the hearing aid is turned on; how the REUG is altered. Some think of this as "insertion loss."
■ **REAG**—What the hearing aid gives the patient when turned on—but not accounting for what might have been taken away, or what the patient had before the instrument was inserted.
■ **REIG**—What the patient has when he walks out of the office (relative to gain at the eardrum) that he didn't have when he walked in. If the output of the hearing aid (REAR) does not exceed his REUR (what he walked in with), it's possible that he could walk out with less than what he came with (and then you have to write *him* a check—very embarrassing!).
■ **RESR**—The maximum output of the hearing aid in the real ear
■ **RECD**—Difference between the *output* in the coupler and the *output* in the real ear.
■ **CORFIG**—Difference between the *gain* in the coupler and the *gain* in the real ear.
■ **RETSPL**—Difference between the audiometer dial setting and the output in a coupler.
■ **REDD**—Difference between the audiometer dial setting and the output in the real ear (equal to the RETSPL added to the RECD).

Matching Prescriptive Targets

Now that we've reviewed the basic probe-mic measures, let's talk about how we can use these measures as part of hearing aid verification. Recall that prescriptive targets are available for a wide range of input levels. Think back to our discussion of WDRC: you do not want the same amount of gain for each input level (the softer the signal, the greater the gain). It's only logical then, that this is reflected in the fitting targets.

As we've already discussed briefly, fitting targets can be displayed in either "desired gain" or in "desired ear canal SPL." Therefore, when it comes to matching prescriptive targets, and ensuring audibility has been achieved with hearing aids, there are two different types of *verification* measures we can conduct with probe-microphone equipment. Both types of measures have some advantages and disadvantages related to how they are displayed, and how they are used to make fitting adjustments, and for patient counseling.

Using the REIG for Verification

The first measurement which can be used for target verification is the REIG, which is really a calculation, not a measurement. The measurements are the REUR and the REAR; your equipment will automatically subtract the UR from the AR. Insertion gain measures look at the difference between the unaided ear canal and the ear canal when a hearing aid is *inserted* and turned on. The REIG calculation can be obtained by either using the measured REUG, or by using an average REUG that is stored in the software of the probe-mic equipment. Because the REIG is the difference between the aided and unaided conditions, it's a measure of *gain*. Prescriptive methods have gain targets, and therefore, these calculations easily can be used for verification. Some advantages of using the REIG for verification include:

- The REIG is similar to functional gain, which was used prior to the introduction of probe-mic equipment.
- Most of the commonly used prescriptive methods of the past several decades used insertion gain for verification (e.g., Berger, Libby, POGO, and the NAL-family).
- Everything is referenced to HL, which is more familiar than ear canal SPL.
- When selecting or programming a hearing aid, it is easier to think in terms of gain, rather than ear canal SPL (e.g., "that patient needs about 30 dB of gain at 4000 Hz").
- When talking to other dispensers, it's easier to talk in terms of gain (e.g., "Are you sure you want to give that patient 30 dB of gain in the low frequencies?")
- When talking to manufacturers, it's easier to talk in terms of gain (e.g., "It seems that whenever I have an OC fitting and I reach 25 dB of gain or so, your product starts to feed back.")
- The selection of the input signal is not as critical if both the REUR and the REAR are measured using the same signal.
- The position of the probe tip is not as critical if the REUR and the REAR are both measured with the probe tip in the same position.

**TIPS and TRICKS:
Measure the REUG?**

If you choose to use the REIG for verification, you will need to subtract the REUR from the REAR. Most probe-mic equipment has a "stored" average REUG that you can use. Or you can measure the patient's individual REUG, and use that. Both will work, and if the patient is "average" it doesn't really matter. If a patient has a really unusual REUG (e.g., a peak of 20 dB at 2000 Hz, which you will see on occasion), and you use measured, you'll find that you'll have to program in a pretty bizarre REAR to obtain the desired REIG. For this reason, we prefer to routinely use the stored REUG, but if you really like to measure it, that's okay too!

Using the REAR for Verification

A second type of probe-microphone verification of fitting targets concerns only observing the absolute sound pressure level (SPL) generated at the eardrum with the hearing aid turned on—this is the REAR. In other words, we're not really concerned with the *gain* of the hearing aid per se, but rather, if the speech signal is being delivered to the TM at the appropriate level. Of course, there is a close relationship between the desired insertion gain (REIG) and the desired ear canal SPL (REAR), so if the REIG tells us that it's a good fitting, the REAR usually is in agreement.

In the past few years, it has become common to use the REAR for verifica-

tion, and use a calibrated speech signal as the input. This is now commonly referred to as "speech mapping," a term that was originally coined by Bill Cole of Audioscan back in the 1990s. It also is possible to use "live speech," that is, the dispenser (or a family member) can provide the input signal live. Live speech might be helpful for demonstrations, and perhaps adding a little "show" to the fitting, but we do not recommend it for target-matching, as fitting targets need to correspond to a given input signal to be accurate—there are no validated targets for live speech.

There are many advantages to the REAR/speech mapping SPL-O-Gram approach of fitting hearing aids:

- The graph is more logical—big numbers on the top, small numbers on the bottom.
- The relationship between the patients hearing loss, fitting targets, and hearing aid output are displayed logically, facilitating counseling.
- The display of both the audiogram and the amplified speech output in ear canal SPL facilitates verification of speech audibility.
- The use of real speech allows for evaluating the hearing aid in its normal use condition, including effects of multiple channels and advanced signal processing.
- The use of real speech clearly illustrates the effects of wide dynamic range compression, including visualization of effective ratios and influence of time constants.
- The SPL-O-Gram mode is effective for assessing and displaying directional and DNR function

■ The use of real speech adds face validity to the overall fitting process.

Targets and Target Matching

At the time of the fitting, using either the REIG or REAR/speech mapping, the general goal is to "match" the target. How close of a match is necessary? In general, we suggest that you attempt to have a match within ±5 dB of the fitting target for all key frequencies, at least through 3000 Hz. Also, attempt to follow the general slope of the fitting target, that is, you wouldn't want to be 5 dB over target at 1500 Hz and 5 dB below target at 2000 Hz.

In particular, it's useful to observe the target for soft speech, and not fall too far below this mark, as one of the primary benefits the patient will obtain is audibility for soft sounds (although they might not thank you for it for several weeks). Recognize, of course, that these targets are only a "starting point." Research has shown that about 60% of patients have preferred gain within ±3 dB of the target for average inputs. This means that nearly half will have preferred gain levels that are significantly higher or lower—but you have to start somewhere!

As discussed in Chapter 9, a bilateral fitting results in a summation of loudness. The degree of summation varies from person to person, and also is dependant on input level (usually more summation for higher inputs). Research has shown this summation can be as small as 1 to 2 dB, or as large as 6 to 8 dB or higher. Your prescriptive algorithm (e.g., NAL-NL2 or DSL 5.0) will account for *average* summation (assuming that you told the software you were conducting a bilateral fitting). But even if its accounted for in the software, the variability among patients is such that you will still want to conduct some bilateral loudness measures just to ensure that average signals are at or near the patient's MCL, and that loud inputs are not too loud.

When on a busy trip through the airport, there is nothing like a "picture" to help out when you're trying to find something quickly. We think that "pictures" help with understanding probe-mic measures too, so we've included several figures to illustrate the points that we've been making.

Over the next few pages you will be taking a little visual tour of some common probe-mic measures. Here is what we have provided for you:

■ REURs from four different adults (Figure 10–6). Note that although they are similar, significant differences do exist. This is why some people use the "average" REUR for REIG calculations.

■ The REOR of an open earmold versus a closed earmold for the same patient (Figure 10–7). Remember that the REOR is a useful measure to asses the tightness of the fitting.

■ Figure 10–8 shows the match to NAL-NL2 REAR target for speech mapping for a 65 dB SPL real-speech input signal. In general, we like to see a REAR curve that is matched within 3 to 5 dB of target for all frequencies through 4000 Hz.

■ The match to soft, average and loud REAR (ear canal SPL) targets using a calibrated speech signal

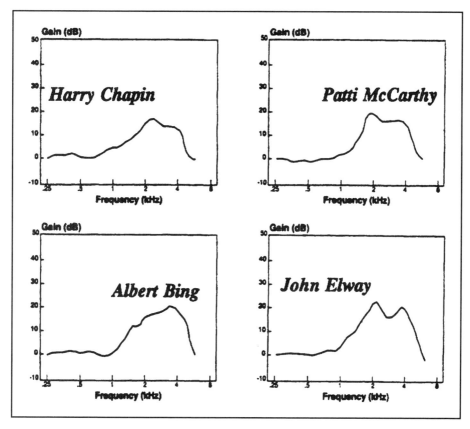

Figure 10–6. The REUG from four famous people. Reprinted from *Audiologists' Desk Reference*, Volume II, Gus Mueller and James Hall III. Copyright © 1998 Singular Publishing, Inc. All rights reserved. Used with permission (p. 296).

(Figure 10–9). Remember the importance of fitting to all three levels.

■ The effects of using two different live voice speech signals (male versus female); note that the difference is quite large at some frequencies (Figure 10–10). This illustrates the importance of using a calibrated speech signal when verifying fitting targets.

■ Example of the measurement of real-ear directional effects

(Figure 10–11). This should also be checked on repeat visits as the port openings easily can become plugged with dirt and debris, which will alter the directivity.

■ Example of the measurement of real-ear DNR effects using an unmodulated noise signal (Figure 10–12). This measure should be conducted at different input levels, as the degree of DNR will likely vary (e.g., greater DNR for higher levels).

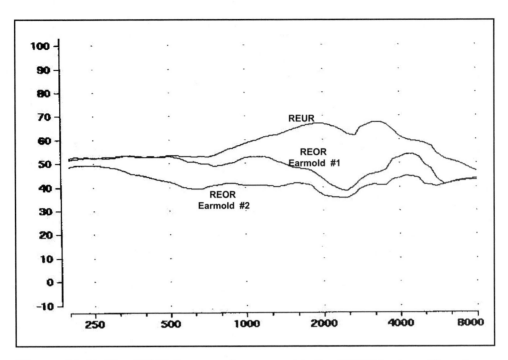

Figure 10–7. The REUR (*top curve*) compared to the REOR for two different earmolds. Earmold #1 (*middle curve*) has a larger vent compared to earmold #2 (*lower curve*).

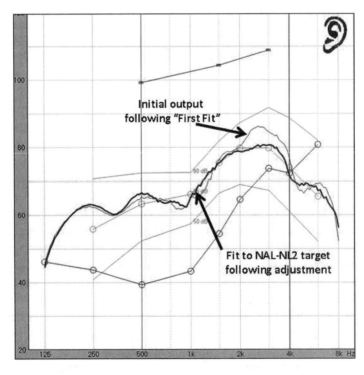

Figure 10–8. The match to the NAL-NL2 REAR prescriptive target using a real-speech 65 dB SPL input.

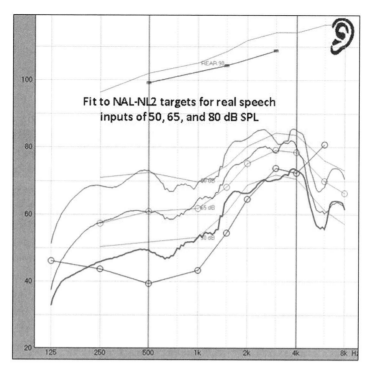

Figure 10–9. The match to the REAR target using a calibrated speech signal at three input levels, soft, average, and loud. The patient's thresholds, unaided LDLs, and aided MPOs are shown.

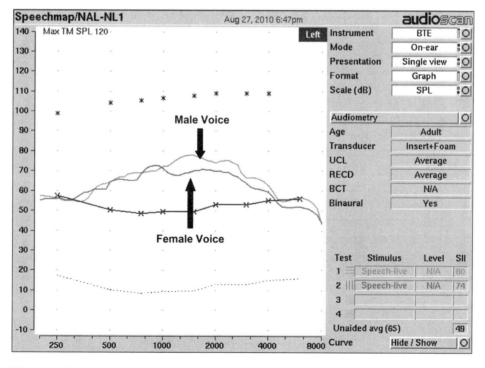

Figure 10–10. The effects of two different live voices on speech mapping (*male vs. female*).

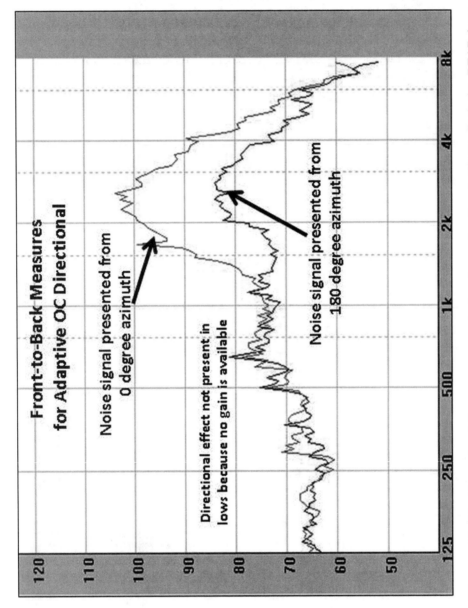

Figure 10–11. Example of the measurement of real-ear directional effects. Both the REAR front and REAR back were obtained with the hearing aid in the directional mode.

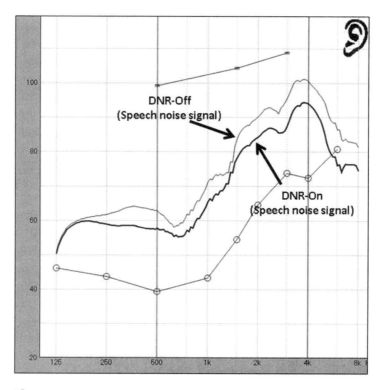

Figure 10–12. The effects of digital noise reduction (DNR) measured with the REAR. The top curve is with the DNR turned off and the bottom curve is with the DNR turned on.

Some Step-By-Step Guidelines

Rather than travel one their own to a foreign destinations, some people like to go on a guided tours. If you're the type of person who likes to have everything planned in advance with minimal preparation and stress, the following cook book approach to hearing aid verification might be for you.

Fitting hearing aids and the verification process is a systematic process. If you follow the steps outlined below, you will be able to successfully to fit and counsel your customers during a 60- to 90-minute appointment.

Step 1. Before the patient arrives for the appointment, run the hearing aids in the test box, using the 2-cc coupler. Check to ensure the hearing aids are functioning properly, and agree with ANSI specifications. This also is a good time to check the function of the directional microphones.

Step 2. Preprogram the hearing aids using the manufacturer's fitting software. Do this by entering threshold and UCL (LDL) data into the fitting software.

Step 3. Once the patient arrives, with the hearing aids turned off, insert them into the ear and check the fit. Ensure that the hearing aids or earmolds are not too loose or too tight.

Step 4. Establish realistic expectations. Mention the universal side effects of initial hearing aid use:

■ Annoyance of soft environmental sounds—hearing things the patient hasn't heard for years
■ Loud sounds being somewhat annoying (remember that even when the AGCo is set appropriately below the LDL, many patients, especially new users complain that loud sounds are too loud).
■ Hearing in noise—it is unlikely that the damaged cochlea will allow for speech understanding in noise equal to that of someone with normal hearing.
■ The occlusion effect.

Step 5. Using your probe-microphone equipment, run the REOR test. Ensure that the fitting has the desired "tightness" or if it is an OC fitting, the desired venting. For example, if you are fitting an OC fitting (and it truly is "open,") the REOR should be very similar to the REUR. Some software will ask you the "tightness" of the fit—better to measure than to guess.

Step 6. Verify the performance of the hearing aids using probe-microphone measures—either through REAR speech mapping, or REIG calculations. Ensure that soft sounds are audible, and that average and loud sounds are consistent with desired targets. Ensure that the MPO does not exceed the RESR targets. Conduct aided LDL testing using environmental noises. Check with your probe-microphone manufacturer's instruction manual for the details of conducting this testing.

Step 7. Counsel the patient on expectations, limitations, insertion/removal, care, and use. It should take you at least 30 minutes to do this.

Step 8. Schedule an appointment for the patient to return for a hearing aid check in one week.

Step 9. Call the patient 24 to 48 hours postfitting to check their current status. If they are having considerable difficult have them return sooner for a follow-up appointment.

Aided Sound-Field Testing

This is your lucky day. You have an appointment to have dinner with Todd Ricketts from Vanderbilt University to discuss a little clinical research study that you have designed. You board your plane in Minneapolis at 10:00 a.m., giving you plenty of time to get to Nashville. But . . . there is fog in Nashville and your flight is diverted to Knoxville. The only way you can fly to Nashville from Knoxville is to go through Memphis—you'll arrive too late for the important dinner. What do you do? You rent a car and drive to Nashville—it's only a two-hour drive. Not your desired or planned method, but it will get the job done and you will make your dinner appointment on time.

A somewhat antiquated method for verifying hearing aid performance is aided sound-field testing. Like driving a car rather than flying, it won't be your preferred method, but it might get the job done. There are cases when probe-mic testing just isn't feasible (e.g., excessive gooey cerumen in the ear canal), and aided sound field testing will at least give you an idea if you are making soft sounds audible (much better than taking a guess based on what you're seeing in the fitting software).

Aided sound-field testing can be used to determine something referred to as "functional gain." The patient is tested in the sound field both unaided and aided, and the aided thresholds are subtracted from the unaided thresholds, and the difference is the function gain. In theory, this should be quite similar to the probe-mic REIG—but ONLY for soft inputs.

Sound-field audiometry is conducted using an audiometer and loudspeakers attached to the audiometer. The patient is placed 1 meter from the speaker at a 0-degree azimuth. The speaker is at ear level. The distance and azimuth needs to be the same for both the unaided and aided measurements if you are conducting functional gain. For monaural testing, the nontest ear is plugged with a noise reduction plug, or preferably, air-conduction masking is applied. The gain of the hearing aid(s) is set at preferred user setting.

Rather than calculate functional "gain," it also is possible to only use the aided results. In this case, you probably would want to plot the findings on the count-the-dot audiogram to assess if soft inputs are being amplified appropriately for the different speech regions. Remember—there is no need to obtain aided thresholds better than 20 dB, as in the real world (with amplified ambient noise) this is about "as good as it gets."

Aided sound-field testing has several limitations and should only be used if probe-microphone measures are not available or cannot be conducted. Some of the problems with this measure include: poor test-retest, it can be influenced by room noise, circuit noise, compression or expansion circuits, head positioning and room reflections, and insufficient masking. At best case, it only provides an indication of gain for soft inputs—but yes, it's better than no verification at all.

A Summary Wine Analogy

We've talked a lot about prescriptive fitting methods, hearing aid verification and probe-mic measures. Many people seem to think that probe-mic measures are a *way* to fit hearing aids. This isn't true. They simply are a way for you to verify *your way* of fitting hearing aids. That means that you must have a way, a gold standard—something to verity.

Many wine drinkers prefer to consume a good Cabernet Sauvignon at 60 degrees. That is their gold standard. Many of these same people have a wine cooler with a thermometer. The job of the thermometer is to ensure that the wine is at 60 degrees. It's a way to measure if the wine meets the gold standard of the wine drinker.

Your probe-mic system is your thermometer. It's not there to think, or to make decisions about the fitting—that's your job. It doesn't have a gold standard. It simply tells you very accurately if the fitting meets *YOUR* gold standard!

Hearing Aid Orientation

All carry-on luggage should be safely stowed in the overhead lockers or under the seat in front of you. In preparing for takeoff, make sure your seat back is straight up and your tray table locked away. Seatbelts must be worn at all times when seated. When the seatbelt sign is turned off, you may move freely around the cabin. Return to your seat immediately if the seat belt sign is switched on and fasten your seat belt. No smoking is allowed on this flight in any part of the cabin, including the toilet areas . . .

An orientation is important when you're taking a flight somewhere, especially if you're a first-time flyer. The same is true for hearing aids.

After you have taken the time to carefully adjust the hearing aid parameters so that you have a reasonable match to prescriptive fitting targets (using your probe-mic equipment), and you've ensured that loud sounds are not too loud (using environmental sounds), you will need to spend considerable time and energy orienting the patient to his or her new hearing aids. This is a laborious, but critically important, process. Research has shown that when you spend quality time with your patients, methodically orienting and instructing them on the use, care and expectations of their hearing aids, that overall patient satisfaction is high. To make things flow a little smoother, we have organized the orientation phase of the fitting appointment into three easy-to-follow steps:

Step One: Hearing Aid Use

■ Instruct the patient on insertion and removal of the devices. Have them attempt to conduct this task in your office in front of you. You will have to show the patient how to hold the hearing aids during the insertion process (conduct this training over something "soft," as the hearing aids *will be* dropped). You will have to instruct them on adjusting the volume control, the remote, and any additional switches the hearing aids may have. Additionally, you need to demonstrate to the patient how to use the telephone with their new hearing aids. It's important to create a real-world situation, for example, they answer a ringing telephone.

■ Instruct the patient on care and maintenance. The patient needs to be shown how to clean the hearing aid. This will involve showing the patient how cerumen is removed from the end of the hearing aid. Part of care and maintenance is instructing the patient on how to change the battery and how to store the instruments when they are not being worn.

Step Two: Establish Realistic Expectations

■ If you are fitting a new hearing aid user, you will want to be sure to place him on a wearing schedule. A wearing schedule allows the patient to become acclimated to the new sounds they will be hearing. As a rule of thumb, new hearing aid users should start out wearing their hearing aids at home in a relaxed and quiet situation for a few days before wearing them in more demanding listening situations, like a restaurant. There is no reason the average new user needs more than a week to begin full-time use. The bottom line is that the patients need to give themselves a few days to get up to speed with their new devices, going from relatively easy to more difficult listening situations.

■ We know that new users tend to be bothered by louder noises when they start using their hearing aids, even if you have programmed gain for loud sounds correctly. Encourage them to attempt to adjust to these sounds, as over time, the annoyance level will be reduced.

■ We know that many new users expect the hearing aids to provide improved speech understanding in all listening environments— including extreme background noise. We recommend that you remind them during this initial orientation that there are certain situations where improvement will be limited.

Step Three: Offering Reassurance

■ Thinking back to Chapter 1 recall that we discussed the potential negative emotions surrounding hearing loss. Many of these emotions are still present on the day of the fitting. It's important to be patient and offer support for each individual, especially during their initial foray with hearing aids. No matter how frustrating you may feel regarding those patients who are just "not getting it," you will need to remain patient.

TIPS and TRICKS: Web Site Content

It's easy to create a Web site for your practice these days. One idea that works well is add hearing aid orientation and instructional material to your Web site. When patients need a refresher or forget something, you can simply have them go to your Web site for additional information. This is easy for most patients and it saves them a trip to your office.

Using a Checklist

Before you send the patient home with their new hearing aids, it is helpful to review a simple checklist with them. This will ensure that you have covered all the main points that often cause confusion or unnecessary stress for the patient. In case you might think that you've already told the patient what they need to know, here are some data about informational counseling, provided by our colleague, audiologist Bob Margolis:

■ Only about 50% of the information provided by health care providers is retained. Depending on conditions, 40 to 80% may be forgotten immediately.

■ Of the information that patients do recall, they remember about half *incorrectly*. So half is forgotten immediately, and half of what is remembered is wrong. Consider that if you remove 50% of the facts you told the patient about their hearing loss and hearing aids, and then distort half the remaining information; the result can be a highly misunderstood message.

■ Patients often forget their medical diagnoses. One study reported that patients could not recall 68% of the diagnoses told to them in a medical visit. When there were multiple diagnoses, patients couldn't recall the most important diagnosis 54% of the time. Another study found that after counseling, patients and the health care provider agreed on problems that required follow-up only 45% of the time.

These disturbing data about informational counseling certainly point out the importance of sending information along home with the patient. A hearing aid checklist is a good starting point. Here is a sample of what you can include:

☐ Verified prescriptive match of gain/output target using probe-microphone measures

☐ Ensured that loud sounds were not uncomfortably loud

☐ Ensured that patient found the quality of the programmed gain and output "acceptable"

☐ No acoustic feedback in typical use conditions

☐ Hearing aids fit properly (not too loose or too tight)

☐ Instructed on insertion and removal of hearing aids, and patient can now put hearing aids in and take them out

☐ Demonstrated how to use hearing aids with telephones

☐ Instructed on properly use of volume control and/or remote control

☐ Counseled on initial use of the hearing aids and realistic expectations (reviewed wearing schedule for the first week to 10 days)

☐ Instructed on care, cleaning, proper storage, and batteries

☐ Given phone number to call with questions or problems

TAKE FIVE:
Internet Friendly

CounselEar is a Web-based company that allows you to design your own patient counseling materials. As patients forget so much of what we tell them, CounselEar allows you to provide them with memorable printed material that has your name, logo, and contact information.

Short-Term Follow-Up Procedures

One tactic you can use to ensure that your patients are adjusting to their new hearing aids is to phone them a day or two after the initial fitting. This small gesture is an excellent way to uncover any problems, such as, are they having trouble inserting the hearing aids into their ears? At the same time, it sends positive messages to each patient by showing them that you care, and that you are going the extra mile to serve them. Ask them questions like how long they are using the hearing aids, what situations, and what problems they might be having.

Remember your pretesting procedures from Chapter 7? You might want to note those patients who have a large

ANL, unusually low LDLs, or a poor score on the QuickSIN and target them for additional attention the first week or two after the fitting.

Troubleshooting Common Problems

You're sitting at the gate waiting to board a flight for a long-anticipated family reunion. Five minutes before boarding, there is an announcement that the flight has been canceled due to "mechanical failure." Most passengers rush to the gate agent for re-boarding, and a 50-person line quickly forms. Others pull out their laptop to look for the next flight to their destination. You simply take out your cell phone and call the Delta priority number you have programmed for such an occasion. Within five minutes, you are re-booked on a flight leaving in two hours, sitting in the bar across from the gate, sipping your favorite beverage (the line for the gate agent is still getting longer). Some problems are easy to solve if you approach them correctly.

We end this chapter on fitting procedures by talking about how to address common problems often associated with first-time hearing aid use. As you have already gathered, fitting hearing aids successfully is a series of compromises. This means that when you solve one notorious problem often you open the door to another. Don't be too alarmed by this statement, as we'll help you to avoid creating new problems (like standing in line, when you simply could have called the airline).

First, not all patients present with the problems that we will describe. If you take the time to do all the clinical procedures outlined in previous chap-

ters, things usually fall into place quite nicely. Second, even when patients arrive at your door with one of these common problems, if you follow the guidelines here, there is a pretty good chance you will solve the problem the first time. Our goal is to familiarize you with some of the more common problems associated with hearing aid use, especially during the first few weeks after a new fitting.

The Occlusion Effect

We've discussed this briefly in previous chapters, but let's talk about it again. The occlusion effect can be best described as an echo or hollow sensation occurring when the patient is speaking or chewing. Your older patients may describe it as sounding like they are "talking in a barrel" (young people don't talk in barrels so much). This sensation can be highly annoying and it is more likely to be annoying for patients having better than 30 to 40 dB HL thresholds in the low frequencies.

Here is how it works. When we talk, sound energy from vocalizations in the back of our throat travels to the ear canal through via bone conduction through the mandible (jawbone). These bone-conducted sounds cause the cartilaginous portion of the ear canal to vibrate, which creates an air conduction sound in the ear canal (primarily low frequency). Normally, this sound energy escapes laterally through the open ear canal. But if the ear canal is closed off by the hearing aid shell or earmold, the energy cannot escape, and is transferred through the middle ear to the cochlea. Thus, the patient with this problem often complains that their own voice sounds loud, hollow (because it primarily enhances the low frequencies) or unusual when they talk. With some probe-mic equipment, you can attach earphones, and listen to this yourself from your patient's ear.

There are two common ways to solve the occlusion effect problem. The first is to fit an earmold or hearing aid shell that fits deeply into the ear canal. By sealing the earmold or shell beyond the second bend of the ear canal, the vibration of the cartilaginous portion of the canal is held to a minimum and the occlusion effect is mostly prevented from occurring. Although tackling the problem in this manner is an earnest goal, the side effects of a deep fitting earmold or shell can cause significant amounts of pain and discomfort for some patients. The hearing aid also can be difficult to insert. Therefore, this solution, although theoretically sound, is not very practical.

The second, and by far more popular, way to fix the occlusion effect problem is through venting. When a vent of 2 mm or more is created, sound energy can readily escape. The larger you make the vent the more likely you are to solve the occlusion problem. Not all occlusions effect problems have the same peak frequency—if the peak of the effect is around 200 Hz, this will be much easier to solve with venting than if the occlusion peak is around 750 Hz (in case we forgot to tell you in an earlier chapter, it's quite easy to measure the effect across frequencies with your probe-mic equipment). Once the vent reaches 3 mm or so, most occlusion effects are minimized. The problem of course, is with some fittings, such as a CIC, it usually isn't possible to create a vent this large.

Today's OC fittings don't have a vent per se, but their "openness" (using the smallest dome) certainly creates the venting of a very large traditional vent. As we've discussed before, this if one of the primary advantages of this type of fitting. However, making the vent bigger is also likely to bring in other problems, namely, the problem we'll talk about shortly, acoustic feedback.

What Doesn't Work Very Well

It is important to talk about what *doesn't* reduce the occlusion effect. Recall that the effect is produced by a signal traveling along the mandible to the ear canal, *NOT* a signal traveling though the hearing aid. Hence, it is only logical that changing the programming of the hearing aid, reducing low frequencies for example, will *NOT* reduce the occlusion effect. In fact, this approach could have a negative effect if the person needed the low-frequency amplification to understand soft speech. If you have a patient and turning down low-frequency gain made the occlusion effect go away, then the problem probably wasn't the occlusion effect in the first place—it probably was "too much gain for the low frequencies"—a different problem.

Some have suggested that you *add* low-frequency gain to fix the occlusion effect. The thought is that the gain of the hearing aid will sound more "natural" than that produced by the occlusion effect (and this might be true, as the occlusion effect is different for different vowels). The extra low frequencies from the occlusion would still be there, but the "effect" would be masked. However, the added low frequencies from the hearing aid might work against speech understanding in background noise, so again, this isn't the preferred solution.

TIPS and TRICKS: Occlusion Effect, Or Not?

When a patients says that there voice sounds "hollow" or "booming" we usually assume it's the occlusion effect, but the complaint could be related to too much programmed low-frequency gain. A quick test is to have the patient read a passage with the hearing turned on, and then again with the instrument off. If the hollow sound goes away with the hearing aid turned off, it's *not* the occlusion effect.

Acoustic Feedback

There are many types of feedback associated with hearing aids. The type that we are concerned with here is called acoustic feedback, and it occurs as a result of sound leaking around or through the earmold or shell, going back to the microphone inlet, and then getting fed back through the hearing aid. When this sound gets fed back through the hearing aid it is amplified with other sounds arriving at the input. This results in an audible squealing sound that is very annoying to the user, and to others, and contributes to poor sound quality for the user. Also, it often prompts the user to use less gain, which then, of course, reduces overall hearing aid benefit. And, in some cases, the patient will simply stop using the hearing aid.

Any hearing aid has the potential to feed back or whistle from time to time.

In fact, all hearing aids will create feedback when a hand is cupped around them tightly while they are being worn on the ear, or the hearing aid is being inserted and removed from the ear and it is turned on. Even when worn, there is always sound leaking out of the ear, which competes with the sound coming into the ear through the same air spaces. When the sound trying to get out exceeds the sound trying to get in feedback occurs. This usually happens when the input is low, and the gain is high, which is why some patients don't notice feedback unless they are sitting quietly in their living room. Consider that for this setting, the input is very low (ambient noise) and if it's a WDRC instrument, gain is probably at its peak. The software from several manufacturers allows you to measure this relationship, often referred to as "open loop gain."

There are a couple of reasons that make some hearing aids more prone to acoustic feedback. Hearing aids with high output are more likely to produce feedback, if the earmold or shell is not sealed tightly into the ear canal. The simple way to fix this problem is to tighten the fit of the earmold or shell. The earmold and shell need to be modified or completely remade. Feedback is especially likely to occur when a high-output hearing aid has a larger (>1 mm) vent. This often causes a fitting dilemma, as the vent may be needed to release some pressure and low-frequency energy.

Another factor which can encourage acoustic feedback is an obstruction in the ear canal, which is likely to be cerumen (earwax). Occluding cerumen causes the sound to be pushed back through the vent and tiny slit leaks of the ear canal or shell, resulting in feedback. Once the occluding cerumen is removed the problem with feedback is solved. A similar event can occur with a RIC device if the receiver is pushed up against the earcanal wall.

A final cause of acoustic feedback occurs because a part of the sounds transmission system is failing. Remember that in most BTE devices amplified sounds travels from the receiver through the earhook and tubing. If there is a crack or split in the earhook or tubing, sound can leak through and cause feedback. Table 10–2 is a checklist outlining common leakage points, which can result in feedback in a BTE instrument.

In modern hearing aids, acoustic feedback problems can be alleviated in two ways. One is mechanical and the other electronic. Mechanical solutions include minimizing the vent size, changing the tubing or removing cerumen from the ear canal. Acoustic feedback

Table 10–2. Common Causes of Acoustic Feedback in a BTE Hearing Aid

- Microphone or receiver is loose within the BTE case

- Earhook is too loose on the hearing aid

- Earhook is split

- Tubing is too loose on the earhook

- Tubing is cracked or split

- Earmold fits into ear too loosely

- Vent is too large

- Cerumen pushed earmold away from the canal wall

- Cerumen directs sound into vent or slit leak

can also be fixed electronically by activating an "anti-feedback" algorithm, also referred to as automatic feedback reduction in the fitting software of the hearing aid (a feature we discussed in Chapter 9). Although each manufacturer uses an automatic feedback reduction algorithm, there are variations in how the algorithms are implemented. All of them can effectively reduce mild feedback problems, but there is a fairly big difference among manufactuers (~8 to 10 dB) regarding the added stable gain each device provides. Today's feedback algorithms, however, on average allow you to use 10 to 15 dB more gain with an open fitting than was possible a decade ago before these algorithms were developed.

Automatic feedback systems are extremely helpful, and as mentioned, allow for patients to enjoy more useable gain, especially in the high frequencies in OC products. They simply don't solve all feedback problems, however, and when overused cause hearing care professionals to cut corners on getting a high quality earmold or shell fit; also, if the feedback suppression circuit is running continuously, battery drain will be increased. Even though some hearing aid features are designed to automatically fix some problems, you still have to think (and sometimes do a little extra work)!

Loud Sounds Are Too Loud

The first two common problems reviewed in this chapter mainly dealt with mechanical solutions requiring the clinician to make some physical change in the earmold or shell to solve it. We now turn our attention to some other common problems that require an electronic solution. An electronic solution simply means that the clinician has to change one or more acoustic parameters to solve the problem by using the hearing aid software to adjust the acoustic parameters of the hearing aid.

When a loud sound amplified by the hearing aid is perceived as being too loud by the user, this can result in a "tolerance" problem. In Chapter 6 we reviewed why and how loudness discomfort levels (LDLs) can be measured. Although measuring the LDL will assist you in setting the output of the hearing aid (AGCo thresholds), and you will conduct aided loudness measures before the patient leaves your office, some patients still may complain that loud input sounds are uncomfortably loud when they begin their real-world experiences. Studies have shown this to be a fairly serious problem, as about 40% report that these sounds are uncomfortable, and 15% of hearing aid users report that loud sounds are uncomfortable enough to prevent them from wearing their hearing aids.

Even if you have measured unaided LDLs and verified that aided LDL are below the output of the hearing aid when you conducted probe-mic testing, there still may be times when you need to reduce the output of the hearing aid slightly in order to eliminate a comfort problem with loud sounds. First, however, it is important to determine if the sound is truly "uncomfortable" (#7 on the Contour Anchor List— see Chapter 6), or if the sound is just louder than what the patient is accustomed to, but is really still okay (#6 on the Contour Anchor List). If loud environmental sounds are rated #6, then your treatment might simply be coun-

seling: the patient simply needs to know that the world is louder than what they remember. If, however, a patient is complaining about loud sounds being too loud, and the loudness ratings indeed are #7, you have three choices regarding how to fix the problem:

- The preferred method is to lower the AGCo kneepoint(s). Do this in 2 dB increments while presenting a loud signal to the patient, until the patient gives you a #6 rating.
- In some instances, even when the AGCo is at its lowest setting, the patient still states that loud sounds are #7 (uncomfortable). Before going any further and potentially messing up the entire fitting, turn the hearing aid off and present the same signal. In some cases, if it is an open fitting, and the patient has an unusually low LDL, the direct sound to the TM is what is causing the discomfort. Obviously, in these cases, changing the hearing aid setting will not make things better. Assuming this is not the case, another method to lower the output for high inputs is to increase (make larger) the WDRC ratio (e.g., go from 2:1 to 3:1). Unfortunately, this also will lower the output for average speech, and now average speech might not be at the patient's MCL, something you will need to check out.
- Finally, lowering gain will decrease the output for loud sounds. This is the least desirable option, and this will likely pull average speech down below the MCL, and could very well make soft speech inaudible. However, if you do not do either choice #1 or #2 above, the patient may be left with no option than to

lower gain, reducing overall benefit simply because of an unsolved loudness problem.

We have included a very helpful chart (Table 10–3) to assist in navigating the many possible adjustments associated with gain, output, and compression. The patient's possible judgments for soft, average, and loud sounds are listed in the columns. The possible adjustments recommended to address the problem are listed at the bottom of the table. The column on the far right of Table 10–3 lists the suggested adjusted you should make for each patient complaint respectively.

Difficulty Understanding Speech in Noise

Many if not most patients complain of an inability to understand speech in the presence of background noise. Many normal hearing people have this same complaint. This is probably the most common problem you will encounter and it is likely to be the most challenging. This is because there are many underlying components to the problem as well as some possible solutions.

A good rule of thumb for solving any of the problems listed is to always do things right during the prefitting selection and subsequent fitting appointments. Cutting corners and failing to complete certain tests and procedures is more likely to increase the likelihood of patients returning with problems. In this case, you will have a printout of the real-ear SPL, which will provide some guidance regarding what has (or has not) been accomplished. If you conducted speech-in-noise testing as

we recommended (e.g., the QuickSIN described in Chapter 6), you already have a fairly good idea of how well a given patient will perform in background noise. For example, if his SNR loss was 12 dB, you should not be surprised that he is having problems, as most all group social activities have an SNR more adverse than 12 dB. If his QuickSIN SNR loss was only 3 dB, you might wonder if you have the hearing aids programmed optimally, or if maybe the patient has unusually high expectations, or is using the wrong program.

When to Leave the Mouse Alone

That leads us to a common challenge associated with solving hearing aid fitting problems, especially the one associated with understanding speech in noise. This is, knowing when to make an adjustment to the acoustic parameters of the hearing aid with the fitting software and knowing when *not* to grab your mouse, but simply to counsel the patient on expectations and acclimatization. Often, clinicians have to do some combination of counseling and fine tuning of the hearing aids to get things right. As a general rule, patients do need to be given ample time to allow the central auditory mechanisms of their brain to adapt to sounds not heard for several years. "Wear it a while and you'll probably get used to it" is a phrase many experienced hearing care professionals rely on when working with new hearing aid users. Or, when it comes to annoying background noise, you might try this line:

"You have to hear what you don't want to hear to know what you don't want to hear."

Table 10–3. A General Guideline for Providing Adjustments in Gain, Output, and Compression Based on Patient Complaints for Soft, Average, and Loud Inputs

Speech (45 dB SPL)	Average Speech (65 dB SPL)	Loud Speech (85 dB SPL)	Adjustment
Okay	Okay	Okay	A
Okay	Okay	Too Loud	D
Okay	Okay	Too Soft	E
Okay	Too Loud	Okay	D, F
Okay	Too Soft	Okay	E, G
Okay	Too Loud	Too Loud	D
Okay	Too Loud	Too Soft	D, G
Okay	Too Soft	Too Loud	E, F
Okay	Too Soft	Too Soft	E
Too Soft	Okay	Okay	C, D
Too Soft	Okay	Too Loud	C, D, G
Too Soft	Okay	Too Soft	C, D, F
Too Soft	Too Loud	Okay	C, D, G
Too Soft	Too Soft	Okay	C, D
Too Soft	Too Soft	Too Soft	C
Too Loud	Okay	Okay	B, E
Too Loud	Okay	Too Loud	B, E, F
Too Loud	Okay	Too Soft	B, E, G
Too Loud	Too Loud	Okay	B, E, F
Too Loud	Too Soft	Okay	B, E
Too Loud	Too Loud	Too Loud	B

A: Pat yourself on the back!

B: Decrease overall gain by 5 dB.

C: Increase overall gain by 5 dB.

D: Decrease compression kneepoint by 5 dB (if kneepoint is already set at "min" dB, increase compression ratio by one step).

E: Increase compression kneepoint by 5 dB (if kneepoint is already set at "max" dB, decrease compression ratio by one step).

F: Decrease compression ratio by one step (if ratio is already set at "min" level, increase compression kneepoint by 5 dB).

G: Increase compression ratio by one step (if ratio is already set at "max" level, decrease compression kneepoint by 5 dB).

As you will soon see, knowing when to counsel a patient and when to make an adjustment to the hearing aid is as much as art as a science.

Problems Talking on the Telephone

The last common problem we address is difficulty hearing conversations on the telephone. Using the telephone might seem like a fairly routine task, but for many hearing aid users talking on the phone is a huge challenge. Adding to the depth of the challenge is that most patients have several land-line telephone as well as at least one mobile phone. Before reviewing some of the common solutions to problems associated with telephone use, you want to review that related material on telecoils in Chapter 8.

As nearly everyone now uses a cell phone it's important to make sure patients have access to hearing aid technology that's compatible with cell phones. It's actually a fairly complicated process, but we have included some things to remember when troubleshooting problems with hearing aids and cell phones.

When using a cell phone, the telephone conversation is transmitted over a wireless network using radio waves. The radio waves emitted by the cell phone are referred to as radio-frequency (RF) emissions. The RF emissions create an electromagnetic (EM) field around the phone's antenna. This EM field has a pulsing pattern. It is this pulsing energy that may potentially be picked up by the hearing aid's microphone or telecoil circuitry and perceived by the hearing aid wearer as a buzzing sound.

To complicate matters, the technology for transmitting calls over a wireless network differs depending on the carrier or service provider. For example, Verizon Wireless and Sprint PCS use CDMA technology, Nextel uses iDEN technology, and AT&T Wireless, Cingular Wireless, and T-Mobile use GSM technology. Of course, cell phone technology changes very quickly, so this information may be outdated by the time you are reading this book! The interference generated by these various technologies has different characteristics, some of which may cause more annoying interference for hearing aid users than others. The amount of interference experienced by hearing-aid users depends on the degree of RF emissions produced by a particular digital cell phone, and how immune his or her particular hearing aids are to these emissions.

In 2003, the Federal Communications Commission (FCC) partially lifted the exemption to hearing aid compatibility (HAC) requirements for digital wireless phones. For acoustic coupling to a hearing aid's microphone, the new rules require each digital phone manufacturer and carrier to have two commercially available handsets for each transmission technology with reduced RF emissions. For hearing aids with a telecoil, digital phone manufacturers and carriers have to make available two handsets that provide telecoil-coupling capability for each transmission technology they offer. The new ruling also requires a standard method for measuring digital cell phone emissions (i.e., ANSI C63.19) and product labeling on the outside packaging of the phone. Volume control is not part of this new requirement. However, most cell phones do have a volume control, although there is a standardized upper limit on the sound level that cell phones can produce.

There are two Web sites that you and your patients can use to sort out capability issues related to hearing aid and cell phone use: http://www.wirelessadvisor.com and http://www.phonescoop.com provide information on cell phones that are compatible with various types of hearing aids.

These days many people use two or more landline telephones. Remember from Chapter 8 that the leaking electromagnetic energy from the telephone is picked by the telecoil and amplified by the hearing aid. The strength of this leaking electromagnetic varies from phone to phone; therefore, it's difficult to gauge success with telecoils when you demonstrate how it works to a patient in your office phone during the initial fitting appointment. To get you started with have included some telecoil troubleshooting advice in Table 10–4.

Finally, each year hearing aid manufacturers introduce new wireless telephone solutions; many incorporating Bluetooth technology. Refer back to Chapter 9 for a review of these features and devices. These systems seem to improve every year, both in quality and ease of use, and we predict that the "problems on the telephone" complaint soon will be reduced significantly.

In Closing

By now we hope you have reached your destination. All your careful planning has enabled you to have a smooth and relatively stress-free journey to you becoming a dispensing professional. You are almost ready to settle in and enjoy the experience of providing hearing health care to patients. You should notice that the hearing aid fitting procedure is a systematic process requiring a blend of art and science. The first

Table 10–4. Common Problems Associated with Landline Telephone Use Plus Possible Solutions

Common Problems	Possible Solutions
Even after several adjustments, the patient complains he or she can't talk on the phone.	1. Have the patient bring the phone to the office. Evaluate their telecoil use along with their actual phone. Patient may need to purchase phone with better coupling capabilities. 2. Talk to your patient about special amplified telephones available from Oaktree or Warner Technologies.
Patient has difficulty switching to telecoil program.	1. Reinstruct patient on using the programming button. 2. Go to switchless telecoil.

phase of the fitting process involves a lot of science. You need to know how prescriptive fitting procedures work, how to check the hearing aid in the coupler, and, then, how to verify that you are at a reasonable starting point through the application of probe-microphone measures.

The second phase of the fitting appointment requires you to be an effective communicator and troubleshooter. You will need to go through many details of use, care, and maintenance in a methodical fashion. This guidance will need to be repeated, and repeated.

The bottom line is that fitting hearing aids correctly requires a lot of thinking and attention to detail—sometimes problem-solving. Once you become comfortable with the entire process, you will ensure that each patient you see is off to a good start with his or her new hearing aids. Let's hope that they too experience little turbulence, and have a safe and enjoyable journey.

11

Outcome Assessments and Postfitting Issues

> *You don't have to subscribe to* **Consumer Reports** *to appreciate a high-quality hearing aid fitting. Find out how buying a car is like fitting hearing aids and assessing outcomes.*

Let's say that you recently have undergone knee replacement surgery, and are concerned about the success of the procedure. Your physical therapist is likely to put you through a series of simple tests that measure your success, and this will be compared to others who have had the same surgery. Some of the measures might include a questionnaire in which you rate the quality of care that you received from the entire organization; everyone from the front office receptionist to the nurses to the surgeon. Today, if a business has obtained your E-mail address when you did business with them, it is common for you to receive a request to rate your satisfaction for their goods or services. Therefore, it's not surprising that measuring success (or "outcomes" as they are commonly called) is also an important part of the service hearing

care professionals provide. It seems like every sort of business measures satisfaction using a questionnaire, including the automobile industry. We're betting the last time you purchased a car you had to complete some type of satisfaction survey shortly after you bought it that asked you questions about the car and the service you were provided. And you know what . . . it's very possible that you were more satisfied simply because they asked you if you were satisfied! More on that later.

Throughout this book, we've emphasized that the selection and fitting of hearing aids needs to be a careful step-by-step procedure. This final step in this hearing aid fitting process is ensuring in some tangible (and documented) way that favorable results from the use of hearing aids have been achieved by the patient during real-world use.

Outcome Measures: Some Background

The measurement of hearing aid outcomes commonly is referred to as *validation* of the fitting. This is an important step because it allows both you and the patient to know how much benefit and/or satisfaction has been attained from the use of amplification. Unlike verification, which we discussed in Chapter 10, validation is not related to whether the hearing aids are meeting a specific standard; validation is related to how the patient "likes" the hearing aids. That highly scientific term "likes" can mean a lot of different things. We show that there are several dimensions of hearing aid use that really should be measured and/or validated. In fact,

we can take this one step further and say that today's well-informed savvy patients actually expect you to systematically measure the results of the fitting, and report your findings to them in clear language.

Another reason measuring hearing aid outcomes is important is because you systematically can compare results across patients. For example, if you work in a busy clinical setting, the use of a couple of outcome measures systemically can show you how hearing aid benefits compare across your entire patient population. The effective professional knows that the only way to improve performance is to measure it. Using a couple of different outcome measures during the postfitting period allows you to find areas in your clinical practice to improve.

TAKE FIVE: Verification Versus Validation

Ever try to make chocolate chip cookies that taste just like your mom's? If you're lucky you have her recipe (if she used one), and you very carefully could follow all the same directions. You, of course, would ensure that the flour, sugar, chips, butter, and other ingredients were mixed together in perfect portions—that's *verification*, just like you use probe-mic measures to ensure that your prescriptive fitting

"recipe" is mixed correctly. But, as you know, the only way to really know if the cookies are as good as mom's is to take a few good bites just as they come out of the oven— that's *validation*! Like chocolate chip cookies, we know that with hearing aid fittings, a good verification procedure *should* lead to a successful outcome, but we really don't know for sure, however, until our patients take a few "bites" in the real world.

Assessing Treatment

The use of outcome measures more or less is a measure of the success of the hearing aid and aural rehabilitative "treatment." In regard to hearing aids,

the treatment can be organized into three different areas:

■ Treatment effectiveness: Do hearing aid improve audibility and speech understanding?

TIPS and TRICKS: Practical Uses of Outcome Measures

Outcome measures can be used to answer this important question posed by patients: "Can I hear any better since I purchased my hearing aids?" Essentially, there are two ways you could answer this question with an outcome measure.

1. Document that hearing aids have improved the quality of life or reduced hearing handicap in everyday listening conditions.

A questionnaire or self-report would be used.

2. Demonstrate to the patient that hearing aids improve speech intelligibility in noise, improve overall listening comfort, or some other important aspect of communication. A comparison of the unaided to the aided condition using a test conducted in your sound booth or a questionnaire could be used.

- Treatment efficiency: Do certain hearing aids and fitting algorithms work better than others for improving audibility and speech understanding in different listening situations?
- Treatment effects: Does the use of well-fitted hearing aids improve the patient's social and emotional well-being, and overall quality of life?

Guidance From the WHO

Outcome measures relate to the different aspects related to having a hearing loss, and the hearing aid treatment of a hearing loss. Many of these measures relate to terms that have been used and standardized over the years by the World Heath Organization, and are reviewed in Table 11–1. To expand on these basic terms, consider that disability is an outcome of interactions which includes the person's health conditions and contextual factors, both personal and environmental. The outcome of disability can be described at three levels:

- Impairment of body function or structure
- Activity limitations measured as capacity
- Participation restrictions measured as performance

This terminology is meant to be generic; it applies to a wide range of health issues—keep these terms in mind however, as we talk about disease-specific outcome measures throughout this chapter.

Unfortunately, the majority of hearing care professionals do not take the time to systematically measure the results of their hearing aid fittings. You're lucky—as you are just getting started it makes good sense to begin the habit of measuring outcomes from your treatments. The goal of this chapter is to give you the tools to measure hearing aid fitting, counseling, and auditory rehabilitative outcomes so that you can monitor results and improve your delivery of services to patients.

Table 11–1. Terms Used by the World Health Organization

> _Disorder:_ Occurs as a result of some type of disease process or malformation of the auditory system (e.g., presbycusis).
>
> _Impairment:_ Any loss or abnormality of psychological, physiologic, or anatomic structure or function (e.g., high-frequency hearing loss).
>
> _Disability:_ Any restriction or lack of ability to perform an activity in the manner or within the range considered normal (e.g., unable to understand average speech in background noise).
>
> _Handicap:_ A disadvantage for a given individual, resulting from an impairment or a disability, that limits or prevents the fulfillment of a role that is normal, based on their age, gender, social, and cultural factors (e.g., unable to continue coaching basketball because of speech-in-noise understanding problems).
>
> _Activity Limitations:_ Difficulties an individual may have in executing activities (e.g., unable to understand television when there is background noise).
>
> _Participation Restrictions:_ Problems an individual might experience in individual life situations (e.g., avoids gathering with friends at neighborhood tavern to watch football on TV).

Types of Outcome Measures

Technically speaking, an outcome measure is a measure of the impact of the management or treatment plan. In prac-tical terms, it is more or less the results of your hearing aid fitting and counseling efforts. There are several dimensions or domains of hearing aid outcome. They include the following:

- Daily use
- Sound quality
- Speech understanding
- Loudness normalization
- Listening effort
- Quality of life
- Social interaction
- Reduced burden of significant other

TAKE FIVE: Quality of Life and Hearing Aids

If we simply say "quality of life," you have a pretty good idea of what we are referring to. It often refers to freedom of choice, peace of mind, family, friends, living conditions, and so on. But of course, your quality of life can be impacted by a medical condition, such as a hearing loss. When quality of life is considered in regard to the impact of a disease, illness, or injury, we are referring to an individual's health-related quality of life which is abbreviated HRQoL. HRQoL can be considered a concept that encompasses the physical, emotional, and social components associated with an illness (such as hearing loss) or treatment (such as hearing aids). There are five major areas that are commonly mentioned in regard to HRQoL: physical status and functional abilities; psychological status and well-being; social interactions; economic and/or vocational status; and religious and/or spiritual status.

The first thing you should notice about this list is that some of the dimensions are directly related to the performance of the hearing aids. For example, sound quality, speech understanding, and loudness normalization are directly related to the quality of the product, and how it is programmed. These are commonly referred to as device components of hearing aid outcomes. On the other hand, there are other dimensions of outcome that measure the impact the hearing aids have on issues related to improving the hearing handicap that often results from the hearing loss. Domains like social interaction, quality of life, and reduced burden on significant others are examples of these nondevice components. Indirectly, of course, they all could be device related; if you do not program the hearing aids correctly. it's very unlikely that quality of life will improve.

For the professional fitting his or her first pair of hearing aids, the important point to remember is that there are several dimensions of outcome (we only listed a few of them), and each dimension can be measured. When it comes to appreciating the importance of hearing aid outcome measures, a good first step is to understand the difference between being satisfied with hearing aids versus benefiting from them.

Benefit Versus Satisfaction— What You're Measuring

You recently purchased a new Hummer H3. You purchased it because you'd like to do more off-road driving in the mountains. Because of its horsepower and size the Hummer excels at off-road trekking. From a benefit standpoint it is excellent. However, *the Hummer has very poor gas mileage and it's incredibly noisy when driving it down the highway—the 95% of the time you're actually using it. Therefore, you are very unsatisfied with the outcome of your purchase. This is an example of having a great benefit (in this case it's benefit in one situation) with poor overall satisfaction.*

A common occurrence with hearing aids is that patients give high praise to the professional and the great service they receive (highly satisfied) but struggle achieving benefit (still cannot hear well in background noise). As we'll mention again later, benefit and especially satisfaction are tied to expectations. A patient who thought he would be understanding about 50% of what is said in background noise with his new expensive hearing aids would be very satisfied if he ended up understanding 75%. On the other hand, a patient who thought he would be understanding 100% in this listening environment would have a low satisfaction rating for the very same benefit.

Measuring Benefit

The difference between a patient's unaided performance and aided performance is called benefit. Any time we administer a test in the unaided condition and compare it to the aided condition we are measuring benefit. Hearing aid benefit can be defined as the difference between unaided and aided performance measured either objectively or subjectively.

After reading the first 10 chapters of this book, you probably can think of several tests you could conduct in both the aided and unaided condition. Each one of these tests, including hearing thresholds, speech-in-quiet, speech-in-background noise, and so forth, are measures of hearing aid benefit when aided results are compared to the unaided condition. For example, a patient's QuickSIN's SNR loss might improve by 5 dB when he is aided. Hearing aid benefit also can be measured subjectively through the use of self-report measures, commonly called questionnaires—for example, a person may have reported 70% problems in background noise without hearing aids, and then a month after the fitting, the problems may be reduced to only 30% using amplification.

Because objective tests usually are completed using a predefined external standard, almost exclusively they are tests taking place within the laboratory (research studies), clinic, or office. Although this type of testing can provide meaningful results, the test environment often does not reflect the actual use conditions for the patient. Therefore, self-report measures of outcome are a useful method of determining real-world benefits of hearing aid performance. It is tempting to believe that a benefit measured in your office or clinic will also be present in the real world, but this only is true if the patient experiences a very similar listening situation.

Measuring Satisfaction

Another separate dimension of a hearing aid fitting outcome is satisfaction. Satisfaction differs from benefit in that satisfaction is not necessarily performance driven. For example, a patient can have a significant degree of benefit as measured on any comparative aided and unaided tests, but be reporting dissatisfaction as measured on a satisfaction scale. The opposite also can happen, although this is less likely.

Most hearing care professionals would agree that satisfaction is a nebulous dimension of outcome because it can comprise many variables, such as professionalism of the staff, cleanliness of the office, and wait time in the reception area. Satisfaction is also highly correlated to expectations: to state the obvious, people who have fairly low expectations are the easiest to satisfy. People who receive free hearing aids tend to be more satisfied, although the difference isn't as much as you might think. Even though satisfaction does comprise many dimensions, just like benefit, it can be measured using a questionnaire.

In the remainder of the chapter we review clinical tests that can be used to measure outcome, and self-reports of hearing aid outcomes and the various questionnaires used to measure it. The important thing to remember for now is that both self-reports and clinical measures are important to conduct.

Clinic Versus Real World—How You're Measuring Outcome

There are two different ways we can measure hearing aid outcomes. The first is laboratory or clinical (office) measures. These consist of any type of measurement you would conduct in your office or clinic, typically in the test booth. As a general rule, laboratory measures are objective in nature and engage the patient in some type of quantifiable task. This means the patient is required to complete some type of test, and results are scored as a percent correct (or incorrect) and compared to

---

TAKE FIVE: When Is It Benefit and When Is It Satisfaction?

This quiz will help you understand the difference between satisfaction and benefit. When a patient who you fitted with hearing aids two weeks ago comes back to your clinic and says the following, is it a statement about satisfaction or benefit. The answers are at the bottom.

1. "I love my new hearing aids."
2. "I sure notice a difference with these hearing aids in noisy places."
3. "When I put these hearing aids on I can turn the TV down low."

4. "I told by friend that he should come in and see you for getting new hearing aids."
5. "I wear these hearing aids 12 hours per day without any trouble. They really help me understand speech."
6. "These hearing aids don't help me all that much, but you have been so helpful"

Answers:
1. *Satisfaction*   2. *Benefit*   3. *Benefit*
4. *Satisfaction*   5. *Benefit*
6. *Satisfaction*

---

normative data. The objective nature of laboratory tests makes them valuable because you can quickly compare scores to an average, or use the patient as their own control. Additionally, the test can be specifically designed to collect important information regarding the functioning of the hearing aids (e.g., does the directional microphone technology improve speech understanding when there is a talker in front and noise originates from behind?). The downside to laboratory tests is that they often are conducted in contrived listening environments that are not reflective of everyday listening conditions. Or, the listening task itself is something that the listener will rarely experience.

Although they are considered subjective in nature, self-assessment inventories or questionnaires of hearing aid outcome capture patients' judgments of hearing aid benefit and satisfaction in real-world listening conditions. For this reason, self-reports of outcome usually are considered to be the gold standard when it comes to measuring hearing aid outcomes because they are capturing success (or lack of) in everyday listening places. However, there are a couple of pitfalls associated with self-reports. First, if the questionnaire does not capture situations the individual patient is familiar with, the information you are gathering is essentially meaningless because the measure does not reflect that individual patient's daily experience. A second issue is that the questionnaire may not be specific enough: general questions about understanding in background noise might not reveal the benefit of directional microphone technology, even though lab findings show that the algorithm is working effectively.

A final limitation is associated with variability. The way you administer (hand it to the patient or mail to them), the personality of the patient (do they want to please you?), and even when you administer it (the day of the fitting or 6 months after) all affect the results.

Do not, however, equate those pitfalls with a lack of validity. Self-reports, when properly standardized and validated, are accurate and reflective of the patient's experiences. Your job is simply to choose the best self-report for the patients you typically see on a daily basis. What self-assessment inventory answers the questions that you are the most concerned about?

Clinic (Office) Measures of Outcome

Before purchasing your next car, you go to the Internet and meticulously review gas mileage, crash ratings, and emissions standards. All of these characteristics are measured objectively in a contrived condition designed to simulate real-world use, and allow you to make some educated decisions about what car is best for you. When you fit hearing aids there are a host of objective measures you can rely on to make some critical decisions regarding hearing aid use for your patient.

Let's first focus on the clinical measures of hearing aid outcome. These outcome measures often are conducted on the day of the fitting, although testing at follow-up visits also can provide useful information. There is a wide array of clinical measures of outcome we could use. Many of them, however, are not very useful because they are time consuming, or because the results do not relate directly to patient counseling. The procedures we discuss here are intended to provide you with a general idea of how much benefit the patient may be experiencing at any given point in time following the fitting. Because we are talking about benefit, we imply that the aided result of our clinic or office testing is being compared to some unaided results. These unaided results sometimes are gathered before the fitting of hearing aids, and sometimes they are gathered on the same appointment that the aided testing is conducted.

Measure of Audibility: Using the Count-the-Dots Audiogram

Conducting aided thresholds in the test suite and charting these thresholds on the count-the-dots audiogram is a handy way to show the patient the benefit provided by the hearing aid, and how appropriate gain for soft inputs might be contributing to speech understanding. The count-the-dots audiogram (Figure 11–1) can be useful for demonstrating to patients if audibility for quiet speech sounds has been achieved. Although maximizing audibility does not always equate to an improvement in speech intelligibility, it is a well established fact that speech intelligibility is impossible without sufficient audibility. Here's how the procedure works:

Step 1. Place the patient in the calibrated sound field, 1 meter from the speaker at 0-degrees azimuth.

Step 2. We recommend conducting this test monaurally (otherwise you only will know the results of the "best" ear). Decide what ear you are going to test first. Then apply adequate masking to the non-test ear.

Step 3. Using a blank count-the-dots audiogram, conduct sound field threshold testing in the

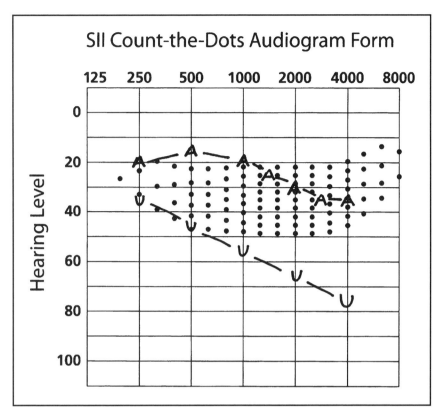

Figure 11–1. Example of the SII count-the-dots audiogram comparing the unaided to the aided condition in the sound field.

unaided condition. Chart the results on the form.

Step 4. Fit the hearing aid and adjust gain to the patient's expected (or known) use condition

Step 5. Conduct the threshold test in the aided condition and chart on the same form

Step 6. Count the "audible dots" for both the unaided and aided conditions.

Step 7. Repeat the procedure for the other ear.

Step 8. Compare the unaided to the aided scores and discuss the

results. Your conversation with the patient should focus on the improvement in audibility with hearing aids, and how it relates to intelligibility with the patient.

Speech Audiometry

One could argue that aided speech audiometry falls better under the *verification* stage of the hearing aid fitting. That argument is a good one. If verification implies determining if all of our fitting goals (audibility, comfort, etc.) were met, then it might be more logical to consider speech testing as part of the verification process. The problem, however, is that it is difficult to use speech results as verification tool, as it is difficult to predict each persons "optimum" performance. For example, if your Monday morning patient scores 82% on your favorite speech test with hearing aid A, how do you know that they wouldn't score 94% with hearing aid B, or maybe even better with hearing aid C? What if you raised the gain at 2000 Hz by 3 dB for hearing aid C? Would your outcome be better or worse? Our verification process would never end.

Another issue related to verification vs. validation is that many clinicians believe that any measure of speech perception ability can only be obtained after some period of practice with the newly fitted hearing aids. That practice is often termed adjustment or acclimatization. Although adjustment to the device may involve getting used to the feel, the pressure in the ear canal, the louder sounds in ones environment, and so on, the term acclimatization (which we discuss later in this chapter) refers to improvement in speech-recognition performance over time, presumably as a result of the introduction of amplification and the learned use of newly available speech cues. This term is frequently used erroneously to mean an adjustment to the hearing aid itself.

To date, there is little evidence that *significant* changes in speech-recognition performance with current signal processing schemes actually occur over time—assuming that the gain and output of the hearing aid is held constant. In fact, one of the greatest weaknesses of clinical measurement of speech recognition lies in the fact that many of

the tests are not sensitive enough to detect small differences in performance that may be due to acclimatization to novel signal processing strategies.

Nonetheless, we often feel obligated to assess speech perception ability pre- and post fitting of hearing aids in an effort to show benefit. If for no other reason, the patient walked in the door describing a problem understanding speech; it is reassuring for them to know that there performance indeed is better when using hearing aids. Recent data from MarkeTrak VIII survey also shows that aided objective speech testing helps improve satisfaction, so there may be an indirect benefit of conducting the testing.

Monosyllabic Speech Tests

If you plan on using a speech test for validation, we recommend using sentence material, and including some type of background noise for at least part of the testing. Audiologists, however, have had a love affair with monosyllables since the 1950s, and despite the availability of several good sentence tests, monosyllabic tests continue to be commonly used for hearing aid validation purposes. For that reason, we review them briefly.

> **W-22:** The CID W-22 test consists of four lists of 50 words each, for a total of 200 words. A male voice recites the test. Each word is preceded by the carrier phrase, "You will say . . . " The words included in the CID W-22 are among the 400 most common words of English writing of 1932. The test is considered to approximate the

---

TIPS and TRICKS: General Guidelines for Conducting Monosyllabic Speech Tests for Hearing Aid Validation

1. Seat the patient in a calibrated sound field, approximately one meter from the loudspeaker located at zero-degrees azimuth
2. We recommend conducting this test monaurally (otherwise you only will know the results of the "best" ear). Decide what ear you are going to test first. Then apply adequate masking to the nontest ear.
3. Present the speech material from CD (*not* live voice), using the standardized versions of the test (e.g., the Auditec of St. Louis version for most tests). Deliver complete 50-word list.
4. Deliver the material at a "soft-average" level, around 35 to

40 dB HL (50 to 55 dB SPL). Unlike earphone speech testing, where the purpose of the test is to find PB-Max, your question at this point is whether the hearing aid provides benefit for the patient's primary area of difficulty, which is most likely soft-speech inputs. Some dispensers make the mistake of conducting this testing at a relative loud level (e.g., 50 dB HL). If the patient has a mild hearing loss, it's probable that no benefit with amplification will be observed, as the patient will have already reached PB-Max in the unaided condition.
5. Repeat the procedure for the other ear.

---

phonetic balance of spoken English. A 1000-Hz calibration tone precedes the recorded test. Per Auditec (supplier of the recorded version of this test), the calibration tone matches the peak of the word "say" in the carrier phrase. The word to be repeated by the patient is allowed to "fall naturally."

NU-6: The NU-6 test consists of four lists of 50 words each, for a total of 200 words. A male voice recites the test. Each word is preceded by the carrier phrase, "Say the word . . . " The NU-6 is designed phonemically, with each word being a CVC monosyllable. A 1000-Hz calibration tone precedes the recorded test. Per Auditec, the

calibration tone matches the peak of the word "word" in the carrier phrase.

CCT: The California Consonant Test (CCT) consists of a single list of 100 words. The test was designed for analyzing consonant confusion in patients with hearing loss. For each presentation, the patient is given four options and is instructed to select the one matching the word they heard. A male voice recites the test. Each word is preceded by the carrier phrase, "Check the word . . . " 1000-Hz calibration tone precedes the recorded test. Per Auditec, the calibration tone matches the peak of the word "word" in the carrier phrase.

Speech Validation Tests for Children. For the younger listener, there are a number of recognition tests available. The Phonetically Balanced Kindergarten (PBK-50) test consists of 4 phonetically balanced lists of 50 words each. The words were chosen from the lexicon of the average young child. A male voice recites the test. Each word is preceded by the carrier phrase, "Say the word . . . " A 1000-Hz calibration tone precedes the recorded test. Per Auditec, the calibration tone matches the peak of the word "word" in the carrier phrase.

The Word Intelligibility by Picture Identification (WIPI) test was designed to assess the speech discrimination ability of hearing-impaired children. The test consists of four lists of 25 words. A male voice recites the test. Each word is preceded by the carrier phrase, "Show me . . . " The child is instructed to point to a picture corresponding to the target word. A 1000-Hz calibration tone precedes the recorded test. Per Auditec, the calibration tone should be within 2 dB of the peak of the target word.

Recently, the CASPA 4.1: The Computer-Assisted Speech Perception Assessment (CASPA) word lists have been used for speech recognition testing in children. The CASPA has 20 phonetically balanced 10-word lists. Each word is CVC, with each phoneme worth 1 point. Within each list there are 10 vowels and 20 consonants, constructed without reference to consonant position (pre- or postvocalic), frequency of word occurrence, or lexical neighborhood size. They are, however, intended to be scored phonemically (i.e., one point for each phoneme correctly recognized). This approach to scoring minimizes the contributions of linguistic factors and reduces confidence limits relative to the more traditional whole-word scoring.

Sentence Length Speech Tests for Validation

As discussed earlier, we recommend the use of sentence (usually with background noise) when speech testing is used for hearing aid validation. In general, there are four tests that have been used in research, and we summarize them briefly.

SPIN: The Speech Perception in Noise (SPIN) test is one of the older sentence tests. It was revised in the mid-1980s and now often is termed the "revised SPIN." The revised SPIN test consists of 8 lists of 50 sentences. Unlike other sentence tests, the task for the patient is to repeat only the last word of each sentence. Half of listed sentences contain a "last word" that has high predictability, indicating that the word is very predictable given the sentence context. The other half of the sentences contain "last word" classified as having low predictability, indicating that the word is not predictable given sentence context. The test is conducted using a background babble noise, with a standard SNR of +8 dB, although other SNRs can also be used.

CST: The Connected Speech Test (CST) consists of 48 passages of connected speech. A female voice recites the test sentences. Multitalker babble is used as the background noise. Subjects are expected to repeat each sentence of the passage, and are scored on 25 key words in each passage. The test is available from Robyn Cox's Hearing Aid Research Laboratory (http://www.umemphis.edu). The test is preceded by a speech-shaped calibration noise.

QuickSIN: The QuickSin consists of 12 standard equivalent lists, with six sentences in each list (female talker), based on the original IEEE sentences. Five key words in each sentence are scored (i.e., 30 key words for each list). Usually, two lists are presented for each test condition (unaided versus aided). Accompanying the sentences, recorded on the same track, is background four-person babble. The babble becomes 5 dB louder for each subsequent sentence on each list, with SNRs ranging from +25 to 0 dB in 5 dB steps. The test can be scored in percent correct, but typically it is scored in "SNR Loss" —the dB for 50% correct for the patient compared to that of normal hearing individuals.. There is a pediatric version of the QuickSIN termed the BKB-SIN. It has a simpler vocabulary, the sentences are shorter, there are 10 sentences in each list, and the background babble ranges from +21 to −6 dB for the 10 sentences in 3 dB steps. The same background babble as used with the QuickSIN is employed. This test is also used with adults.

HINT: The Hearing-in-Noise Test (HINT) consists of 25 phonemically balanced and equivalent 10-sentence lists. Speech-spectrum-shaped noise is presented at a fixed level, and the sentence level changes adaptively (e.g. if the patient correctly repeats a sentence, the next sentence is presented 2 dB softer; if the patient misses the sentence, the next sentence is presented 2 dB louder). A 1000-Hz calibration tone is used to adjust the VU-meters (speech and noise signals) of the audiometer. A speech-spectrum-shaped noise is used to calibrate the sound-field speakers in the test booth, other background noises can be used. Unlike the QuickSIN, individual key words are not scored. Rather, the patient must correctly repeat all key words within the sentence for the sentence to be scored correct. If only one word is missed, the sentence is scored incorrect. The final score for the patient is an RTS (reception threshold for sentences): the difference in dB between the 50% correct point for sentences and the level of the background noise (similar, but not the same as the SNR Loss scoring for the QuickSIN).

Picking a Test to Use

When making the decision on which speech-in-noise tests to use in your own clinic there are several considerations. It's important to choose a test that has been normed, and is easy to administer and score. Next, the presentation level of both the speech and the noise need to be taken into consideration. If the test is too easy (very favorable SNR) or too difficult (very aversive SNR) it's not going to give you very much useful information. Finally, the type of noise and type of speech used are important variables. In the case of the speech signal, there are some good reasons to use sentences, but also some good reasons to rely on words or phonemes.

All things considered, the QuickSIN would be a reasonable choice for the most clinicians, as it provides useful information about how patients perform in everyday types of listening situations quickly and accurately. Because the SNRs range from 0 dB to +25 dB, it's unlikely that you will experience ceiling or floor effects for a wide range of patients. Because the six different SNRs are pre-recorded on a single channel, calibration also is less of an issue.

TIPS and TRICKS: Using the QuickSIN to Validate Audibility

As the count-the-dots audiogram lacks face validity, other lab procedures can be used to validate aided audibility. Speech in noise tests can be used to demonstrate the effects of improved audibility with hearing aids. The QuickSIN works very well for this.

When the QuickSIN is conducted at a low intensity level (e.g., 35 or 40 dB HL; 50–55 dB SPL), it provides you and the patient with meaningful information on how improved audibility usually translates into improved speech intelligibility in noise, and how this relates to different signal-to-noise conditions. To conduct this test, do the following:

Step 1. The patient is placed approximately 1 meter from a single speaker at 0-degrees azimuth. Using the QuickSIN (two lists), unaided scores are obtained and charted for a presentation level of 35 to 40 dB HL (See scores indicated by squares in Figure 11–2). If the patient has a severe hearing loss, and the sentences are completely inaudible at this presentation level, raise the intensity until audibility is present.

Step 2. In the aided condition, the sentences are presented at the same level as for the unaided condition (e.g., 35–40 dB HL for most patients). As before, the noise level is increasing for the six sentences using the adaptive procedure of the QuickSIN. Plot these aided findings on the same graph as the unaided results as shown in Figure 11–2.

Step 3. Relate the results of this test to real-world listening conditions that the patient experiences (e.g., a crowded bar is around 0 dB, a busy restaurant is about +5 dB, a "coffee session" at work is about +10 dB, etc). Note the poor scores in the unaided condition; and how significantly the scores improve as a result of restoring audibility with the hearing aids. To better understand the concept find the 50% point on the y-axis and draw a horizontal line across the graph at this point. Notice the 50% correct point for the unaided condition is about 11 dB SNR loss, and the 50% correct point for the aided condition is about 5 dB SNR loss. By improving audibility you have improved this patient's ability to hear in noisy places 6 dB. Conducting speech in noise tests at low intensity levels is an effective way to demonstrate to patients the effect audibility has on speech intelligibility in background noise.

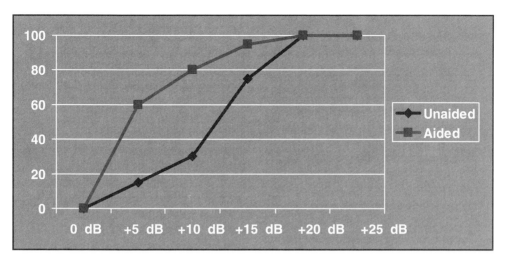

Figure 11–2. Example of QuickSIN in sound field conducted at 35 to 40 dB HL as lab measure of aided audibility for soft speech in noise for patient with unaided SNR loss of 10.5 dB. SNR loss is plotted on the *x*-axis and percent correct for each sentence is plotted on the *y*-axis.

Aided Measures of Sound Quality

When it comes to fitting and assessing hearing aids, the term "good sound quality" is rather vague. We know, for example, that aided speech intelligibility can be excellent and patients still struggle with issues related to sound quality, especially when listening to music. Aided sound quality can be best defined as attributes in the auditory perception that describe naturalness and timbre. Speech intelligibility is not part of sound quality. Getting sound quality "right" can be a tricky process, as in some cases, when you make sound quality better, you make speech intelligibility worse. This may not be obvious to the patient if only informal measures are used.

There are a number of ways that sound quality can be evaluated in the clinic. The method we recommend is a modification of that originally reported by Gabrielson and Sjogren in 1979. It is reasonably easy to administer, and has been demonstrated to be a valid procedure for recording sound quality judgments. It requires the patient to listen to a recorded conversational speech passage at a comfortable listening level and favorable signal-to-noise ratio of around +10 dB SNR.

This sound quality rating procedure can be used to validate sound quality of speech or music. This measure should only be completed once audibility for quiet and average levels of speech has been verified using probe-mic measures. In other words, we do not suggest you use subjective clinic measures of sound quality to determine initial gain and output settings, but rather, it can be used to tweak the hearing aids fitting in order to maximize (or improve) sound quality.

Step 1. The patient is placed in the sound field 1 m from the loudspeaker while wearing his or her hearing aids in the "on" position.

Step 2. A one to two minute passage of either conversational speech or music is played through the speaker. Using the Cox loudness anchors (Table 11–2) and using an ascending procedure, obtain a "comfortable" (#4) level.

Step 3. The patient is asked to rate the following dimensions of sound quality on a 0 (very poor) to 100 (very good) scale: clearness, background noise and overall impression. The scale shown in Figure 11–3 can be given to the patient as a guide.

Step 4. Once the patient has been instructed to provide his or her rating for those dimensions, the patient listens to the passage for approximately one minute, or until he can make a subjective rating— some patients are quite confident in the first 15 seconds or so. The patient uses the scale in Figure 11–3 to make their rating.

Table 11–2. The Cox Loudness Anchors

Loudness Chart from Cox Contour Test
• #7 Uncomfortably Loud
• #6 Loud, But Okay
• #5 Comfortable, But Slightly Loud
• #4 Comfortable
• #3 Comfortable, But Slightly Soft
• #2 Soft
• #1 Very soft

Source: Adapted from Cox, 1995.

Step 5. For ratings less than 70, further adjustment of the acoustic parameters of the hearing aid may be needed. We suggest using a different memory for this comparison so that you can return to the original settings for a direct comparison. Given the subjective nature of this procedure, you must carefully discuss ratings with the individual. For patients with good audibility of speech as documented on probe-microphone measures and the count-the-dots audiogram, counseling may be needed to address expectations.

When sound quality ratings in the aided condition are compared to ratings, using the same passages, in the unaided condition, a reasonably good indication of the impact that amplification has on sound quality can be demonstrated to the patient. Because sound quality and speech intelligibility are thought to be two separate dimensions of hearing aid performance, taking the time to conduct sound quality ratings may help to systematically measure outcomes. For this reason, they should be used as part of a comprehensive hearing aid validation protocol. We also know, as with other clinical validation measures, the simple act of conducting sound quality ratings will help to improve overall patient satisfaction.

Measures of Directional Microphone Benefit

Speech-in-noise tests can also be used to assess directional microphone benefit in the clinic. When using speech in noise testing for evaluating directional

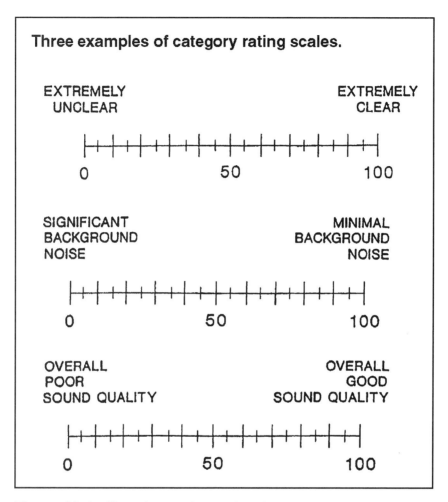

Figure 11–3. Chart that can be used to obtain the dimensions of sound quality. From Mueller and Hall, *Audiology Desk Reference*, Volume II, Singular Press, 1998. Reprinted with permission.

microphones, the speech and noise need to be delivered via separate channels to two different speakers. Because speech and noise are recorded on separate tracks, the QuickSIN easily can be used for this test. In a pinch, you could use monosyllables and a background speech noise from your audiometer.

In order to simulate real-world listening conditions, the loudspeaker delivering the primary speech to the patient should be placed 1 meter from the pa-

tient at 0-degrees azimuth. The speaker delivering the noise should be placed directly overhead, 1 meter above the patient. If it's not possible to use an overhead speaker in your clinic or office, place the noise-speaker directly behind the patient. This condition, however, will likely show directional benefit that is better than what the patient would obtain in a real-world diffuse field noise condition. When using the QuickSIN, speech should be delivered around 50 to

60 dB HL, and the noise automatically varied in 5 dB steps, starting at a signal-to-noise ratio of +25 dB).

Step 1. With the hearing aids in the omnidirectional mode, a score is obtained for the QuickSIN at six different signal to noise ratios (using two or three lists).

Step 2. With the hearing aids switched to the directional mode, a second score on the QuickSIN is obtained. The difference score is the directional benefit. It's best to use the true "directional mode" setting for this testing. In the automatic mode, depending on the input signal that you use, switching into directional might not occur. Your results in the "fixed directional" mode will be the same as if the hearing aid had switched using the "automatic directional" mode.

Step 3. Results can be compared to self-reports of benefit and satisfaction in noise and discussed with the patient. Because of the manner in which the speech and noise are delivered in the sound field, this lab test is a good estimation of the amount of directional benefit the patient is likely to receive in a typical noisy listening situation. The instruction manual for the QuickSIN has some examples of how to conduct this test (http://www.etymoticresearch.com).

Measures of Loudness Discomfort

As discussed earlier (Chapter 6), you've already used unaided measures of loudness discomfort levels (LDLs) to set the AGCo kneepoints correctly, and as we just discussed in Chapter 10, you've conducted the RESR to assure that the MPO was below these LDLs. It is nonetheless beneficial to also conduct aided LDLs for identifying discomfort associated with high hearing aid outputs. This is especially true during the initial adjustment period, after the patient has been subjected to common loud environmental sounds. Factors enter into the aided loudness perceptions that were not present in the earlier earphone and probe-mic measures:

- Monaural summation: The monaural summing of broad band signals such as speech versus loudness perceptions for pure tones.
- Binaural (bilateral) summation: Prior testing only has been conducted monaurally. The bilateral LDL does not seem to be too different from the unilateral one, but it remains important to account for this.
- Channel summation: There can be a summing of the signal when multiple channels are used in the processing. The exact degree varies depending on the setting of the instrument and, therefore, this is difficult to predict.

All three of these factors have the potential to affect loudness discomfort with hearing aids (even though to some extent they are accounted for in the prescriptive fitting, this is for the *average patient*).

Aided loudness testing usually is conducted in a test booth, but it also easily can be conducted in the hearing aid fitting room or an office. In order to complete aided loudness discomfort level testing outside of the test booth, you will need a portable CD player with an external speaker system (affectionately referred to as a "boom box"), an inexpensive sound level meter (SLM; about $49.95 for a digital one at Radio Shack), a CD with recordings of common noises, and the Cox contour 7-point loudness anchors printed on a large chart. Because you frequently will be making hearing aid adjustments at the same time that you are conducting these measures, we have found that it is much more efficient to conduct this testing in the fitting room. The procedure is conducted in the following manner.

Step 1. Before conducting the test, calibrate the CD through the stereo system. This is done by placing the SLM approximately 1 m from the speaker (at the place of the patient's head) and setting the volume of the stereo system (or intensity dial of the audiometer) so that the reading on the SLM reaches 85 dBA. If you're using a boom box, mark this point for future reference.

Step 2. Place the patient 1 m from the speaker while wearing the hearing aids with the gain adjusted a little higher than their "average use level". Using the Cox loudness anchors (see Table 11–2), ask the patient to rate the loudness of various signals (both speech and environmental noises) that have been calibrated to reach 85 dBA on the SLM.

Step 3. Patient listens to the passage and rates the loudness level on the Cox scale. Patients should rate the passage to be a #5 or #6 on the chart. If the patient

rates a given sound as #7, and this is verified on retest, the output (AGCo kneepoint) of the hearing aids (or at least one hearing aid) needs to be adjusted downward.

Step 4. Following the AGCo adjustment, repeat testing until a consistent #6 rating is obtained. If this cannot be obtained using the AGCo setting, it might be necessary to make the compression ratio larger for the WDRC. Finally, for open fittings, it is important to assure that the unaided signal is not uncomfortably loud—simply conduct testing with the hearing aid turned off to check for this.

TIPS and TRICKS: Validation of Maximum Loudness

We recommend a method of using a portable CD player for loudness validation. However, you can also use your probe-mic system or your fitting software to deliver the signals. If you use your probe-mic system, the regulating mic will ensure that you have the signal at the correct output. If you use the loudspeakers of your computer with the fitting software, you again will need to use the sound level meter.

Self-Reports of Hearing Aid Outcome

Ever hear of J.D. Power and Associates? You could possibly be a member of their panel. Many of us rely on Consumer Reports *or a "rating" agency when buying a car. Reports on car satisfaction are done by experts using questionnaires that evaluate a wide range of car characteristics, including quietness of the engine and smoothness of the ride. Questionnaires are a valuable way to measure subjective judgments are many things and when a questionnaire has been properly designed it can be very useful in make decisions about hearing aid success.*

Self-reports (questionnaires) of hearing aid outcome have been developed and utilized over the past few decades. Patients have always provided clinicians with real-world assessments of outcomes from their hearing aids, and frequently these reports were used for counseling and hearing aid adjustments. Until quite recently, however, most real-world assessments of outcome involved informal discussions between the patient and the professional.

As recent as the 1980s, rather than formally measuring real-world outcomes, professionals relied more heavily on clinical measures of fitting outcomes. These measures included speech recognition in quiet and in noise, functional or insertion gain measures, and aided loudness judgments. In the past 20 years, however, there have been several well-designed and validated self-assessment inventories introduced. The goal now is to make these inventories part of the routine hearing aid fitting protocol. Self-report outcome measures with known psychometric properties are useful for determining the effectiveness of hearing aids. Effectiveness with amplification can be measured across several dimensions, including handicap reduction, acceptance, benefit, and satisfaction. Several different self-report measures of hearing aid outcome have been developed over the past two decades address-

ing each one of these dimensions. Because they comprise two of the most significant components of a patient's experience with hearing aid, we focus primarily on self-report measures of hearing aid benefit, satisfaction, and handicap reduction.

Three Reasons for Self-Report Outcomes

An important question to address at this time is, "Why do we need self-report measures of real-world outcome?" We can think of at least three reasons. First, for largely economic reasons, health care is becoming more consumer driven. In this evolving system, the consumer decides what treatment is selected and when it is complete. The major index of quality of service is self-report outcome and satisfaction. Consumer driven health care places an added emphasis on the patient's point of view. Therefore, it is critical to measure the real-world benefit and satisfaction of hearing aid use. Because today's patients, on average, are more savvy and better informed than our grandparents, they want to know how much benefit they are receiving in everyday listening situations. Using a self-report of hearing aid outcome allows you to measure and report to the patient how they are doing compared to an average.

A second reason self-report measures of outcome are gaining importance is related to the fact that many of these real-world experiences simply cannot be measured effectively in laboratory conditions. The traditional hearing aid outcome measures clinicians have used in the past like speech recognition in quiet and in noise, do not capture the true experiences of hearing aid use in everyday listening situations. Consider our discussion in Chapter 9 concerning hearing aids with automatic and adaptive directional technology, coupled with different types of noise reduction, signal detection and automatic feedback reduction. The effectiveness of the combination of features such as this depends heavily on the lifestyle and listening conditions of the individual patient. In order to quantify the true impact hearing loss and its associated treatment have on activity limitations, lifestyles, and so forth, self-report measures outcome can be used. Some would say they are necessary.

Third, even when laboratory conditions are used to simulate real-world listening situations they do not always resemble the patient's impression of the actual real-life situation. Self-report outcome measures are increasing in

---

TIPS and TRICKS: Some Practical Applications of Self-Report Outcome Measures

1. Comparison of different dispensing sites or personnel: You're the manager of a hearing aid dispensing practice that has two different offices. You fit the same hearing aids in both offices. Are the patients in Office A as satisfied with their hearing aids as the patients fitted at Office B?

2. Comparison of different fitting procedures: You always fit your hearing aids to the NAL-NL2 targets with careful verification and adjustment using probe-mic measures. Your partner simply uses the manufacturers' first-fit setting. Will both group of patients have the same benefit and satisfaction with hearing aids in the real world?

3. Comparison of circuitry: Your favorite manufacturers just added a new noise reduction feature, which adds several hundred dollars to the cost of the hearing aids. If your patients were fitted with that feature, would they observe improved speech understanding in noise in their everyday use situations?

4. Counseling effectiveness: You have decided to conduct a free morning counseling session each Saturday for all of your patients who have a high ANL test score and poor QuickSIN performance (e.g., patients considered "at risk"). Will this extra effort result in improved real world satisfaction and benefit with their hearing aids?

5. Documentation of service effectiveness: You know you do a good job, but do you have data to prove it? Are your patients more satisfied than the average person fitted with hearing aids? How often do their IOI-HA scores exceed national norms? How often are their COSI goals obtained?

Bonus Reason: Research has shown that patients are significantly more satisfied with their hearing aids when they have been given a formalized outcome measure asking them if they are satisfied with their hearing aids.

use because they give us a scientifically defensible way to validly measure the real-life success of the hearing aid fitting.

Finally, something called "evidence-based practice" has become a standard component in the clinical decision making process. An evidence-based practice paradigm requires that clinicians demonstrate their hearing aid fittings are providing benefit in real world conditions. For this reason, self-reports of outcome are the new "gold standard" for measuring and reporting success.

We review some sample self-report measures of hearing aid benefit and satisfaction. There are two major types of self-reports or questionnaires that can be administered. One is open-ended and the other is closed-ended.

Open-Ended Self-Report Measures of Outcome

Open-ended self-report measures are those that allow the patient to nominate and target their own areas of expected improvement with amplification. The assumed advantage of an open-ended scale is that it can be tailored to the true communication needs of the individual patient. That is, if you and the patient work together carefully, the items selected will represent true difficult listening situations for that patient, rather than arbitrary listening situations collected from "average" patients. The downside of these open-ended questionnaires is that it makes it difficult to compare your patients performance to a large pool of other hearing aid users, as the specific listening situations they nominated might be quite unique.

Client Oriented Scale of Improvement (COSI)

The Client Oriented Scale of Improvement (COSI) was developed by the National Acoustic Laboratories in 1997. The COSI is an open-ended scale in which the patient targets up to five listening situations for improvement with amplification (e.g., listening to television when there is background noise, talking on the phone with my grandchildren, etc). The COSI was normed on 1,770 adults with hearing loss in Australia. The goal of the COSI is for the patient to target specific listening situations when the hearing aids are fitted, and to report the degree of benefit obtained after a few weeks of hearing aid use. It is important to have patients nominate situations that are common and long-standing, as many times they will want to focus on "current events." The first two items (in importance) will probably give you the best "read" regarding the success of the fitting. The findings then can be generally compared to that expected for the population in similar listening situations. It can be scored as "Degree of Change," "Final Ability," or both.

Many hearing aid manufacturers now include the COSI in their fitting software. The COSI can also be downloaded from the NAL at http://www.nal.gov.au . The COSI has become one of, if not the most commonly used real-world measures of benefit among dispensers. This is partly because of the "personalization" that we have discussed. It's popularity is also because it is very easy to administer and score, and is quite "low tech" (in desperation, you could get by with a pencil and bar napkin!)

TIPS and TRICKS: Measuring Outcome with the COSI

In Figure 11–4 you see an example of a COSI completed during the prefitting appointment. This patient has returned to your clinic for his second postfitting appointment. As it's been about 30 days since he was fitted and he is reporting few problems with his new hearing aids, you take out your prefitting COSI (Figure 11–4) and ask him to measure his success on two scales.

Degree of change is how much relative benefit he is reporting in the aided condition relative to the unaided condition (or his old hearing aids if he's an experienced user you recently fit with new hearing aids). You ask him to place an X in the box that corresponds to his experience with the new devices for each of the five listening situations he targeted for improvement with hearing aids during the prefitting appointment. Your goal should be for the patient to rate the degree of change for all five situations "better" or "much better" compared to the unaided condition. If you don't receive a "better" or "much better" you

may need to spend more time counseling the patient or perhaps doing some tweaking, and giving the patient more time before re-measuring benefit on this scale. If the patient reports "better" or "much better" (2 or 3 categories of improvement relative to the unaided condition) you can pat yourself on the back and assume that you have just documented a "successful" fitting.

Next, you can ask him to rate his "final ability" in each of the five listening situations he targeted for improvement with amplification. You can document final ability or absolute improvement by asking the patient, "When you are in this situation (each of the five areas targeted for improvement) you can communicate: hardly ever, occasionally, half of the time, most of the time, or almost always. Allow the patient to self-rate their ability on this scale. If the patient reports "most of the time" or "almost always" for the majority of listening situations, you have documented improvement.

Glasgow Hearing Aid Benefit Profile (GHABP)

The GHABP examines six dimensions of hearing aid outcome: disability, handicap, hearing aid use, benefit, satisfaction, and residual disability. The GHABP consists of four predetermined and four patient-nominated items. Therefore, the GHABP could be considered a combination open-ended and closed-ended measure of outcome. This is an advan-

tage for patients who have trouble thinking of specific situations on their own. The GHABP was normed on 293 adults. Based on the normative findings, it is an appropriate instrument for clinicians who want to use self-report data to measure improvement in audibility. The Hearing Aid Benefit Interview, a completely open-ended questionnaire, is the precursor to the GHABP (Gatehouse, 1994). The GHABP can be downloaded at http://www.ihr.mrc.ac.uk .

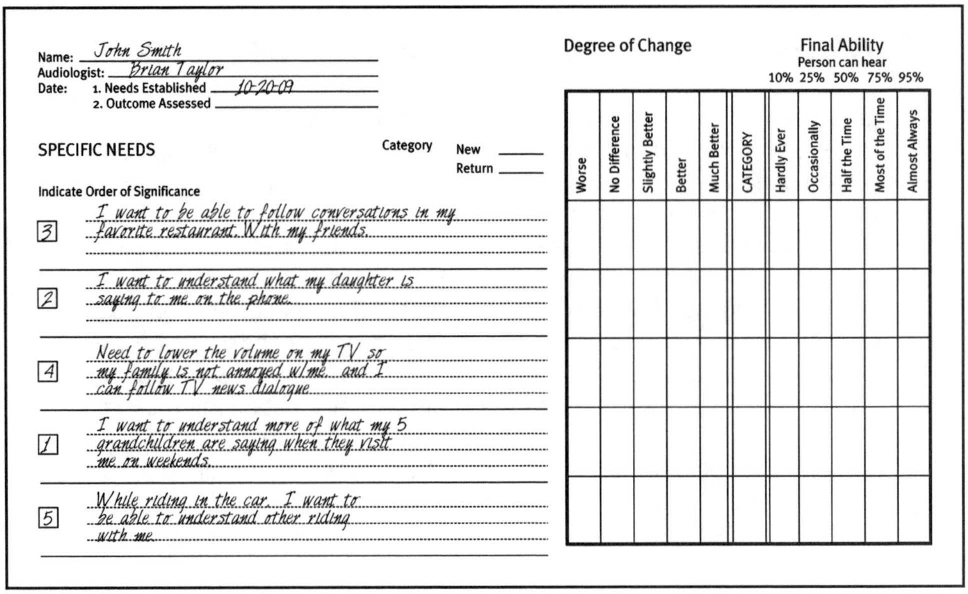

Figure 11–4. The COSI completed in the unaided condition. Thirty to 45 days following the fitting, use this form to document degree of change and final ability.

Closed-Ended Self-Report Measures of Outcome

Closed-ended self-report measures allow the patient to complete a self-report scale using a predetermined list of areas of concern. The primary advantage of the closed-ended scale is that the scores can be more readily compared to normative data. That is, your patient sitting in Nome, North Dakota, Athens, Texas, or Paris, Tennessee, is answering the very same questions as a new hearing aid user sipping his Spotted Cow in New Glarus, Wisconsin. This provides a large database, allowing for comparisons with considerable hearing aid and demographic data. One of the disadvantages of a closed-ended measure is that individual communication preferences cannot be accounted for. In an era in which outcome measures are gaining importance, this is an impor-

tant consideration. Closed-ended outcome measures, although outstanding tools for conducting clinical research are sometimes difficult to use to address the unique needs of all individuals seen in the clinic. Here is an overview of some of the more popular closed-ended surveys.

Abbreviated Profile of Hearing Aid Benefit (APHAB)

In an attempt to develop a more clinic friendly measure of outcome, the APHAB was developed; the term "abbreviated" refers to the fact that it is a shortened version of the PHAB, a more detailed scale sometimes used in research, but seldom in the clinic. Like the COSI, which we discussed earlier, it is a measure of benefit rather than satisfaction. The goal of the APHAB is to quantify the disability (percent of problems) caused by

---

TIPS and TRICKS: Daily Journal of Hearing Aid Use

Even the best self-report measures of outcome may not be sensitive enough to document hearing aid benefit. One way to gauge the effectiveness of hearing aids with several advanced features is to have the patient keep a daily journal of hearing aid use. This can be an especially helpful tactic to use with an experienced hearing aid users that are already receiving "okay" benefit from their existing devices.

Here's how it works:

■ Have the patient record on page 1 of the their journal the 5 to 10 situations where they expect to hear better with hearing aids. (You can take some of this information directly from the prefitting COSI).

■ At the end of each day, encourage the patient to record his or her comments in the journal as they relate to communication in these areas.

■ If you plan to use a use a daily journal with your patients here are some suggested questions:

■ How many hours did you wear the hearing aids? (4 hours or less is usually a bad sign)

■ On a scale of 1 to 10 (10 being the best) how much are the hearing aids helping you in your most important listening situations: (Anything higher than 6 is probably okay)

■ On a scale of 1 to 10 (10 being extremely noticeable) how much did you notice the effect of (name a special feature here): (Anything higher than 6 is probably okay)

■ Describe the situations where your new hearing aids were helpful today:

■ Describe anything you didn't like about the hearing aids

Daily journaling is not a replacement for measuring hearing aid outcome with one of the several tools we mention in this chapter. It is, however, a great way to gather more detailed information about how successful the hearing aids are working in real world listening conditions.

---

hearing loss, and the reduction of that disability that was then achieved with the use of hearing aids. The APHAB uses 24 items covering 4 subscales: ease of communication (listening in quiet), reverberation, background noise, and aversiveness to sounds. It can be used to measure unaided or aided "percent of problems" or hearing aid benefit (the difference between unaided and aided. The APHAB has been normed on 128 adults with mild to moderate hearing loss.

The APHAB is the most commonly used outcome measures in hearing aid research. It is probably the most commonly used closed-set outcome measure used among dispensers too, although the overall use rate is disappointingly low. The administration and scoring is relatively simple and is computerized, although it is more detailed than some of the other scales. Several hearing aid manufacturers have the APHAB and the automated scoring as part of their fitting software. The APHAB can be downloaded by going to http://www.ausp.memphis.edu/harl/aphab.html .

TIPS and TRICKS: Use of the APHAB

Choosing an outcome measure that has published norms, and critical difference values is important to the clinical management process. The norms tell you how your patient compares to other patients of similar demographics. The critical difference values will allow you to make a statement of true difference in scores. For example, the APHAB) provides for both pretest and posttest administration, norms for different groups for both aided and unaided, and critical differences. The prefitting and postfitting items are identical; the patient is simply instructed to respond (initially) as though they are not using amplification. Alternatively, some clinicians use the pretest administration to determine the status with current or old hearing aids to compare to newly acquired hearing aids.

Examples of items include:

- Traffic noises are too loud . . .
- When I am talking with someone across a large empty room, I understand the words . . .
- When I am in a small office, interviewing or answering questions, I have difficulty following the conversation . . .

Responses to the items are:

A Always (99% of the time)
B Almost Always (87% of the time)
C Generally (75% of the time)
D Half the time (50% of the time)
E Occasionally (25% of the time)
F Seldom (12% of the time)
G Never (1% of the time)

The prefitting scores might look like this: EC: 65, RV: 80, BN: 90, AV: 15.

By looking at the table of norms (Table 11–3), it readily can be discerned that the patient is at about the 50th percentile for EC, RV and AV subscales, but closer to the 90th percentile for the BN subscale. Translated to language that would be useful in counseling and management planning: The patient performs similarly to others with her degree of hearing loss in three of the subscales (EC, RV, and AV) but has considerable more trouble with background noise than her comparison group. According to the normative table, her percent of problems would place her at the 80 percentile; that is, 80% of her peers have less trouble in background noise. Stated another way, only 20% of her peers have *more* trouble in background noise.

Now, following the issuance of hearing aids and several weeks of adjustment, you repeat the APHAB (the aided version). For this administration you obtain scores of: EC: 15, RV: 30, BN: 30, and AV: 50. Again, referring to the table of norms Aided Condition, these scores indicate that the patient is at approximately the 35th percentile for EC, RV, and BN, and the 50th percentile for AV. Translated to language that would be useful in counseling and management planning: The patient has less problems in the listening situations (EC, RV, and BN) than 65% of her peers (100 *minus* 35 *equals* 65) but has about the same amount of trouble with aversive sounds as about 50% of her peers (i.e., scores at the 50th percentile). The difference between the unaided and aided scores will derive the benefit score: EC: 50, RV: 50, BN: 60, and AV: –35.

One more time, looking at the table of norms for *benefit* it is obvious that our patient's benefit scores put her at approximately the 80th percentile for EC and RV. Interpolating the percentile for the BN subscale suggests that she is actually up at the 90th percentile for benefit obtained in noisy environments. Pat yourself on the back for doing a "Good Job." But wait. The AV subscale puts her at approximately the 25th percentile for benefit with aversive sounds. That subscale can be a bit tricky to interpret. Most hearing aid users tend to have a "worse score" (negative benefit) when the aided scores are compared to unaided. This score might simply imply that she is now hearing some of those louder sounds as loud sounds (they should be!), compared to the unaided condition where they might have been less annoying. On the other hand, it might indicate the MPO is set too high for real-life aversive sounds. It probably something you should look into, and this is when you'll want to compare these results to some of your other findings—like the RESR results when you conducted probe-mic measures.

Profile of Aided Loudness (PAL)

Up to this point, we have discussed outcome measures that primarily have been designed to measure hearing aid benefit, that is, do the hearing aids help the patient communicate in the real world? A related, but different aspect of the hearing aid fitting is providing the appropriate gain for soft, average, and

Table 11–3. Published Norms for the APHAB (developed at the University of Memphis)

APHAB Norms for WDRC-Capable Hearing Aids			
Percentile	EC	RV	BN	AV
Users of WDRC-capable hearing aids—Unaided				
95	99	99	99	70
80	83	87	89	35
65	75	81	81	21
50	63	71	75	14
35	56	65	67	9
20	46	58	58	3
5	26	47	41	1
Users of WDRC-capable hearing aids—Aided				
95	86	79	82	82
80	39	57	58	64
65	29	46	49	53
50	23	37	40	38
35	17	29	32	23
20	12	21	22	14
5	5	12	14	2
Users of WDRC-capable hearing aids—Benefit				
95	76	70	56	16
80	52	52	47	0
65	46	41	39	−8
50	38	34	33	−13
35	29	27	23	−25
20	19	16	12	−41
5	−10	−3	−1	−61

Source: Adapted from Cox, 1995.

loud inputs: making soft sounds soft, average sounds comfortable, and loud sounds loud, but not too loud. Recall that we talked about this in our discussion of WDRC, and matching probe-mic targets. It also is reasonable, therefore, to conduct a real world subjective measure to determine if indeed aided loudness perceptions are appropriate. That is the purpose of the PAL.

The PAL consists of 12 items, all relatively common environmental sounds, four each in the soft, average and loud categories. The patient scores the loudness rating for each one of these sounds (usually aided, but could be conducted both unaided and aided) using the 7-point loudness anchors of the Cox Contour Test (see Table 11–2). The patient also rates their satisfaction for the loudness on a five-point scale (1 = very satisfied). For example, your patient might rate the "beep" of a microwave #4 for loudness, but only a #3 for satisfaction. The loudness rating of #4 is great (just like normals), but why isn't he satisfied? Probably, because for the past 20 years the loudness perception of the beep was only a #2, and now at #4 it's annoying. This clearly is now a counseling issue, not a "turn down the gain" issue. But how would have you known without the PAL findings? If a patient simply said, "My microwave is too loud" some dispensers would be tempted to make hearing aid adjustments.

The PAL is easy to administer and score, and provides information not available from other self-assessment scales (although, the AV scale of the APHAB should agree with the four loud items of the PAL). See Figure 11–5 for the PAL instructions and form that can be copied and administered to patients.

Hearing Handicap Inventory for Adults (HHIA) and Hearing Handicap Inventory for the Elderly (HHIE)

So far, we have mostly discussed measuring the benefit of hearing aids (reduction of disability) but we also are concerned with the reduction of handicap. Although the two usually go hand in hand, it certainly is possible to have a handicap without a disability. There are two scales that commonly have been used to measure hearing handicap, and the resulting effects of hearing aid treatment. The original scale was the HHIE (elderly meaning people over the age of 65) that was then modified for younger adults and called the HHIA (administered to people under the age of 65). The HHIE/HHIA were designed to both quantify handicap and also assess benefit by measuring change in perceived handicap after the fitting of hearing aids. Both scales have a 25-item version, and a 10-item screening version. They both also have two subscales: emotional consequences and social and situational effects. The goal of these scales is to measure the perceived effects of hearing loss. Both the HHIE and the HHIA allow the patient to answer "yes," (4 points) "no," (0 points) or "sometimes" (2 points) to all 25 items on the questionnaire. The higher the total score, the greater the hearing handicap. The scale is designed so that even people with normal hearing may answer "sometimes" for some items (e.g., Do you have difficulty hearing when someone speaks in a whisper?).

Some dispensers have used this tool in the unaided format to gain insight whether a patient is a candidate for amplification. If a person has a 30 to 50 dB hearing loss, but their self-reported HHIE score is only 8, one might question is they need (or are ready to accept) hearing aids. Usually, a score of 12 or higher would suggest communication problems significant enough to at least consider the use of amplification.

We have provided the screening versions of both HHIE and HHIA. See Figure 11–6 for the screening version of HHIA for patients and their significant other. The HHIA can be administered to the patient and his or her significant other during the prefitting appointment in order to gather baseline hearing handicap information, and can be readministered 30 days postfitting to obtain the reduction in handicap resulting from hearing aid usage. You may copy Figure 11–6 and use it in your clinic.

Satisfaction with Amplification in Daily Life (SADL)

The SADL was designed to quantify satisfaction with hearing aids using 15 items in four subscales. It is a companion test to an expectations questionnaire titled the ECHO (Expected Consequences of Hearing Aid Ownership). The four subscales of the SADL consist of positive effects, service and costs, negative features, and personal image. Each item is rated on a 5-point scale ranging from A = Not At All, B = A Little to F = Greatly, and G = Tremendously.

The SADL was formed on 126 to 225 adults (depending on the subscale), and can be downloaded at http://www.ausp.memphis.edu/harl/sadl.html .

International Outcome Inventory— Hearing Aids (IOI-HA)

You've decided to buy a new car. Your brother can get you a good deal on a Jeep, *so that's what you're getting. But wait . . . there are a lot of different Jeeps. Let's see, you want to look cool when you head down to the Missouri River to unload your kayak—okay, the Wrangler soft-top sounds like the winner. But . . . what about all the trips to Lowe's in the spring, bringing back shrubs, plants, pots, and so forth? Not enough room in a Wrangler. Hmm. The Liberty might be a little more practical. But what about those evening out for dinner at the Country Club—do you really want to drive up in a Liberty? Maybe you're really the decked-out Grand Cherokee kind of person. But how does that look with a kayak on the roof? It does sort of cry out "old, but trying to look "young." You're not really as cool as cruising with the top down in a Wrangler. But . . .*

As you see from the above example, trying to find the best car to buy often involves thinking about several different areas where potential use, benefit and satisfaction might occur. We have discussed various scales that have been designed primarily to assess a specific aspect of hearing aid outcome: benefit, reduction of handicap, loudness normalization, satisfaction, and so forth. It is cumbersome and time consuming to conduct five or six different inventories and some experts have suggested that a single "screening" inventory could be used to cover many areas in one single form. Maybe one doesn't have to ask 10 or more questions about benefit to determine if someone indeed is obtaining benefit? Consisting of eight questions on a five-point rating scale, the goal of the IOI-HA, therefore, is to assess benefit, satisfaction, and quality of life changes associated with hearing aid use. The creators of the IOI-HA determined that the questions could be grouped into two separate factors.

PROFILE OF AIDED LOUDNESS

Name: _____
Date: _____

Status: ___ unaided ___ previous hearing aids
___ current hearing aids

Instructions: Please rate the following items by both the level of loudness of the sound and by the appropriateness of that loudness level. For example, you might rate a particular sound as "Very Soft." If "Very Soft" is your preferred level for this sound, then you would rate your loudness satisfaction as "Just Right." If, on the other hand, you think the sound should be louder than "Very Soft", then your loudness satisfaction rating might be "Not Too Good" or "Not Good At All." The Loudness Satisfaction rating is not related to how pleasing the sound is to you, but rather, the appropriateness of the loudness. Here is an example:

The hum of a refrigerator motor:

Loudness rating	Satisfaction rating
0 Do not hear	(5.) Just right
1 Very soft	4. Pretty good
(2) Soft	3. Okay
3 Comfortable, but slightly soft	2. Not too good
4 Comfortable	1. Not good at all
5 Comfortable, but slightly loud	
6 Loud, but OK	
7 Uncomfortably loud	

In this example, the hearing aid user rated the loudness level of a refrigerator motor running as "Comfortable, but slightly soft" and rated his loudness satisfaction for this sound as "Just right." This satisfaction rating indicates that the person believes that it is appropriate for a refrigerator motor to sound "Comfortable, but slightly soft."

Circle the responses that best describe your listening experiences. If you have not experienced one of the sounds listed (or a similar sound), simply leave that question blank.

1. An electric razor:

Loudness rating	Satisfaction rating
0 Do not hear	5. Just right
1 Very soft	4. Pretty good
2 Soft	3. Okay
3 Comfortable, but slightly soft	2. Not too good
4 Comfortable	1. Not good at all
5 Comfortable, but slightly loud	
6 Loud, but OK	
7 Uncomfortably loud	

2. A door slamming:

Loudness rating	Satisfaction rating
0 Do not hear	5. Just right
1 Very soft	4. Pretty good
2 Soft	3. Okay
3 Comfortable, but slightly soft	2. Not too good
4 Comfortable	1. Not good at all
5 Comfortable, but slightly loud	
6 Loud, but OK	
7 Uncomfortably loud	

3. Your own breathing:

Loudness rating	Satisfaction rating
0 Do not hear	5. Just right
1 Very soft	4. Pretty good
2 Soft	3. Okay
3 Comfortable, but slightly soft	2. Not too good
4 Comfortable	1. Not good at all
5 Comfortable, but slightly loud	
6 Loud, but OK	
7 Uncomfortably loud	

4. Water boiling on the stove:

Loudness rating	Satisfaction rating
0 Do not hear	5. Just right
1 Very soft	4. Pretty good
2 Soft	3. Okay
3 Comfortable, but slightly soft	2. Not too good
4 Comfortable	1. Not good at all
5 Comfortable, but slightly loud	
6 Loud, but OK	
7 Uncomfortably loud	

5. A car's turn signal:

Loudness rating	Satisfaction rating
0 Do not hear	5. Just right
1 Very soft	4. Pretty good
2 Soft	3. Okay
3 Comfortable, but slightly soft	2. Not too good
4 Comfortable	1. Not good at all
5 Comfortable, but slightly loud	
6 Loud, but OK	
7 Uncomfortably loud	

6. The religious leader during the sermon:

Loudness rating	Satisfaction rating
0 Do not hear	5. Just right
1 Very soft	4. Pretty good
2 Soft	3. Okay
3 Comfortable, but slightly soft	2. Not too good
4 Comfortable	1. Not good at all
5 Comfortable, but slightly loud	
6 Loud, but OK	
7 Uncomfortably loud	

Figure 11–5. The Profile of Aided Loudness. Adapted from Palmer, Mueller, and Moriarity.

7. The dryer running:

Loudness rating	Satisfaction rating
0 Do not hear	5. Just right
1 Very soft	4. Pretty good
2 Soft	3. Okay
3 Comfortable, but slightly soft	2. Not too good
4 Comfortable	1. Not good at all
5 Comfortable, but slightly loud	
6 Loud, but OK	
7 Uncomfortably loud	

8. You chewing soft food:

Loudness rating	Satisfaction rating
0 Do not hear	5. Just right
1 Very soft	4. Pretty good
2 Soft	3. Okay
3 Comfortable, but slightly soft	2. Not too good
4 Comfortable	1. Not good at all
5 Comfortable, but slightly loud	
6 Loud, but OK	
7 Uncomfortably loud	

9. Listening to a marching band:

Loudness rating	Satisfaction rating
0 Do not hear	5. Just right
1 Very soft	4. Pretty good
2 Soft	3. Okay
3 Comfortable, but slightly soft	2. Not too good
4 Comfortable	1. Not good at all
5 Comfortable, but slightly loud	
6 Loud, but OK	
7 Uncomfortably loud	

10. A barking dog:

Loudness rating	Satisfaction rating
0 Do not hear	5. Just right
1 Very soft	4. Pretty good
2 Soft	3. Okay
3 Comfortable, but slightly soft	2. Not too good
4 Comfortable	1. Not good at all
5 Comfortable, but slightly loud	
6 Loud, but OK	
7 Uncomfortably loud	

11. A lawn mower:

Loudness rating	Satisfaction rating
0 Do not hear	5. Just right
1 Very soft	4. Pretty good
2 Soft	3. Okay
3 Comfortable, but slightly soft	2. Not too good
4 Comfortable	1. Not good at all
5 Comfortable, but slightly loud	
6 Loud, but OK	
7 Uncomfortably loud	

12. A microwave buzzer sounding:

Loudness rating	Satisfaction rating
0 Do not hear	5. Just right
1 Very soft	4. Pretty good
2 Soft	3. Okay
3 Comfortable, but slightly soft	2. Not too good
4 Comfortable	1. Not good at all
5 Comfortable, but slightly loud	
6 Loud, but OK	
7 Uncomfortably loud	

Take an average score for soft, average, and loud sounds and compare the scores to the average scores of normally hearing individuals. The patient summary sheet is used for this type of scoring. In this manner, the clinician may compare unaided loudness perception to aided loudness perception as well as having a numeric target for the aided condition.

PATIENT SUMMARY
Profile of Aided Loudness (PAL)
Unaided Performance

Soft sounds	Q3	Q4	Q5	Q8	Category average
Loudness	___	___	___	___	___(target = 2)
Satisfaction	___	___	___	___	

Average sounds	Q1	Q6	Q7	Q12	Category average
Loudness	___	___	___	___	___(target = 4)
Satisfaction	___	___	___	___	

Loud sounds	Q2	Q9	Q10	Q11	Category average
Loudness	___	___	___	___	___(target = 6)
Satisfaction	___	___	___	___	

Aided Performance

Soft sounds	Q3	Q4	Q5	Q8	Category average
Loudness	___	___	___	___	___(target = 2)
Satisfaction	___	___	___	___	

Average sounds	Q1	Q6	Q7	Q12	Category average
Loudness	___	___	___	___	___(target = 4)
Satisfaction	___	___	___	___	

Loud sounds	Q2	Q9	Q10	Q11	Category average
Loudness	___	___	___	___	___(target = 6)
Satisfaction	___	___	___	___	

Figure 11–5. *continued*

HEARING HANDICAP INVENTORY FOR ADULTS - SCREENER

INSTRUCTIONS: The purpose of this questionnaire is to identify the problems your hearing loss may be causing you. Circle Yes, Sometimes, or No for each question. DO NOT SKIP A QUESTION IF YOU AVOID A SITUATION BECAUSE OF A HEARING PROBLEM.

E-1	Does your hearing problem cause you to feel embarrassed when meeting new people?	Yes	Sometimes	No
E-2	Does a hearing problem cause you to feel frustrated when talking to members of your family?	Yes	Sometimes	No
S-1	Does a hearing problem cause you difficulty hearing/understanding co-workers, clients or customers?	Yes	Sometimes	No
E-3	Do you feel handicapped by a hearing problem?	Yes	Sometimes	No
S-2	Does a hearing problem cause you difficulty when visiting friends, relatives or neighbors?	Yes	Sometimes	No
S-3	Does a hearing problem cause you difficulty in the movies or theater?	Yes	Sometimes	No
E-4	Does a hearing problem cause you to have arguments with family members?	Yes	Sometimes	No
S-4	Does a hearing problem cause you difficulty when listening to the TV or radio?	Yes	Sometimes	No
E-5	Do you feel that any difficulty with your hearing limits or hampers your personal or social life?	Yes	Sometimes	No
S-5	Does a hearing problem cause you difficulty when at a restaurant with relatives or friends?	Yes	Sometimes	No

HEARING HANDICAP INVENTORY FOR ADULTS - SIGNIFICANT OTHER SCREENER

INSTRUCTIONS: The purpose of this questionnaire is to identify the problems your hearing loss may be causing you. Circle Yes, Sometimes, or No for each question. DO NOT SKIP A QUESTION IF YOU AVOID A SITUATION BECAUSE OF A HEARING PROBLEM.

E-1	Does a hearing problem cause your spouse to feel embarrassed when meeting new people?	Yes	Sometimes	No
E-2	Does a hearing problem cause your spouse to feel frustrated when talking to members of your family?	Yes	Sometimes	No
S-1	Does a hearing problem cause your spouse difficulty hearing/understanding co-workers, clients or customers?	Yes	Sometimes	No
E-3	Does your spouse feel handicapped by a hearing problem?	Yes	Sometimes	No
S-2	Does a hearing problem cause your spouse difficulty when visiting friends, relatives or neighbors?	Yes	Sometimes	No
S-3	Does a hearing problem cause your spouse difficulty in the movies or theater?	Yes	Sometimes	No
E-4	Does a hearing problem cause your spouse to have arguments with family members?	Yes	Sometimes	No
S-4	Does a hearing problem cause your spouse difficulty when listening to the TV or radio?	Yes	Sometimes	No
E-5	Do you feel that any difficulty with hearing limits or hampers your spouse's personal or social life?	Yes	Sometimes	No
S-5	Does a hearing problem cause your spouse difficulty when at a restaurant with relatives or friends?	Yes	Sometimes	No

Figure 11–6. The Hearing Handicap Inventory for Adults Screening Version. Adapted from Newman and Weinstein.

Factor 1, which are questions 1, 2, 4, and 7 is interpreted as encompassing introspection about the hearing aids ("me and my hearing aids"). Factor 2, comprising questions 3, 5, and 6, is interpreted as reflecting the influence of the hearing aids on the individual's interactions with the outside world ("me and the rest of the world"). Question 8 was included to allocate patients into two groups based on the severity of subjective hearing problems.

The IOI-HA was primarily designed to be used as a supplement with other self-report tools and, because from the onset, it was made available in over 20 different languages, it also would serve as a way to compare hearing aid outcomes around the world using the same self-assessment tool. Many dispensers, however, use it as a stand-alone measure of the quality of the fitting, as it does cover many important aspects (and is short and easy to score). As the IOI-HA is an international scale, it is available in several languages at the University of Memphis Hearing Aid Research Laboratory (HARL) Web site. We've provided you with the English language version (Figure 11–7) which you may copy and administer in your clinic.

The TELEGRAM

Dr. Linda Thibodeau of the Callier Center at the University of Texas at Dallas created the TELEGRAM several years ago. Originally devised to be an outcome measure for pediatrics, the TELEGRAM can be used with adults. TELEGRAM is an acronym. Each letter stands for the following listening situation: T = telephone (cell and land line), E = employment (school or job), L = legislation (communication in public places where the 1990 ADA might be of concern), E = entertainment (TV or movies), G = groups (church, parties, meetings), R = recreation (left open ended on the TELEGRAM form), A = alarms (doorbell, smoke, clock), and M = members of family (description of people most often communicating with the patient on a daily basis).

Using the 1 (no difficulty) to 5 (great difficulty) scale, the TELEGRAM is first completed in the unaided condition and following 30 to 45 days of hearing use re-administered to the patient. Figure 11–8 shows a blank TELEGRAM form. Like the open-ended COSI, the TELEGRAM has a section for the patient to write in specific communication problems to be addressed. The TELEGRAM also has a section for the clinician to write in specific recommendations for each of the eight distinct listening situations it measures. This is especially helpful with the growing number of wireless accessories and integrated assistive listening devices that interface with many of today's hearing aids. To our knowledge, normative data have not been collected on the TELEGRAM, but we still think it's a practical way to measure benefit across several listening situations. There is an article on the TELEGRAM archived at the Hearing Journal Web site published in March, 2008.

Acclimatization: The Effects on Outcome Measures?

Should you think about acclimatization when you conduct outcome measures? Just exactly how long a hearing aid user has to wait to be sure amplification is providing its maximum benefit in everyday listening situations does not have a clear answer. Hearing care professionals have wrestled with the question of hearing aid acclimatization for many years. Conventional wisdom suggests that the adult hearing aid user needs anywhere between one month and one year to receive maximum benefit from amplification.

<u>International Outcome Inventory for Hearing Aids (IOI-HA)</u>

1. Think about how much you used your present hearing aid(s) over the past two weeks. On an average day, how many hours did you use the hearing aid(s)?

	less than 1	1 to 4	4 to 8	more than 8
none	hour a day	hours a day	hours a day	hours a day
☐	☐	☐	☐	☐

2. Think about the situation where you most wanted to hear better, before you got your present hearing aid(s). Over the past two weeks, how much has the hearing aid helped in those situations?

helped not at all	helped slightly	helped moderately	helped quite a lot	helped very much
☐	☐	☐	☐	☐

3. Think again about the situation where you most wanted to hear better. When you use your present hearing aid(s), how much difficulty do you STILL have in that situation?

very much difficulty	quite a lot of difficulty	moderate difficulty	Slight difficulty	no difficulty
☐	☐	☐	☐	☐

4. Considering everything, do you think your present hearing aid(s) is worth the trouble?

not at all worth it	Slightly worth it	Moderately worth it	quite a lot worth it	very much worth it
☐	☐	☐	☐	☐

5. Over the past two weeks, with your present hearing aid(s), how much have your hearing difficulties affected the things you can do?

affected very much	affected quite a lot	affected moderately	affected slightly	affected not at all
☐	☐	☐	☐	☐

6. Over the past two weeks, with your present hearing aid(s), how much do you think other people were bothered by your hearing difficulties?

bothered very much	bothered quite a lot	bothered moderately	bothered slightly	bothered not at all
☐	☐	☐	☐	☐

7. Considering everything, how much has your present hearing aid(s) changed your enjoyment of life?

worse	no change	slightly better	quite a lot better	Very much better
☐	☐	☐	☐	☐

8. How much hearing difficulty do you have when you are **not** wearing a hearing aid?

severe	moderately-severe	moderate	mild	none
☐	☐	☐	☐	☐

Figure 11–7. The International Outcome Inventory for Hearing Aids (IOI-HA). Adapted from Cox and the University of Memphis Hearing Aid Research Laboratory.

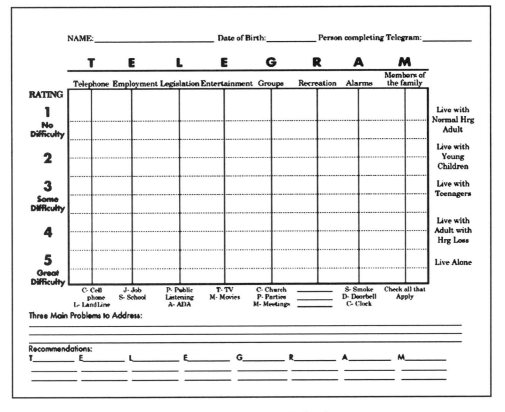

Figure 11–8. The TELEGRAM. Adapted from Thibodeau.

TAKE FIVE:
Device Oriented Subjective Outcome Scale (DOSO)

Just when you thought you had read about every self-report outcome tool, the DOSO was created by Robyn Cox and her team at the University of Memphis. In addition to its memorable name, the DOSO questionnaire is designed to measure the device-only component of outcome. As we mentioned earlier in this chapter, there are many things, like personality of the patient, motivation, and attitude that influence the outcome of a fitting. The aim of the DOSO is to minimize those variables in order to measure the impact of the device on outcome. The DOSO is composed of 40 questions along six subscales: speech cues, listening effort, pleasantness, quietness, convenience, and use. Each of the questions can be scored on a 1 to 7 scale. Before you go to your computer and try and download a copy, please note that the DOSO is not yet commercially available. However, it's been used in a couple of studies and would seem to have some appeal for clinicians. For those of us that like to measure outcome, the DOSO is something to look forward to.

TIPS and TRICKS:
Practical Issues Related to the Use of Outcome Measures

In order to make this review of self-reports more useful for the busy clinician, two commonly asked questions are posed, along with recommendations. Recommendations to each question are based on the best available clinical evidence.

When Should Outcome Measures Be Conducted?

The question of exactly when a self-report of outcome should be administered to a patient is important for two reasons. One, if the self-report is completed too soon, the patient may not have had enough time to become familiar with the fundamental daily care and maintenance of the devices, like cleaning and insertion/removal into the ears. At least one study concludes that administering self-reports too soon results in artificially lower than expected outcomes because patients were not given ample time to learn how to use their hearing aids.

On the other hand, if a clinician waits too long to conduct self-report measures, the entire fitting process is unnecessarily prolonged. Both the patient and the clinician are needlessly waiting to put closure to the fitting process. Recent evidence-based reviews of hearing aid acclimatization suggests that hearing aid benefit is

optimized approximately thirty days postfitting for the typical patient. The clinical evidence suggests that self-reports of outcome should be administered about 3 to 4 weeks postfitting—See our section on acclimatization for detailed information on this.

What Outcome Measures Should Be Used?

Due to the abundance of self-reports available to the clinician, it is difficult to know which ones work the best. When making this decision, it is important to examine exactly what dimension of real world outcome you are trying to capture in the most time-efficient manner. In one large scale study with several variables examined the relationship between self-reports of outcome and personality. Analyses of the collection of outcome measures produced a set of three components that were interpreted as a Device component, a Success component, and an Acceptance component. Results suggest that personality is more closely linked to self-reports of hearing aid outcome than conventional laboratory measures, like the audiogram. How personality affects outcome needs to be taken into consideration when selecting a self-report questionnaire.

Knowing when maximum hearing aid benefit is achieved also has commercial significance. The savvy consumer wants to know when he can expect to be "getting the most" from his new purchase. In a consumer age of

instant gratification, informing patients that they may need to wait up to one year to become fully acclimatized to their new purchase may result in dissatisfaction (remember, many consumers think of hearing aids like eyeglasses, which in many cases provide maximum benefit the moment they are placed on the head). It is common for new hearing aid users to ask, "How long do I need to wear these things until I get used to them?" Consumers have a vested interest in knowing when peak hearing aid benefit is achieved, and it is the responsibility of professionals to answer this question using the best available evidence.

Acclimatization has been referred to as the *process of adjustment* and *accommodation* in the literature. One can "acclima-

tize" to many aspects of amplified sound ranging from hearing ambient noise for the first time in 20 years, to the harshness of a church bell that once sounded dull.

Improvements in Speech Understanding?

One dimension of acclimatization which has been the most heavily studied and discussed, relates to improvements is speech understanding over time resulting from the use of amplification.

TIPS and TRICKS: Practical Issues Regarding Acclimatization

The understanding of the hearing aid acclimatization process has several important clinical implications.

■ Most clinicians make one or more adjustments to the hearing aid during the adjustment period, which usually comprises the first 30 to 60 days of initial use with new hearing aids. If acclimatization occurs over months rather than days, clinicians might be better off waiting to make these adjustments until after peak benefit for a given setting has been achieved.

■ If benefit peaks at a specific point in time, patients might be best advised to "wear it and get used to it" before returning for any additional office visits in which adjustments to the hearing aid parameters are made. Is it the brain that needs adjusting, or the hearing aid? But what if, without adjustments, they don't wear the hearing aids?

■ If acclimatization takes place over a specific time frame, patients

should be provided with programmed gain and output that will lead to the best performance, rather than being fitted with hearing aids tailored to the patient's preference (e.g., "sounds good" on the day of the fitting).

■ If there is a point in time when peak benefit is reached, the clinical evaluation of hearing aid benefit (e.g., speech in noise testing) would not be considered valid unless it was performed after this time period.

■ Regarding documenting self-reports of outcome, the same holds true, as real world benefit should be measured around the time that benefit is at its peak. Most states, however, require a hearing aid trial period as part of the purchase agreement. The patient is able to return the hearing aids for full or partial credit if dissatisfied for any reason. If maximum benefit is achieved only after a long period of use, states might be inclined to extend trial periods beyond the customary 30 days.

Because of the debate surrounding this area, the Eriksholm Workshop on Auditory Deprivation and Acclimatization convened in 1995, and subsequently released a consensus statement. In summary, the Eriksholm Workshop held that acclimatization does occur, and that it is a phenomenon with importance to clinical practice. Consequently, several investigators began to examine the acclimatization more closely. Two separate meta-analysis were published in the late 1990s. Both of these meta-analysis concluded that acclimatization (related to improved speech understanding over time) does occur to a small extent but *these improvements in benefit over time cannot be measured or observed to any noticeable effect in the clinic.* Many of these findings, as they relate to clinical practice were summarized in a special issue of *The Hearing Journal* published in 1999 and edited by Dr. Catherine Palmer. In the dozen years since that special issue, more studies, using modern hearing aid technology have been published on acclimatization. Given the recent advent of evidence-based practice, and the evolution of hearing aid technology, an update on this clinically relevant subject is warranted. The focused questions to be investigated using an EBP paradigm is related to how long a typical patient must wear hearing aids before maximum benefit it achieved.

Hearing Aid Orientation: One More Time

Recall that we devoted a section in Chapter 10 to *hearing aid orientation*. This is something that usually is conducted after verification—and *before* validation. We have found, however, that as you are conducting your postfitting outcome measures, and talking to your patients regarding their responses, you often have to go back and repeat part of the orientation, So, to help you remember this point, we thought we'd give you a reminder on the topic.

If your clinic is anything like the ones we have managed, there is not a lot of time to spare, so here is a handy acronym to help you remember the nine topics for discussion: HIO BASICS (hearing instrument orientation BASICS); an excellent tool developed by audiologist Ron Schow. We think you'll find this a great way to remember all the essentials ingredients of the hearing aid orientation process. There is probably even a few tidbits here that we forgot to tell you Chapter 10.

H = Hearing expectations: Unfortunately, hearing aids do not work just like eyeglasses. Everything will not be perfectly clear once you start to use them. Additionally, adjustment to amplification requires days, weeks, and even months for some patients. The patient needs to know this.

I = Instrument operation: The patient should be able to turn the hearing aid on and off, change programs (if necessary), adjust volume, activate telecoil (if present), function of automatic telecoil (if present), use with remote (if there is one), use with telephone, demonstrate use of hearing aid on telephone, connectivity with Bluetooth (if available), discuss assistive telephone listening devices. Important to conduct as much of this as possible with patients own personal phone.

O = Occlusion effect: Have the patient talk with the hearing aids in their ears, <u>but turned off</u>—see if an occlusion effect is present. If so, and if it is bothersome, conduct treatments for reducing the occlusion effect (e.g., increase venting, lengthen canal, use more open fitting tip) or explain why you can't make it go away (assuming that you can't).

B = Batteries: Discuss different battery types and sizes, what batteries they use, how they obtain batteries, how long a battery lasts, and what to do with those sticky tabs (don't put them back on the battery!). Have the patient demonstrate proficiency in opening and closing the battery door, and inserting and removing the battery.

A = Acoustic feedback: Demonstrate what acoustic feedback sounds like (if the patient can hear it), what causes it, when it is "okay" and when it is not "okay." Demonstrate some typical patient activities that my induce feedback (e.g., learning against a wall, putting your hand to ear, etc). Provide a general idea of how much additional gain (realistically) is available before feedback is present.

S = System troubleshooting: Provide the patient with a trouble shooting chart (this chart is often found in the user manual)

I = Insertion and removal: Demonstrate insertion and removal on an artificial ear, then have the patient practice in front of mirror. Continue until he or she can complete the task. If the hearing aid has fitting tips that need to be exchanged, also have the patient complete this task.

C = Cleaning and maintenance: Show patient where wax accumulates in the earmold or receiver tubing, demonstrate wax cleaning tool, show how hearing aid itself can be wiped clean. Talk about taking the battery out when storing the instrument, using the battery recharger (if there is one), use of a dry-aid kit if moisture is a problem, keeping the instrument away from water, excessive heat, hair spray, avoid dropping hearing aid on hard surface, and other potential hazards.

S = Service, warranty and repairs: Explain warranty and repair policies, give patient warranty card, explain how repairs are handled in your office. Discuss your walk-in policy, and discuss charges for postfitting visits.

TAKE FIVE:
Hearing Aid Orientation 2.0

Due to the wonders of the World Wide Web, it's now really easy to upload instructional videos of the hearing aid orientation process to your clinic's Web site. With a digital recorder and some basic video production knowledge you could even record your own version of the hearing aid orientation procedures mentioned here. If you're not into making your own instructional videos, there are a couple of places offering this service. John Greer Clark at the University of Cincinnati has produced a 15-minute instructional DVD that provides supplemental information to patients.

Postfitting Follow-Up

"Counseling won't make a bad fitting a good one, but it will make a good fitting a more successful one."

After the hearing instruments have been delivered and verified, and your self assessment scales have been administered (and maybe you repeated a little of the orientation), we begin postfitting care. A synonymous term is rehabilitative audiology, or the more historic term, aural rehabilitation. Aural means ear, rehabilitation means, well, rehabilitation. Obviously, a big part of the aural rehabilitation process involves the hearing aids themselves. The fitting of a pair of excellent hearing aids, however, rarely is the complete solution for helping the hearing impaired. A hearing impairment has multifaceted effects on the user. Complete "aural" rehabilitation may involve other aspects of the patient's life: medical, social, economic, psychological, and biological.

Total aural rehabilitation of the patient is multifaceted:

- It may involve the family physician or otolaryngologist, if the case history suggests progression of a medical condition of known or unknown symptoms.
- Family counseling and involvement of the family is always important in that the family needs to support the efforts of use and care of the hearing aids, and to properly manage expectations of the patient and the entire family.
- Psychologically, the patient must learn to live with the limitations the hearing impairment. In extreme cases, a psychologist may be needed.

- Biological and genetic counseling may be indicated for expected congenital issues.

During postfitting aural rehabilitation sessions, we continue to counsel the patient of maintenance of the hearing aid, as well as to continually monitor (verify) the fit of the hearing aids, by using both subjective (subjective listening scales such as APHAB, COSI) and objective measures (ANSI test box and real-ear measurement) to ensure aural rehabilitation is successful. It's also important to monitor the changes in hearing status at least annually.

TAKE FIVE: And Why Not?

Unfortunately, few dispensing professionals conduct any type of formalized aural rehabilitation or auditory training in their daily clinic practice, despite the evidence supporting its effectiveness.

For example, published reports suggest that return for credit rates for participants in group aural rehabilitation (AR) classes is up to three times less than patients who opt not to participate in group AR.

Embrace Rehab?

Historically, aural rehabilitation has failed to become embraced by the wider dispensing community for a number of reasons: First, AR is viewed as time consuming by many practitioners. Even in the face of solid evidence supporting its effectiveness, AR has not been widely used because it has taken time away from the more lucrative and perhaps rewarding task of fitting the hearing aids.

Another factor that has impacted this area, is that as hearing technology has improved significantly in the past decade, many dispensers have believed that the quality of the digital technology was enough to overcome many of the obstacles associated with postlingually acquired sensorineural hearing loss in adults. Another factor is that many traditional aural rehabilitation techniques used in the past had relatively poor face validity. That is, AR exercises often have little resemblance to real-world listening situations, and therefore were not widely embraced by clinicians or patients. Moreover, there was little evidence that long-term benefit would result. Finally, dealing with protocols, circuits, numbers and test scores is easier, and more appealing for many dispensers than working with the person.

New Age Patients

Today, as patients have gained more access to information through the Internet and other sources, they have come to realize there are supplemental exercises and information available to them that will help them improve their listening skills. Additionally, better educated patients seeking these types of services tend to be more demanding, and are willing to shop around for this service until they can find it. For the practitioner this means he or she must be ready to incorporate new and innovative tools into their practice if they want to remain competitive.

Although AR programs have failed to be widely embraced by the profes-

sion and patients' alike, recently published reports indicate that the winds of change may be blowing. In one recent article, audiologists are advised to change the name of the hearing aid evaluation to the "functional communication assessment." The reason for this name change, according to the author is to take the focus off the product and place it on the end goal of improving communication. In other words, communication is a much broader term that incorporates the value of aural rehabilitation and auditory training into a total communication package for the patient. The basic idea being that if you change the name of the procedure to reflect the current thinking, patients and clinicians will be receptive to the benefits of auditory training, and therefore, more likely to embrace it.

Patients are also being encouraged to think beyond the mere product as a solution for their communication deficits. In a recently published open letter to patients they were urged to fully participate in the rehabilitation process if they want to get their moneys worth from their investment of new hearing aids. There also have been recent articles published touting the overall effectiveness that self-guided AR programs have on lowering returns for credit; something that has plagued the entire industry for decades.

To this point, the terms aural rehabilitation and auditory training have been used synonymously. It is important to point out the difference between these two terms. For our purposes, aural rehabilitation (or rehabilitative audiology) is a much broader term encompassing several aspects of nonmedical treatment for hearing loss. Traditionally, aural rehabilitation is offered to patients as a supplemental service when hearing aids are acquired. For example, aural rehabilitation could be general counseling, basic education about the ear and hearing, speech reading classes, assertive training, hearing aid orientation groups, or formal instruction on communication skills.

Auditory Training

Ever been on a vacation or a business trip when you've driven a rental car for an extended period of time? What happened when you came home and drove your own car? A little out of practice perhaps? There was maybe some residual "training" from the rental car?

The term auditory training relates to a much narrower view of the auditory rehabilitation process. Auditory training relates to exercises patients can do to improve listening and communication; the focus of which is on improving various components of auditory memory and comprehension. Even though there is some evidence supporting its effectiveness, auditory training has been thought to be both repetitive and dull. Recently, however, computer-based self-guided tools have been introduced commercially. These tools are thought to be more engaging for the patient, which is likely to result in greater use of the product by patients.

If we focus only on computer-assisted auditory training programs for adults, there are at least five programs available clinically. All of them are designed to take advantage of the plasticity of the auditory system, which hopefully generalizes to improved communication skills. Additionally, there are several anecdotal reports and a couple of research studies showing that the consistent use of an auditory training program can improve hearing aid satisfaction to the point that it results in greater acceptance of hearing aids (fewer in-the-drawer hearing aids, and lower returns for credit).

Although lower returns for credit don't necessarily equate to improved patient satisfaction, all of us can agree that lower returns are a good thing. Considering the clinical evidence of effectiveness for auditory training and its underutilization in most practices, it's obvious that the majority of audiologists are overlooking the value of computer-based auditory training programs. Here are some programs to consider.

1. Computer-Assisted Speech Perception Testing and Training at the Sentence Level, or CASPERSent. CASPERSent is a multimedia program designed by Dr. Arthur Boothroyd. The primary training target is perceptual skill. The program consists of 60 sets of CUNY sentences representing 12 topics and 3 sentence types. Sentences are presented by lipreading only, hearing only, and a combination of the two. Patients are required to hear and/or see a spoken sentence, repeat as much as possible, view the text, click on the words correctly identified, see/hear the sentence again, and move on to the next sentence. The CASPERSent can be either self-administered or administered with the aid of another person. For more information, visit: http://www.rohan.sdsu.edu/

~aboothro/files/CASPERSENT/
CasperSent_preprint.pdf .

2. Computer-Assisted Tracking Simulation (CATS) and Computer Assisted Speech Training. The CATS program, which was developed at the Central Institute for the Deaf in St. Louis and subsequently updated by Dr. Harry Levitt, allows the patient and another person to interact.
It works the following way: the talker says a sentence or phrase, and the listener repeats verbatim the sentence or phrase. If the sentence is correct, the talker goes on to another sentence or phrase. If it is incorrect, the talker repeats some variation of the utterance until the listener correctly repeats it. The computer-based tracking program makes it easier to score the results of each session and monitor progress.

3. Computer-Assisted Speech Training (CAST). Like the previous auditory training programs mentioned, CAST was originally designed for adults with cochlear implants, but, like the other two, it can be adapted for use with adult hearing aid wearers. CAST uses more than 1,000 novel words spoken by four different talkers. The CAST program is adaptive in that the level of difficulty is automatically adjusted according to the patients performance. To learn more about CAST, visit http://www.tiger speech.com/tst_cast.html .

4. Listening and Communication Enhancement (LACE). The LACE program is a user-friendly computer-based program for both patients and clinicians. Patients are required to complete a series of short exercises that are intended to boost their auditory memory and speed of processing. LACE can be completed on any home computer and results can be tabulated and shared with the clinician using the Internet. Recently, Neurotone, the creators of LACE, introduced a DVD version to make it even more accessible. LACE was originally designed to be completed at home by the patient; however, we do know that many clinics around the country are seeing increased patient compliance when at least some of the exercises are completed in the clinic. For more information, visit http://www.neurotone.com .

5. Siemens Hearing Instruments has a computer-based auditory training program called eARena. This training program is similar to LACE in that the level of difficulty of the exercises is automatically adjusted based on the skill level of the patient. Speech-in-noise perception and auditory memory are two of the skills eARena is designed to enhance. Also included in the eARena software is a basic hearing aid orientation, which helps reinforce the individual orientation the audiologist provides each patient during the fitting appointment. Although the data are unpublished, Siemens has presented data at conferences indicating that eARena contributes to better real-world outcomes. For more information, visit http://www.hearing-siemens.com .

TAKE FIVE: Your Place or Mine?

Even though computer-based auditory training programs completed in the privacy of the patient's home seem like a good idea and have been around for several years, their acceptance by both patients and clinicians has been very low. One way to improve acceptance of these programs is to offer the computer-based program at your office. Some clinics have set up a special auditory training room in which patients complete the training exercises in the office, rather than at home. Making computer-based auditory training part of a group hearing aid orientation group also seems to have some possibility for improving acceptance of it.

The Future

Historically, auditory training programs have been viewed by some as largely academic exercises that are conducted in a university clinic. With the evolution of computer technology and the Internet over the past decade or so, audiologists need to reconsider the use of computer-based auditory training. Although an array of questions remain unresolved (e.g. which program is most effective for different adult populations), there is evidence supporting the efficacy of computer-based auditory training programs. Given the relatively steady in-the drawer and return for credit rates plaguing our industry, it is imperative that professionals embrace computer-based auditory training programs. Moreover, as hearing aids become more accessible over the Internet and over the counter, it's probable that you will be evaluated more for your "services" than your "product." Without a doubt, computer-based auditory training needs to be part of a more comprehensive aural rehabilitation program that we offer our patients.

Hearing Aid Follow-Up Appointments

Ever notice that some people's car looks and runs like new after five years or more of use, yet other people's cars, after five years, look and run like something "old?" Think it might have something to do with the care given to the car? The service? The routine maintenance?

We've covered a lot of territory. Clinical tests, real-world measures, and rehabilitative audiology. By now, you probably have realized that it often takes patients anywhere from two weeks to more than a month to become fully adjusted to their new hearing aids. As we're not just talking about the issue of acclimatization, which we discussed earlier—there are many, many other factors related to hearing aid adjustment. Because it does take some time for things to fall into place, you'll need to bring every patient you fit with hearing aids back to your office for routine scheduled follow-up appointments.

Here is a general schedule for when you should bring patients back. Of course, for some difficult-to-fit patients you may need to vary this schedule.

- 24 to 48 hours after the initial fitting, call the patient to see how they are doing with their new devices and if there are any questions.
- 1 week after the fitting, a scheduled follow-up appointment is advised.
- 3 to 4 weeks after the fitting a second routine follow-up appointment is needed. At this scheduled appointment, you will need to measure outcomes using some of the tools we discussed.
- 4 to 5 months after the fitting a semiannual appointment is a good idea. There is some research indicating patient satisfaction declines at six months postfitting. Therefore, bringing your patients in for a checkup prior to 6 months of use is prudent, and may provide them a "shot in the arm."
- 1 year after the fitting a routine appointment should be scheduled, which would include a repeat audiogram.

And remember all those pretests we talked about. If the patient has a large ANL score, a poor QuickSIN score, high expectations, and so forth, your follow-up appointments may need to be more frequent and intense.

In Closing

You don't have to be a car aficionado to appreciate the value of both objective and subjective reports of outcome. This chapter reviewed the essential elements of the postfitting phase of the patient's experience acquiring hearing aids with an emphasis on outcome measures. Your ability to measure the various dimensions of hearing aid outcome, understand acclimatization, conduct some type of aural rehabilitation, and schedule a series a follow-up appointments with your patients are good habits to obtain early in your career. The research shows that all of them will contribute to more satisfied patients.

12

"Selling" Hearing Aids:
It's Not a Bad Thing!

> *"Crazy fans in the stands, a band playing fight songs, cheerleaders, and pom-poms. Yes, we're here to tell you why dispensing hearing aids in a commercial environment can be a lot like college basketball."*

For many patient interactions, effective communication skills can be the most important asset of the overall hearing aid fitting process. In fact, one of the hallmarks of a successful hearing care professional is the ability to be a great listener and communicator. Even the most technically proficient clinician is doomed to fail if he has poor bedside manner. Many audiologists and hearing instrument specialists enter the workforce ill-prepared to meet the common challenges of clinical practice in the real world, such as relating hearing aid features to expected benefits, addressing objections to a hearing aid recommendation, or feeling uncomfortable talking about price with patients.

This chapter outlines a specific system for addressing the needs of hearing impaired patients in a busy commercial environment, where you are likely to be practicing. The tools and tactics described here are designed to add structure to the technical skills you are now acquiring. In the commercial hearing aid business, value is largely created between the interaction of the professional and the patient. The more effectively we can build relationships and solve our patient's communication problems, the more likely we are to succeed both professionally and financially.

Before reviewing the various tools and tactics needed to be an effective consultative selling professional, it is important to clearly define the term *consultative selling*. This is important because in many hearing aid dispensing clinics, the word "selling" has a rather negative connotation—even though most hearing care professionals engage in the practice every day. In fact, to some individuals the term "selling" conjures up the image of fast-talking men in brightly colored checkered sports coats, white belts and pinky rings trying to pressure you into buying something you may not even want. After reading our review on consultative selling, we hope you will agree that hearing care professionals engage in it constantly, and by honing your underlying communication skills it can be improved (no checkered sports coats required).

Consultative Selling

Consultative selling is a way to systematically discover the needs of each patient, and to fulfill their needs so that they can have a better quality of life through our counseling and treatment recommendations. Consultative selling is not about manipulating or pressuring the patient into doing something. It is a system in which the trained professional can apply both his or her technical and interpersonal skills in order to be successful in a commercial environment.

The core of the consultative selling system that we describe is discovering the needs of each patient by executing a series of "next steps." The goal of the consultative system outlined here is to allow the patient to make an informed decision to buy, in an atmosphere in which the dispenser can practice in a professional manner.

Why a Consultative Sales System?

Systems are designed to provide clarity and consistency in your daily work. If you are a college basketball fan, you probably know what we mean. For decades Bobby Knight at Indiana University won several championships even though he didn't have the most talented teams. A few chair-throwing incidents aside, he was successful because his players methodically executed a specific offensive system.

As with coaching basketball, the same is true for hearing healthcare professionals: If you follow a system, you can be more productive. The majority of audiologists and hearing instrument specialists are not natural salespeople. This means that they usually have some discomfort with transacting a sale. For example, they have difficulty asking people for money, or they spend too much time talking about the technical nature of the patient's hearing loss—what they know best. The execution of a selling system is perhaps the most effective way in which professionals with some uneasiness with the sales process can perform admirably. In fact, many professionals that execute a proven selling system flourish with a small amount of practice.

An effective consultative sales system has two core components: Discovery and Fulfillment. Within each core component is a series of tactics you need to execute in order to move from point A (the patient has walked in the door for a prefitting appointment) to point B (the patient has agreed to purchase hearing instruments from you). Figure 12–1 outlines the essential tactics and tools you need to execute both the Discovery and Fulfillment phases of the appointment.

Phase 1: Discovery

The discovery phase of the appointment takes between 30 and 60 minutes

DISCOVERY (70% of the first appointment)	FULFILLMENT (30% of the first appointment)

1. Personal Greeting
 	
2. Establish rapport/build trust
 	
3. Manage expectations by gathering information about:
    a. Reason for visit today ("why am I here?")
    b. Salient event ("why am I here today?")
    c. Cosmetics ("how will it look?")
    d. Lifestyle ("where I want improved communication?")
    e. Performance ("how will they work for me?")
    f. Finances ("what I expect it to cost")
 	
Record all information on COSI
 	
4. Listening intently
5. Complete and thorough evaluation using QuickSIN and ANL Test
 	
6. Assessing motivation to get help ("If we improve your communication in these areas is that what you're looking for?")
	1. Review results: Two key components: COSI and QuickSIN
	
	2. Educate: Review Consequences of Untreated Hearing Loss
	
	3. Demonstrate Technology
	
	4. Discuss Options – Relate technology features to real-world benefits in language the patient understands
	
	5. Offer choices - Make appropriate recommendations using a Top-Down approach and exact price points
	
	6. Overcoming objections as they arise by addressing it directly and Ask for the business
	
	7. Reassure the patient that they made the right choice

Figure 12–1. The essential tools and tactics needed to execute the Discovery-Fulfillment process.

to complete and its singular goal is to build a personal relationship between the patient and audiologist. Although not referred to as the "discovery process," audiologists engage in it many times per day. For example, any time you are learning about the patient, asking good questions and finding out all you can about a patient's communication needs, you are in the discovery phase. There are three essential steps of the discovery phase of the consultative selling model:

Step 1: Establishing Rapport and Building Trust

In order to effectively execute the discovery phase of the consultation appointment, you need to focus on two fundamental skills:

1. Asking good questions to the patient.
2. Being an effective listener.

If you can master these two fundamentals, you will be more comfortable in a commercial environment.

Asking good questions and taking the time to listen is truly an art. Both of these skills can take a lifetime to master. Below is a list of seven essential questions we should ask all patients during the initial evaluation. Please note this is not intended to be a script that is mindlessly read to the patient. That would be insincere, and patients would notice this right away

Establishing Ownership of Visit.

1. "What brings you to the office today?"
2. "How may I help you?"
3. "How long have you noticed this (communication difficulty)?"
4. I'm curious about _____, please tell me more about that . . .

(Don't forget to involve the companion or third party)

Assessing Motivations/Establishing Need to Help.

1. "What situations cause you the most difficulty with your communication?"
2. "On a scale of 1 to 10, 10 being perfect hearing and 1 being a complete hearing loss; how would you rate your hearing?"
3. "How ready are you for hearing aids?" If 1 is "No way I'm ready for hearing aids" and 10 is "I wish I had hearing aids yesterday," how would you rate yourself?

TAKE FIVE: Improve Your Listening Skills

There are two separate and unique types of listening. One type is listening to understand. The second type is listening to respond. During the Discovery Phase of prefitting appointment, we must listen to understand.

As technically trained professionals, our inclination is to respond. There is something called "Inverse Listening/Intellect Law" that says that the more intelligent a person is, the less likely they are to be a good listener. If you think about it, the law makes sense. Really smart and well-educated people want to ensure that their ideas and insights are being heard. They have a natural tendency to want to get their ideas heard—even if they unknowingly and innocently interrupt others in the process.

When we are sitting face to face with a patient for the 500th time, it is easy to anticipate what the patient is going to say. In fact, it is quite common and even expected that we interject our opinions and thoughts throughout the process. In order to improve your ability to listen to understand, take the time to occasionally repeat or paraphrase what the patient just said. This is not always easy to do. We have included a 5-step process designed to help you do a better job of listening to understand.

Those who listen to understand with skill and effectiveness know that the Discovery phase of appointment is the patient's time. They know that they need to allow the patient time to respond in a thoughtful manner, and they must resist all temptation to talk when the patient has the floor.

TIPS and TRICKS: Five Steps for "Listening To Understand"

It might seem obvious, but there are five simple things you can do to improve your ability to listen to understand. These five skills are easy to talk about, but often difficult to execute. If you doubt my words, focus on what you actually are doing during your next appointment with a patient.

1. Square up with your shoulders and face the patient. This sends the message that you are focused on what the patient is going to say. Squaring your shoulders also sends the message of respect.
2. Look him or her in the eyes. When you fail to look the patient in the eyes during the conversation, it sends the message that you are not interested. When you are talking with one person, about 70% of the time you should be looking him or her in the eyes. More than 70% is considered

staring. Less than 50% is perceived as noninterest.
3. Smile. This will send the message that you are open-minded and pleasant to work with. In short, having a smile will break down barriers.
4. Nod your head. This sends the message that you are following the conversation and trying to have a good relationship with the patient.
5. Take Notes. On a blank COSI/ HEAR form, start taking notes. To go one step further, tell the patient that you need to capture as many details as possible and take notes during the conversation. Think about this: People like it (and probably feel more important) when you take notes during a conversation. Finally, you'll quickly realize that taking notes on the COSI allows you to slow down and ask more open-ended questions when needed.

Step 2: Assessing Communication Needs

When a college coach goes on recruiting trips in hopes of building a championshiop team, he begins by assessing his needs. A point guard with speed. A good three-point shooter. A small forward with quick moves. A big guy in the middle. A strong rebounder. Some needs pretty much stay the same, but other needs may shift depending on the situation.

How to Complete a Detailed COSI

We introduced you to the COSI in previous chapters, but we go into a little more detail here. The COSI (short for

Client Oriented Scale of Improvement) is the ideal tool for completing a prefitting assessment of communication needs. It takes one of the things that most providers already do quite well, which is emotionally connect with the patient, and allows you to add some structure to the process.

Because the COSI allows the patient to target as many as five or six specific listening situations for improvement, it is called an "open-ended" prefitting assessment. As it is open-ended, it allows the hearing care professional, the patient, and also significant others to work together during the hearing consultation, building a hearing aid treatment plan.

Below are four practical tips for completing a detailed COSI with all your patients.

List and Target. The first step when completing the COSI is to obtain patient-specific needs. The goal is to obtain at four or five of the most important environments your patient struggles to communicate effectively, and would like to improve with the use of hearing aids. These individualized needs can be, and often are, as diverse as our clientele.

During the initial interview process, you should sit down and engage the patient in conversation as you normally would. The only difference when using the COSI is that you need to record the patient's goals and needs on the form. Notice that on the blank COSI form, there are 5 spaces to record goals.

After collecting the individual's four or five specific needs it is important to rank each area in order of importance to the patient. The specific needs then can be directly targeted as areas of improvement. The COSI allows the hearing care professionals to build a patient-specific counseling agenda, as well as to pinpoint specific areas that are essential when talking about expectations.

Shown in Figure 12–2 is the COSI for a patient, Henry O. His five specific needs are described in detail, then ranked in order of importance to him.

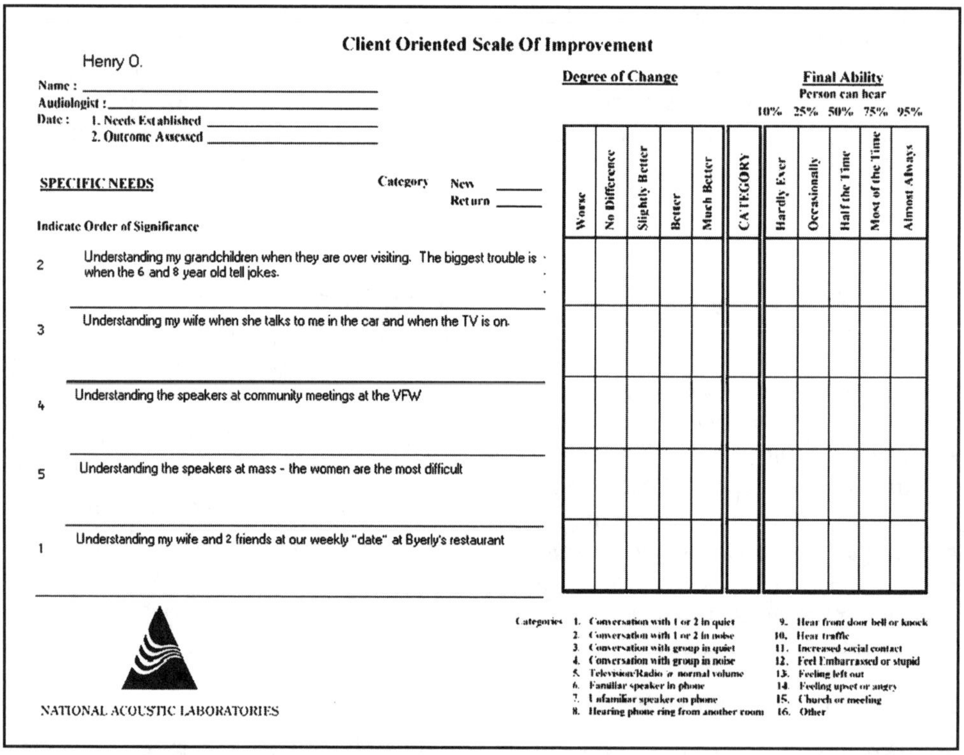

Figure 12–2. A completed COSI. Reprinted, by permission, from Dillon (2001) "Hearing Aids."

Get the Details. When obtaining the specific needs from your patient, it is important to obtain as much information as possible. For example, if the patient states, "I want to hear better in noise" it is important to find out where, when, and with whom. Try to have your patient be as specific as possible.

Below is a list of questions to help delve further.

- What are specific situations that you have trouble?
- When was the last time you had trouble in noise and where was this?
- How frequently are you in these types of noisy situations?
- Who are you trying to communicate with in these noisy situations?
- What kind of rooms are you in when you have these difficulties hearing in noise?
- How many people are typically in this environment?

It is important to make sure the questions are open ended rather than simple "yes/no" questions.

After an extensive discovery period the original statement, "I want to hear better in noise" is more like, "I want to hear my wife and friends better on Sunday mornings when we meet Jim and Aileen for coffee and breakfast at "Johnny's," the local breakfast joint." This statement now provides better information that you will be able to use later for counseling regarding realistic expectations and benefit from amplification.

Pick Two. After the five specific areas are written down and ranked, choose two of the five most important areas to specifically focus on. Circle the two areas on the COSI form and number them #1 and #2. The reason for choosing only two of the areas is based on research that shows most patients will only consistently pick 2 of the 5 original situations targeted for improvement. That is, because the world of communication is not static, different needs occur at different times. The person who listed "understanding my daughter while watching my grandson's basketball games" will probably not have this communication need in the summer.

For our patient, Henry O., we have chosen a situation that involves listening in noise, which is a fairly difficult environment (and fairly difficult to completely fix with amplification) and a situation that involves hearing soft voices in a quiet environment (something that will be easier to fix with amplification). It is important to pick both an easy and difficult environment to specifically focus on and then develop realistic expectations around these areas. It also is important to pick areas to encompass a good portion of the patient's life. Some patients may want to focus on a couple specific difficult listening environments, even though they only encounter those environments once or twice a month. On your COSI (see Figure 12–2) you can even circle the two areas you are going to target for immediate improvement with amplification.

A Tactic for Establishing Realistic Expectations. After choosing the two specific situations to focus on, ask the patient how much benefit he or she expects to receive from their hearing aids in each environment. We do this to discover the patient's expectations. You can do this on a scale from zero to one hundred by asking the patient, "From zero to one hundred, how much do you ex-pect a hearing aid to improve this area?"

Once the expectations have been collected for the various COSI items, it is important to evaluate these expectations relative to his hearing loss and your speech test results. Consider the audiograms and QuickSIN scores for patient A and patient B, shown in Figure 12–3. You can see that both patients have relatively similar audiograms, but vastly different QuickSIN SNR Loss scores

(refer back to Chapter 11 for QuickSIN review). Patient A is able to understand speech in noise at near normal levels, whereas Patient B has significant difficulty understanding speech in noise, and needs an SNR 6 to 8 dB more favorable to understand speech as well as Patient A. Depending on their expectations, there may be vastly different counseling approaches applied for these patients.

If both patients A and B reported that they expected hearing aids to improve their outcome by 70% we know there would be a need to counsel each patient quite differently. Due to Patient

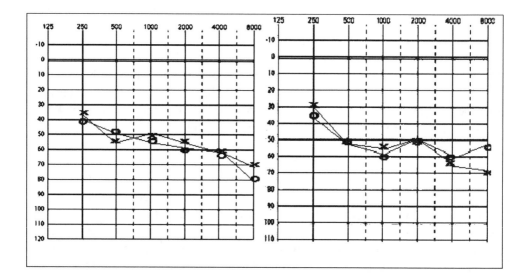

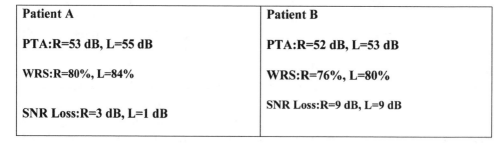

Patient A	Patient B
PTA:R=53 dB, L=55 dB	PTA:R=52 dB, L=53 dB
WRS:R=80%, L=84%	WRS:R=76%, L=80%
SNR Loss:R=3 dB, L=1 dB	SNR Loss:R=9 dB, L=9 dB

Figure 12–3. The pure-tone thresholds, word recognition in quiet, and SNR loss scores for one patient.

A's near normal ability to understand speech in noise we may counsel him that this is very possible to obtain, or maybe we can do even better than 70%. However, patient B will need to be counseled that due to his difficulty to understand speech in noise he may perform a little worse than 70%, maybe even lower than 50% in some situations, especially without directional microphone technology. You can even draw this out on a 0 to 100 scale as shown in Figure 12–4.

We believe that it is important to provide realistic expectations in the beginning, even before the patient listens with the hearing aids. This establishes more real-world expectations and provides for more successful outcomes. Knowing the information contained on the COSI allows the clinician to continue to encourage Henry to wear his hearing aids to obtain maximum results. Also, the clinician can continue to counsel on the use of hearing aids in noise. From Henry's COSI we can see that he is only obtaining a slight amount of improvement in this area. This may be due to using the wrong program (check data logging), directional microphone misuse, unrealistic expectations, or improper positioning in a noisy environment. With further questioning, the clinician will be able to continue to counsel Henry appropriately regard-ing understanding speech in background noise.

Step 3: Audiologic Assessment

The final stage of the discovery process is the comprehensive audiologic assessment. As we've discussed in previous chapters, the primary purpose of this testing is to assure that the etiology of the hearing loss, or other patient conditions, does not warrant medical referral. A secondary purpose is to collect information for the fitting and programming of hearing aids, such as identifying the patient's residual dynamic range. From a consultative selling perspective, however, these tests are used to gather information about the patient's communication ability in order to help them make an informed decision later in the appointment. We consider the following as the essential components of a complete audiologic assessment:

- Air Conduction Thresholds
- Bone Conduction Thresholds
- Immitance Audiometry (tympanomety and acoustic reflexes)
- Speech Audiometry (Quick SIN and ANL test)
- Threshold of Discomfort (LDL) Testing

While it is true that some patients receive little more than an air conduction audiogram prior to the hearing aid fitting, this is highly inadequate. Given that most patients complain about an inability to understand speech in noise, a vital part of the hearing assessment needs to be some type of speech in noise testing. A sentence length test with face validity is a good choice; we recommend the QuickSIN. Speech-in-

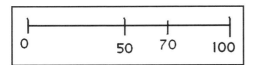

Figure 12–4. Zero to 100 scale used to establish realistic expectations for patients.

noise testing quantifies the degree of problems the patient is having in challenging environment, and if a variety of SNRs are used (as with the QuickSIN), counseling information also can be provided for easier listening conditions. Results of speech in noise tests, moreover, are easy for the typical patient to understand: "Joe, our tests results show that when there is only a little noise present, you understand almost 100% of what is being said, but when there is considerable noise, like that of a typical cocktail party, you probably will only understand about one-half of what is being said." The results of speech in noise testing should be shared with the patient during the Fulfillment stage of the appointment.

Moving to Fulfillment

Once you have completed your discovery work, it is time to move to "Fulfillment," but we cannot move to this stage of the appointment abruptly. It is helpful to transition from discovery to fulfillment by obtaining permission from the patient to move ahead.

An effective way to do this is to simply ask the patient if they are ready to learn about the test results and possible treatment options. Once the patient has granted you "permission" you may move to the second phase of the consultative sales model, which is fulfillment.

Phase 2: Fulfillment

In college basketball, a national letter of intent is a formal agreement between student-athlete and team, stating that the player will attend a given institution in return for an athletic scholarship. Once the student signs a letter of intent, the recruiting process is officially closed. Letters of intent must be signed during specific signing periods for each recruiting year. There is an "early" signing period in mid-November and a "regular" signing period that runs from mid-April to mid-May.

Like college basketball coaches, we also are looking for binding agreements. The single goal of the fulfillment stage is gaining an agreement from the patient to do business with you. Gaining agreement does not necessarily mean that the patient is agreeing to purchase hearing aids. It could mean that the patient has agreed to see another professional you are recommending. It might simply mean that the patient is agreeing to come back and see you for a follow-up appointment in 6 months. Many times, however, we indeed are asking the patient to complete a hearing aid transaction. In most cases, the fulfillment stage is much shorter than the discovery stage. If you have executed the discovery phase effectively, the fulfillment phase should be a natural conclusion to the appointment that often results in a transaction.

The fulfillment stage of the appointment is a 6-step process that should culminate in the patient's decision to do business with you. In order to make the essential steps of the fulfillment stage easy to remember, the acronym RED DOOR is used..

Review

Educate

Demonstrate

Discuss options

Offer choices

Overcome objections

Reassure

Step 1: Review Results

TAKE FIVE: Informational Counseling

It is well documented that when patients understand the information that is presented to them by a health care provider, they are more satisfied, and are more likely to comply with the treatment, such as wearing hearing aids. Although most dispensers enjoy telling the patient about the test results, and may actually spend too much time in this area, it is important to assure that it is conducted effectively. It sometimes is assumed that if a given fact is related to the patient: "You have a high-frequency hearing loss in both ears, and it is probably was caused by damage to the hair cells of the inner ear"—that it is understood and retained. Unfortunately, this is not true. Audiologist Bob Margolis of the University of Minnesota has written on this topic, and here are a few things to remember from his work:

- About 50% of the information presented to a patient is forgotten immediately.
- Unfortunately, to add to this problem, about 50% of what they *do* remember is incorrect.
- In one study, patients could not recall 68% of the diagnosis told to them.
- In another study, patients and their physicians agreed on what needed follow-up only 45% of the time.

Start by asking the patient if they would like a relatively brief review of the results, or if they would like to go into the details. By asking the patient how to proceed the patient will be more receptive to your explanation of the results.

It is important that you use language that the patient understands and relate the test results to the communication difficulties the patient is experiencing on a daily basis. It is up to you to create urgency to get help and the way in which you communicate the results can build the necessary urgency in order for the patient to move to the next step. When reviewing results always use visual aids so that the patient clearly understands what you are saying.

There are many things that you can do to improve the way your information is presented, which will help with retention. We've mentioned the work of audiologist Bob Margolis in this area. Here are a list of tips that he provides:

- Present the most important information first. Patients are best at remembering the first thing you tell them.
- Give advice in the form of concrete instructions.
- Use easy-to-understand language; short words and sentences.
- Repeat the most important information.
- Stress the importance of recommendations or other information that you want the patient to remember.
- Ask for questions and confirm the patient's understanding before moving on to the next category.
- Don't present too much information.
- Present only the information that is important for the patient to remember.

- Supplement verbal information with written, graphic, and pictorial materials that the patient can take home.
- Plan on going slower, and spending more time with older individuals who may have cognitive problems.
- Again, repeat the most important information!

Step 2: Educate (Discuss Consequences of Untreated Hearing Loss)

Most of us would agree that there is a strong stigma associated with hearing loss and the use of hearing aids. In simple terms, most patients do not want to wear hearing aids because they make them feel or appear old. For example, in a MarkeTrak survey of about 10 years ago, when hearing-impaired users who were nonowners of hearing aids were asked if they would wear hearing aids if they "free and invisible," only 35% said yes. We doubt that this opinion has changed significantly today. It is relatively easy for many patients simply to delay their decision to purchase hearing aids, as acquired and gradual hearing loss is normally painless and not a life-threatening condition. Educating the patient on the ill effects of untreated hearing loss can help create urgency to accept your recommendation for new hearing aids (assuming the patient is a candidate for them) in an evidence-based manner.

After you have reviewed test results, ask the patient for permission to move to the next step, which is to educate them about the consequences of untreated hearing loss, and how they can obtain help today from hearing aids. This is an extremely important step because you will need to overcome the reluctance on the part of many patients to overcome the easy decision *not* to obtain help from you. The most effective professionals take the time to build a strong case to encourage the patient to get help today, rather than waiting. Their effectiveness is directly related to their ability to explain the consequences of untreated hearing loss.

The content of your message will vary slightly depending on the test results and the needs of the individual, however, there are consequences of *not* getting the necessary help today, that

---

TIPS and TRICKS: Practice Makes Perfect

Louisville University has one of the most successful college basketball programs in the country. They play a very up-tempo, run-and-gun style of basketball. In order to ensure their players are able to outrun their opponents, head coach Rick Pitino doesn't allow his players to rest more than seven seconds during scrimmages.

Although we are not saying you shouldn't rest during practice, we are saying that it's important to practice the techniques outlined in this chapter. Your "practice" should simulate "game time" situations. Role playing with another staff person or videotaping an appointment with a patient (be sure to get his or her permission first) are two proven strategies for improving your consultative selling skills.

you will need to focus on. One way to convey this message is to simply say, "There are a few consequences of untreated hearing loss that all my patients need to know about . . . " At the least, all patients need a brief explanation of four different factors.

Factor 1. Potential auditory deprivation. Auditory deprivation is the term used to describe a decrease in speech understanding resulting from a hearing loss. You may recall we've talked about this back in previous chapters. Any hearing loss of significant degree reduces the information that reaches the processing areas of the auditory cortex. When it comes to fitting hearing aids, there is some evidence suggesting that patients with hearing loss lose their ability to understand speech more rapidly when compared to people of the same age group with normal or near normal hearing. It, of course, is difficult to determine is this is simply due to the hearing loss itself, or if indeed the central processing system is "forgetting" the correct coding for some speech sounds. If the latter is true, then it's possible that early intervention with hearing aids would help prevent central deterioration of speech understanding. It's also possible that if the patient waits too long to obtain help, hearing aids will provide less benefit."

Factor 2. The bilateral advantage. The discussion of auditory deprivation leads directly into a discussion of the advantage of bilateral hearing provided from two hearing aids. We can also talk about the auditory deprivation effects (unaided ear effects) that occur for patients with bilateral hearing loss who only wear one hearing aid.

That is, research has shown that with many of these patients, the ability to understand speech in the unaided ear becomes poorer after years of unilateral amplification. In some cases, the "deprived ear" will catch up when a hearing aid is fitted in later years. In other cases, there is only partial, or no recovery. It is important, therefore, to utilize bilateral fittings whenever the patient has two aidable ears.

Factor 3. Social and emotional impact of untreated hearing loss. There is also some interesting evidence, much of it archived at The Better Hearing Institute (BHI) Web site, suggesting that patients with untreated hearing loss suffer more from depression and social isolation compared to those of similar age who wear hearing aids. Moreover, struggling to understand speech leads to stress, tension, and often fatigue. Learn more about how untreated hearing loss affects quality of life by reading some of the related studies at http://www.betterhearing.com .

Factor 4. Financial impact of untreated hearing loss. The last piece of evidence to share with patients during this phase of the appointment is the fact that working age people with untreated hearing loss typically earn less than those with hearing loss wearing hearing instruments. One large-scale study, concluded that people wearing hearing aids earned $12,000 more per year on average compared to individuals with the same degree of hearing loss choosing not to use them.

Two Critical Points in Step 2. The tactics described here should be part of the education phase of the prefitting appointment. When you communicate the consequences, in a compelling way you are very likely to create urgency within the patient to get help now. An added benefit is that it takes the focus off product and price. It puts the focus on the needs of the patient.

During this specific phase of the appointment, this technique requires that *you only discuss the consequences of not taking action to get help now and avoid any discussions of product or price*. Once you have built a case for taking action today, you can move to the next step, which is to demonstrate technology and discuss model and price options in a top-down manner.

A second point is that when you are discussing consequences of untreated hearing loss with the patient, you need to focus on the evidence. This means you are citing findings from relevant studies and communicating them to the patient in language they understand, rather than relying on your opinions. You may even want to have some "easy to read" journal articles handy supporting your comments, that you could provide for interested patients. Your clinical experience and opinions are important, but when you include evidence-based thinking into your process, it markedly improves your credibility and professionalism to the patient. Also, remember that many of today's patients are educated and conduct their own "evidenced-based review" on the Internet before their appointment with you. Hence, it's important that you do not embellish the consequences or twist the data to make things sound worse than they are. Not only is this unethical, and possibly illegal, but you will quickly lose all credibility that you have established. Let the evidence speak for itself.

Step 3: Demonstrate Technology

After you have taken the time to educate the patient, emphasizing the consequences of untreated hearing loss, the next step is to demonstrate to the patient how hearing aids can work. Using a pair of programmable hearing aids, take the time to briefly show the patient how modern hearing aids are programmed with computer software and are customized to the individual's hearing loss. Be sure to use a pair of devices that are cosmetically appealing, such as the mini-BTE open-canal products.

During the demonstration process, it is a good idea to show the effectiveness of directional microphone technology and binaural hearing. You will need to prepare for the demo ahead of time by having two hearing aids ready to program and a sound-field listening situation available that has some background noise. In general terms, the demo step is designed to build value and to educate the patient.

Step 4: Discuss Options

The two major points of discussion are hearing aid style (form factors) and level of technology (often determined by features). Using the results of the audiogram and other information you learned about the lifestyle and communication needs of the patients, make a clear recommendation regarding the style that is best for them. Depending on the social style of the patients, you can either inform them regarding what you believe is best for them, or give them a couple of possibilities and allow them to make an informed decision.

When discussing technology it is easy to overwhelm patients on the technical

---

TIPS and TRICKS: Some Thoughts on "Trial Closing"

As you might expect from your own experience as a consumer, it takes some time to make a decision on high-price items and services. Some people might even get sticker shock when you mention the cost of a pair of hearing aids. Others might be fearful of making an investment in hearing aids due to factors such as denial. During the consultative appointment, you need to monitor the motivation and intent of the patient from time to time. The "retail" name for this practice is trial closing. Trial, or preclosing, simply means that you are assessing the motivation level of the patient. Trial closing gives you the opportunity to broach the final decision process without the patient actually having to make a final decision. There are many preclosing tactics you can use. They can be used to move from one step to the next.

Another way to look at trial closing is that it's simply a way to ask the patient permission to move to the next step of the appointment. Getting his or her permission is likely to result in a patient who is engaged in the process.

---

details. Remember to keep things simple, and talk about "what needs to go inside the hearing aid" to maximize their ability to communicate. The emphasis needs to be on what level of technology is needed for their individual needs. As a general rule, you need to discuss technology and advanced features using an evidence-based approach. Relating the items indentified on the COSI to the levels of technology needed to accomplish the goal is another effective tactic for this step of the fulfillment stage.

Step 5: Offer Choices

During this phase you will be recommending between two and four different hearing aid models/styles for the patient to choose from. It is very important to write the options down, including the price, so that the patient can clearly see them. Recommendations should be communicated in a top-down fashion. This means that you begin with the highest technology and work down

from there. Be sure to include price with each level of technology you are presenting. Price points are important. You need to make sure that you are presenting your recommendations at two to four specific price points, corresponding to the level of technology. Price points should be separated by between $500 and $1,000, assuming you are recommending a pair of hearing aids.

Even though you are discussing technology options, you are still educating the patient about how technology will improve *his or her* ability to communicate in everyday situations. Be sure to relate the features at each price point to the expected benefit they should receive. Use the information you wrote on the COSI as a guide. You need to explain how each feature will help them is the areas they nominated as goals on the COSI.

Once you have finished educating the patient, make one recommendation in writing, including the price. To avoid the perception of haggling, ask the patient if they have any other coupons or offers that will help them save some money. Simply wait for the patient to respond once you have made the recommendation. Talking too much during this step can lead to confusion and apprehension on the part of the patient.

Phil Jackson, the current coach of the Los Angeles Lakers, is widely considered one of the greatest coaches in the history of the National Basketball Association (NBA); in total, he has won 10 NBA titles as a coach. Originally from North Dakota and a college star at the University of North Dakota, Jackson is known for his use of a holistic approach to coaching that is influenced by Eastern philosophy, earning him the nickname "Zen Master." You too will find that if you take into account all aspects of the person, not just the hearing loss, and think of your patient as a person first, your ability to connect with his or her needs and to offer appropriate choices will be enhanced.

Step 6: Overcome Objections and Ask for the Business

Chances are great that you will encounter at least one objection, which usually is involving price. You can think of price objections as issues related to value. Perhaps, you have not built enough value into the products or services. Just like everything else, objections can be overcome with a step-by-step process:

- First, acknowledge the objection. "Yes, Mr. Smith, I understand your concern."
- Second, respond to the objection in an unflappable and honest manner. "Mr. Smith, the price of that set of hearing aids is because it has the most sophisticated technology on the market."

- Third, offer the patient something that is agreeable to him or her. "If we stepped down in price and gave up some features, would that be suitable to you."
- Finally, move to the next step. Many inexperienced providers get defensive and actually explain more than they need to. This often results in a lost sale because the patient loses confidence in you.

Objections are as natural as the smell of fresh-cut hay. They are simply requests for more information. Your job is to acknowledge them when they come up, and work to move the patient to the next step. Objections are expected but really are no big deal. In fact, objections can be positive because it means the patient is interested. It is the perfect time for you to demonstrate your knowledge of the products and features, and your concern for finding them the best solution.

Step 7: Reassurance

Once the patient has made a decision on a product and price, you need to take the time to offer some reassurance. Basic psychology tells us that buyers want to feel good about their purchases. During the ear impression phase of the appointment, remind the patient what you want your business to be known for. Offer them something tangible as proof that their decision was the best thing they could have down. For example, you could say, "I am proud of having the most satisfied patients, so I expect you to always leave this office feeling good about your decision to do business with us."

In order for patients to become better educated about what to expect when they visit a hearing aid dispensing office for a consultation, the Hearing Loss Association of American (HLAA), has created a Consumer Checklist. By going to http://www.hearingloss.com you can download a copy of the checklist. The checklist is divided into three sections: testing, dispensing, and full disclosure. We encourage you to study the checklist, making sure you cover each point on the checklist during your appointment with each patient. This will ensure that you are addressing all the details with every patient.

TAKE FIVE: "Feel, Felt, Found" Tactic

One proven way to address most any objection is to use the feel-felt-found principle. It goes something like this, "Mr. Jones, I know how you **feel**. I have had many patients that have **felt** the same way you do right now about this recommendation. But after they have the opportunity to use this technology in everyday listening situations, they **found** out for themselves how well it really works."

Quality and Productivity: Two Keys to Long-Term Success

We spend the second half of this chapter reviewing some of the essential aspects of trying to run a thriving hearing aid dispensing practice. It turns out that many of the skills needed to select and fit hearing aids aren't necessarily the same as those needed to manage a business.

Although we've been focusing on basketball for our sidebars in this chapter, we do recognize that some of you are not basketball fans, so let's turn to music for a moment. In the summer of 1970, the Grateful Dead released arguably their best album, Workingman's Dead. By combining elements of folk, country, and psychedelic rock, the Dead were able to capture a larger audience while garnering praise from even the most ardent critics of the band. You don't have to appreciate the Dead to value their business acumen. By gathering ideas from a wide range of influences, being different from your competitors, catering to your most loyal customers and measuring what's meaningful you can emulate the Dead to improve quality in your practice. (Don't think the Grateful Dead are known for their business prowess; check out an April, 2010 article in The Atlantic Monthly.*)*

As a practice owner or manager it's critically important to focus on the long-term profitability of your operation. The amount of cash flowing into your practice, your ability to control costs and how you differentiate your practice from the competition are just a few of the many components defining a healthy business strategy. Unfortunately, the typical hearing aid dispensing practice owner is too busy taking care of patients (and sometimes lacks the formal training necessary) to think (and act) strategically about their practice.

This section is geared toward those busy owners and managers who unquestionably want to do the right thing for their practice, but lack the time to analyze the details of countless business reports or the resources to implement complex strategies. By distilling practice management into two essential elements, productivity and quality, you can learn how to execute the indispensable drivers of a profitable practice. Part 1 will focus on quality; Part 2 will look at productivity.

Begin with a Self-Assessment

The Rolling Stone's reputation as the greatest rock 'n' roll band in history was certainly not built in a day, and neither is a thriving dispensing practice. A good place to start the building process, however, is by using a self-assessment matrix. The process of evaluating both the productivity and quality, using a 1-to-10 scale can be conducted by ranking your proficiency along two axes, shown in Figure 12–5. A self-ranking of "1" on the scale would suggest very poor performance and a self-ranking of "10" would mean you have a best-in-class practice. Like any self-assessment tool the ratings are somewhat arbitrary, but the value of the self-assessment

matrix is that it helps you prioritize areas of improvement

Does Your Practice Have A Quality Gap?

Over the past few years there have been several reports suggesting there is a quality gap in the way products and services are delivered in a hearing aid dispensing practice. For example, in the July 2009 issue of *Consumer Reports* it was reported that two-thirds of hearing aids are not fitted correctly. The most recent MarkeTrak report suggested that approximately one-third of all hearing aid fittings result in failure when you count the in-the-drawer people, and those users reporting only to wear their devices two hours or less per day. Finally, an April 2010 article published in *The Hearing Review* suggested that there is an important relationship

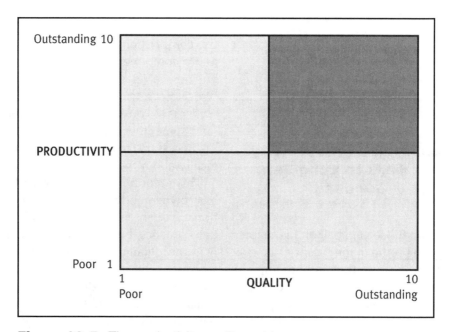

Figure 12–5. The productivity-quality matrix.

between hearing aid satisfaction and the testing conducted during the pre-fitting and fitting appointments. Clearly, there is evidence that there is a gap between knowledge and execution in the typical dispensing office on matters related to *quality*.

Without any knowledge of these recent industry reports, we know that Quality is an important differentiator among practices. Not only are practices that compete on Quality able to command a significantly higher average selling price, practices that differentiate themselves on Quality have another unique competitive advantage: they are able to generate more word-of-mouth referrals. In a low-volume–high-margin industry, like commercial hear-ing aid dispensing, a large number of practice promoters is vitally important to success. For these reasons, managers need to have a passion for improving Quality. Moreover, you will quickly find that you start to like the person you see in the mirror!

The 3-E's of Quality

Quality can be difficult to define, but we know it when we experience it. Most of us would agree that quality as defined in the hearing health care industry is service and product delivery that is effective, efficient, patient-centered and results-oriented. Keeping with our theme of simplicity, let's review the 3-E's of Quality, shown in Figure 12–6.

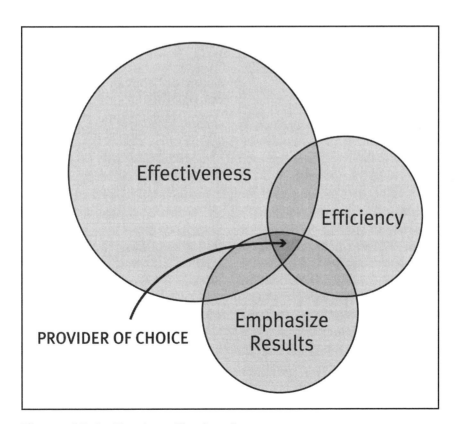

Figure 12–6. The three-E's of quality.

By allocating resources to each of the 3-E's, you can differentiate your practice on Quality, and as Figure 12–6 would suggest become the provider of choice in your market.

TIPS and TRICKS:
What Are Your Priorities?

Once managers begin the process of self-assessing their practice, they can be overwhelmed with the number of areas to target for enhancement. In order to keep the list manageable, rank the top five priorities in your practice requiring additional resources. We've already discussed the COSI, in which patients are asked to rank order their top listening priorities. Managers can do much the same thing with the Practice Oriented Scale of Improvement (POSI). Simply rank order the priorities you think will drive productivity and quality in your operation.

Efficiency. Efficiency is related to patient work flow and time spent with each patient. For each "touchpoint" that your practice engages the patient, it's important to have some idea how much time is needed to optimize satisfaction. Figure 12–4 is an example of how patient work flow can be assessed. Notice that face-to-face contact with the patient is shown at the top of the figure and indirect contact via the telephone or the Internet is listed on the bottom of the time line.

The amount of time spent is also indicated for each "touchpoint." Although there are no data outlining the optimal amount of time for each point of contact, there are data from MarkeTrak suggesting that satisfaction significantly increased when two to three hours of collective time were spent face-to-face with a patient over several office visits. Suggested time benchmarks are shown in Figure 12–7.

Effectiveness. The second "E" of the Quality trinity is effectiveness. Effectiveness is related to how a specific procedure or behaviour contributes to the outcome of the fitting. This is where your knowledge and ability to execute an evidence clinical protocol or a set of "best practices" comes into play. There are several popular clinical procedures that generally *do not* contribute to a

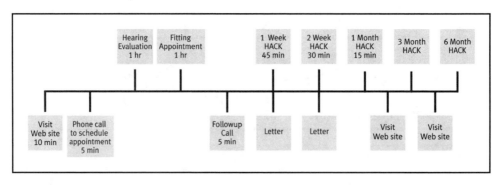

Figure 12–7. The essential points of contact with one patient. The "touch points" above the line are actually office visits. The "touch points" below the line are indirectly interaction with your office via the Internet, phone, or letter. HACK = hearing aid

superior outcome for the patient. One example, is the measure of the patient's most comfortable level (MCL). This is because of its poor test-retest reliability, and the fact the even if you have a reliable value, it doesn't impact on the programming of the hearing aids. It's probably not worth the time conducting this test, although for reasons we don't quite understand, many dispensers do. Tests and other procedures we engage our patients in that don't contribute to a better clinical decision or outcome need to be abandoned and replaced with procedures that have been proven to add value to the decision making process. For instance, there is good clinical evidence suggesting that the acceptable noise level (ANL) test is a pretty good predictor of whether your patient will be a full-time hearing aid user. The ANL, therefore, could replace traditional MCL testing during the prefitting process. Managers can improve the effectiveness of their clinical procedures by conducting an evidence-based review of current procedures and updating any tests that are not supported by research, or do not improve or alter the fitting or patient counselling process.

TAKE FIVE: Taking Action

Once you have established clear priorities to target for improvement in your practice, the next step is to make sure things actually get done. This can be accomplished by establishing clear goals and consistently monitoring progress. For each goal take the time to document the small, actionable steps needed to ensure the goal is met, and then vigilantly following up to monitor progress.

Emphasize Results. The final "E" of the Quality trinity is "emphasize results." The highly influential business management pioneer, Peter Drucker, once said, "When you measure something you begin the process of improving it." Simply put, Quality cannot be improved unless it is measured. Given the fact that most hearing care professionals do not take the time to measure outcome, it is imperative that we use the word *emphasize* when we talk about results. Taking the time to measure various aspects of your practice can have a profound and lasting effect on quality.

Direct Versus Proxy Measures of Quality

Before getting into some of the down-to-earth ways quality can be measured in a busy practice, let's review the two approaches of measurement. Direct measures of quality are any measures that objectively quantify something. For example, 2-cc coupler measures are an objective measure of quality. However, in order to comprehensively measure quality, indirect measures, commonly referred to as proxies, are also needed.

Proxy measures indirectly gauge if something has been completed successfully. Most of you are old enough to remember the Monsters of Rock tours in the 1980s. Van Halen was one headline act, and like most top-notch rock bands from the era, they relied on pyrotechnics to energize the crowd. As you can imagine, these exciting stage shows were difficult to set up and extremely dangerous. Not only the band, but also the crowd was put at risk, if something was not properly set up before the show. Compounding the danger, these expansive concerts were conducted all around the country for days on end; therefore, each city had a group of workers rushing to set up equipment in advance of the band. David Lee Roth, the lead singer of Van Halen, came up with the ingenious idea of using a proxy measure to ensure the pyrotechnics were properly installed. Like all rock stars, the band required a list of specific foods be available prior to the show. This list of demands included one large bowl of M & Ms with all the brown ones removed. Most people think this is obsessive, narcissistic rock star behavior, rather the M &Ms served as a proxy measure. If the band discovered brown M & Ms in the bowl, this was a cue to have the stage checked more carefully, because if the stage crew was not paying attention to the candy, chances are great they were not paying attention to the details of setting up the stage either.

TAKE FIVE: Execution: There Are No Magic Bullets

Establishing a clear strategy, identifying areas of improvement, setting goals, action planning and measuring results are mundane, methodical and downright boring processes that require persistence and attention to detail. Once you have established a clear strategy and plan for improvement, stick to it. Effectively managing your practice is akin to rolling a large boulder up a hill: progress is not immediately noticed. It's only after months of hard work that you sometimes can step away and see that you have made progress toward your goal.

Measuring Seven Dimensions of Quality

Let's leave rock music and get back to basketball for a moment. Like many sports, stat sheets are important in college basket-

ball. While a coach has a "hunch" of who is doing what and how things are going, it is not until he reviews the stat sheets that he knows the precise areas for improvement. Why are our team's turnovers twice as high as the competition? Why does the competition shoot a higher free throw percentage? Why do we average less offensive rebounds than the competition? When these factors are carefully measured, efforts to make things better can be addressed in a systematic manner.

Here are some helpful, easy-to-use tools that busy clinicians can use to measure quality. The seven dimensions of quality shown in Figure 12–8 represent the various phases of the patient's journey from initial contact with the office until initial use of hearing aids. By taking the time to measure these quality dimensions, hearing professionals can manage the entire process and begin to ensure that each patient is highly satisfied with all aspects of his or her experience.

Wait Time and Initial Greeting. Woody Allen once said that 80% of success is simply showing up, and in any customer service business, this is certainly true. Little things, like when the office manager answers the telephone with a friendly voice, go a long way toward improving quality. Armed with this information, managers can train their front office staff to warmly greet every patient over the phone or when they arrive in the clinic. Communication experts agree that standing up, squarely facing the patient, smiling and offering a handshake are components of an ideal greeting, and the ability of front office staff to perform these behaviors can be tracked using a form like the one shown in Table 12–1. As the old saying goes, "You only have one chance to make a first impression."

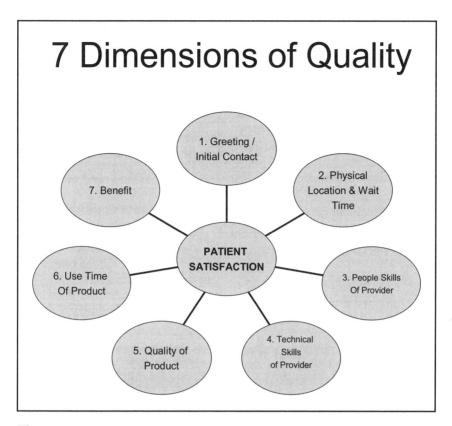

Figure 12–8. The seven dimensions of quality.

Table 12–1. Sample Tracking Form Used When a Patient Checks into Your Practice at the Front Desk

Patient Name	Date & Time	Appropriately Greeted	Wait Time	Notes

Appearance of Physical Location. The reception area or waiting room is one of the most easily overlooked aspects of a practice, but often the most important first impression for patients. It may seem obvious that when patients enter a practice location, they expect the facilities to reflect their perceptions of a professional business. Beyond the reception area, the entire physical location of the practice needs to be routinely inspected. A simple approach to measuring the quality of any physical location is to maintain a checklist with meticulous attention to detail. The physical location checklist is completed each morning by the office manager, and a written copy is shared with the owner or managing director. All deficient areas in need of upgrades or repair are recorded at the bottom of the form (Table 12–2).

Interpersonal Communication Skills. An audiologist's or hearing instrument specialist's effectiveness is largely determined by his or her ability to form strong relationships with patients. Any investment managers can make to improve the relationship building skills of their employees is likely to pay off in improved service delivery. Good listening skills, the ability to ask open-ended questions, and clear and concise explanations of test results are a few of the "people skills" needed to build effective relationships with patients and enhance patient satisfaction.

Interpersonal or relationship-building skills can be directly measured by patients. Using a comment card with five or six important components of interpersonal skills, like the one shown in Table 12–3, patients can directly measure the effectiveness of this dimension of quality. Once you have collected a representative data sample (20 to 30 responses per month for the typical practice), you can begin the process of improving behaviors that have the largest impact on patient satisfaction.

Table 12–2. Physical Location Checklist

Date: _____ Responsible Party: _____	
Restroom is clean and stocked	
Current, tatter-free reading material in reception area	
Floors, walls and windows are clean	
Furniture is clean and properly arranged	
Literature with practice brand is prominently displayed	
Well-lit areas (no burned out bulbs)	
No foul odors	
Equipment is orderly and dust-free	
Staff is properly groomed and wearing appropriate attire	
Deficient areas:	

Technical Skills. The ability of a hearing professional to conduct a comprehensive hearing evaluation, as well as program, fit, and troubleshoot hearing devices can be indirectly measured by assessing the professional's adherence to a clinical protocol. There is no shortage of clinical hearing aid selection and fitting protocols. The most current hearing aid selection and fitting protocol recommended by the American Academy of Audiology incorporates evidence-based practice standards.

Unlike interpersonal skills which patients can directly measure, a hearing professional's technical ability needs to be gauged indirectly by tracking their adherence to a clinical protocol. In Table 12–4 the essential standards for a prefitting hearing aid consultation appointment are outlined. Managers

Table 12–3. Five Important Components of Relationship-Building Skills That Can Be Measured on a Patient Comment Card

I felt the hearing professional really listened to me.	0 1 2 3 4 5 6 7 8 9 10
The hearing professional took the time to thoroughly test my hearing.	0 1 2 3 4 5 6 7 8 9 10
The hearing professional took the time to clearly explain my test results.	0 1 2 3 4 5 6 7 8 9 10
I was given reasonable treatment options.	0 1 2 3 4 5 6 7 8 9 10
The hearing professional solved my problem.	0 1 2 3 4 5 6 7 8 9 10

The rating "0" is highly dissatisfied, and a rating of "10" is highly satisfied.

Table 12–4. An Example of a Prefitting Clinical Protocol Checklist

Standard	Clinical Tool/Procedure
Pretest Communication Assessment	• COSI • COAT • HHIA-E/Screening Version
Testing	• Audiogram • Immittance Audiometry • Speech Audiometry (Quiet and Noise)
Post-Test	• Reviewed Test Results • Demonstrated New Technology • Discussed Options • Offered Recommendation

Once the hearing professional has been given guidance on how to conduct each procedure, she can begin to document that the protocol was followed by using the checklist.

can track the execution of a protocol by requiring hearing professionals to place a completed checklist into each patient's chart notes at the end of the consultation.

Product Quality. A starting point for product quality is to conduct 2-cc coupler measures in the hearing aid test box to ensure that hearing aids are performing at a specific standard developed by the manufacturer. These measures also can be used by the hearing professional before the fitting to ensure that the hearing aid is functioning properly. Prior to the fitting, the hearing professional must take the hearing aids from the packaging material, perform a listening check on them and, finally, conduct a routine electroacoustic analysis of the devices, using the correct 2-cc coupler procedures.

In addition to 2-cc coupler measures, hearing professionals can rely on a hearing aid fitting checklist as a proxy measure of product quality. After the fitting has been completed, the clinician completes the checklist, noting anything unusual or problematic before placing the checklist into the patient's chart. Table 12–5 is an example of a hearing aid fitting checklist.

The final three dimensions of quality can be systematically evaluated using traditional measures of hearing aid outcomes. Studies conducted by Larry Humes and colleagues from the Univeristy of Indiana, using an assortment of more than 20 outcome measures, identified three separate and distinct aspects of hearing aid outcome:

1. Aided and unaided speech recognition performance.

Table 12–5. An Example of a Hearing Aid Checklist Used to Measure the Quality of the Initial Fitting

Patient Name: _____ Date: _____   Manufacturer and Style: _____ Model _____
• _____ Preliminary electroacoustic evaluation satisfactory   • _____ Physical fit is comfortable and without feedback.   • _____ Patient can insert and remove devices.   • _____ Patient can change battery and clean instruments.   • _____ Initial usage of devices and expectations were discussed.   • _____ Verification of desired targets was conducted, results documented.   • _____ Demonstrated special features to the patient.   • Areas of concern:

2. Self-reported hearing aid usage.
3. Subjective benefit and satisfaction.

Given these findings, both subjective and objective measures of outcome should be used to assess quality in clinical practice.

Use Time of the Devices. There is a relationship between patient satisfaction and the amount of time the patients uses the hearing aids; as you would expect, full time hearing aid users are more likely to report higher overall satisfaction scores compared to part time or nonusers. In addition to lower satisfaction, lower rates of usage also are reported for patients with negative attitude towards amplification, and those who consider hearing aid use to be stigmatizing.

Hearing aid use rate can be measured either subjectively or objectively. Subjective measures of use time would be considered to be diaries or questionnaires that the patient completes. Unfortunately, research has found that subjective reports of usage are unreliable. As discussed in Chapter 10, objective measures of usage can be obtained using data logging, which is found in most modern hearing aids. One of the advantages of data logging is that it objectively tracks the total number of hours of hearing aid use. Part-time and nonusers can be managed differently than full-time users. For example, a patient with a low use rate, which has been objectively verified with data logging, might have a problem with annoyance from noise as measured on the acceptable noise level (ANL) test. The low use time combined with the high unaided ANL score might be an indication that the patient needs repeat instruction on the use of the "nosie" program,

a more aggressive noise reduction strategy or perhaps the patient needs to be counseled differently.

Laboratory and Self-Reports of Hearing Aid Benefit. Benefit is simply the difference between the unaided and aided condition. Hearing aid benefit can be measured in a number of different ways, including laboratory measures of speech recognition and self-reports or questionnaires following real-world hearing aid use. A work-day approach to measuring benefit would be to use some combination of laboratory and self-reports. See Chapter 11 for more details on this dimension of quality.

Measuring each of the seven dimensions of quality, using a combination of direct and proxy measures, enables the professional to identify performance gaps and begin the process of eliminating them. Managing today's modern audiology practice requires judicious application of quality metrics that complement traditional productivity measures. Audiologists, hearing instrument specialists and practice managers must all begin measuring quality in order to improve it. By borrowing from other fields you don't have to have an appreciation of early 1970s rock music to create your own version of a Grateful Dead classic.

Productivity: Getting the Most Out of What You've Got

If by chance you can remember back to the first page of Chapter 1, recall that we provided you with a "Hony-Tonk" message. Well, here is another:

I keep my nose on the grindstone, I work hard every day

*Might get a little tired on the weekend, after
    I draw my pay
But I'll go back workin, come Monday
    morning I'm right back with the crew I'll
    drink a little beer that evening,
Sing a little bit of these working man blues*

—Merle Haggard

You don't have to enjoy a beer after work to relate to Merle's classic country tune, "Working Man's Blues." If you've ever owned or managed a practice, you know how difficult it is to keep up with the steady flow of patients, while simultaneously creating a credible marketing plan, paying your bills, negotiating hearing aid prices with manufacturers, and devising a long-term strategy that differentiates your practice from the competition. Our goal here is to arm you, the workaday manager, with tools to increase the productivity of your practice by focusing on a few simple strategies that will stave off the working person's blues. Although these strategies may be simple, it's important not to confuse simple with easy. By rolling up your sleeves, bringing your lunch pail to work, getting some dirt under your fingernails, and taking action, your practice has the potential to experience double-digit growth.

With limited formal business training, the typical hearing care professional often works under the assumption that there are literally hundreds of ways to increase revenue in a practice. When faced with so many options, it's not surprising that many practitioners become paralyzed by the sheer number of choices and fail to take decisive action resulting in revenue growth. The good news is it's not that complicated. No matter what type of practice you own or manage, there are only three things to focus on when trying to increase the overall productivity of your practice:

- Office traffic (patient visits to your clinic)
- Number of units sold
- Average selling price (ASP)

The so-called Productivity Trinity is shown in Figure 12–9 along with the expected result, *IF* the manager shows up everyday and devotes time and resources to improving each of the three dimensions.

Some Simple Math

Before getting into specific actions, you can take to increase the productivity of your practice, let's take a look at some numbers. Just like a construction worker might do some quick calculations of the rise and the run of a specific area in order to determine the correct grade (or slope) of a new road, you can quickly project how much extra revenue you can generate by plugging in some numbers before you begin work. This little exercise is a great way to gain a better understanding how each small improvement along the three dimensions of the Productivity Trinity results in significant top line revenue growth. According to a recent survey, we know the following about an *average* dispensing practice:

Average number of prospects visiting your office per month: 42

Average number of units dispensed per month: 17

Average selling price per unit (ASP): $1800

Projected revenue: **$367,200**

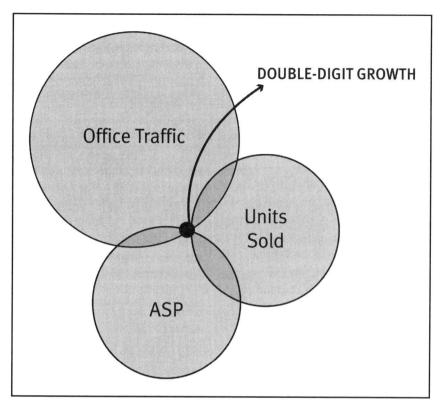

Figure 12–9. The Productivity Trinity. The point in which the three circles interconnect indicates the path to double-digit revenue growth.

Now let's see what happens when we simply increase the number of prospects, units sold, and ASP each by a margin of 15%.

Average number of prospects visiting your office per month: 48

Average number of units dispensed per month: 20

Average selling price per unit: $2070

Projected revenue: **$496,800**

As you can see, a modest increase of just 15% in each of the three dimensions increases annual revenue by over 30%. In other words, six more patients per month walking through your door, and three additional units per month, results in more than $125,000 in revenue at the end of the year. So, the real question becomes, what are you packing in your lunch pail that will provide this boost in productivity?

Office Traffic

Since 1889, Carhartt has been the leader in durable, premium quality workwear. Whether you are looking for a garment in our signature brown duck fabric or one of our innovative, technically advanced fabrics like Waterproof Breathable, we have the most complete line of workwear available.

—From http://www.Carhartt.com

Like the logger's Carhartt jacket, having a steady flow of prospects coming through your door will protect your practice from the elements. In traditional marketing parlance, prospects can become loyal customers through the methodical process depicted in Figure 12–10. The marketing funnel, which looks more like a bullhorn used by a policeman, would indicate that prospects first have to be aware of, interested in, and desire your services before they will take action by calling your office to schedule an appointment. In fact the entire advertising profession uses this funnel to create demand for goods and services. There is no doubt that this approach works. The challenge for the practice manager, however, is that the approach is expensive and inefficient. You can spend significant amounts of cash on advertising

and never receive a reasonable return on your investment, therefore practice managers need to spend time marketing to their existing database.

A sustainable approach to driving more prospects through your door rests with your ability to flip the marketing funnel. Rather than simply relying on advertising to generate awareness, interest and desire in your offerings, use the power of your existing patients to create new ones. There are at least four tactics (shown in Figure 12–10) you can use to gain new prospects by relying on existing loyal patients.

1. Incentivize word-of-mouth referrals:
   All of us would agree that word-of-mouth referrals come to our practice with fewer barriers than the typical prospect responding to

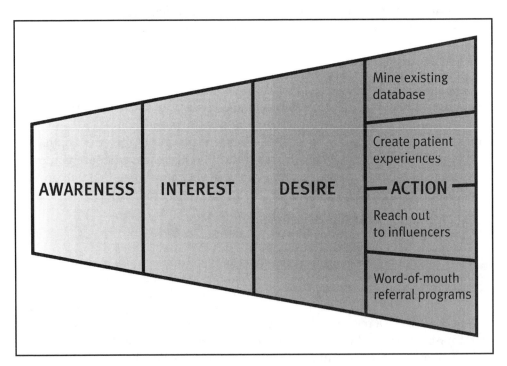

Figure 12–10. The hearing aid dispensing practice marketing funnel.

an ad. Plus, it is essentially no cost from your marketing budget to acquire them. One effective word-of-mouth referral program tactic is to offer gift certificates of a nominal amount (e.g., $25) to any patient who refers another to your office. Also, don't forget what we've mentioned in previous chapters based on the MarkeTrak VIII data—proper verification and validation leads to satisfaction; satisfied patients will provide word-of-mouth advertising without *any* incentive!

2. Provide an impeccable office experience:
   This point is directly related to the one above. In order to generate more promoters, your practice has to have an emotional appeal. You can think of the "office experience" as a higher level, more visceral type of customer service. When you and your staff appeal to the emotions of your prospects you can more readily solidify your practice as the provider of choice. Entire books and Web sites are devoted to improving the office experience in elective medicine. One excellent website is http://www.premiumexperiencenetwork.com . In short, rather than simply focusing on the results of the fitting, you need to focus on the patient's entire experience with your practice—from the time they initially picked up the phone to call you for an appointment until they are a habitual visitor of your practice.

3. Mine your existing database:
   There are two facts that should

motivate you to implement a patient retention program:
(1) Over half of all hearing aid purchasers go elsewhere when it's time to repurchase, and (2) More than 60% of hearing aids are purchased by experienced users. For these two reasons it's imperative to give patients a reason to come back to your office. Each new product and form factor launch is an opportunity to inform your patients about improvements that may provide better communication. There is no shortage of office management tools available to you that can help you target a specific group of patients for a flyer or mailing. Some of the latest product innovations from many of the manufacturers provide opportunities to mine your existing database by offering an interesting form factor or technologic advancement to a precise segment.

4. Reach out to patients and influencers:
   Even the most well-designed flyer mailed to your database is a passive form of marketing, as it is easy for patients to discard them. You truly can turn the marketing funnel into a megaphone, by looking for ways to engage your patients in an ongoing dialogue about your practice. There is no shortage of tools and tactics you can use to actively maintain the conversation with prospects and patients. Here are a few:
   - Measuring patient satisfaction is a great first step. By taking the time to ask your patients and

prospects their opinion about how you conduct business, you are able to foster a deeper relationship with them. (Not to mention that patient surveys and focus groups are really the only way to understand what your practice does well and what it needs to improve from a patients perspective.)

- The Internet can also be used to maintain the conversation with patients and offer deeper levels of customer service; video snippets and blogs can be used to educate your patients; and it allows them to network with other patients dealing with similar issues.

- Another proven tactic for maintaining the conversation with your patient base is through public relations opportunities. One growing industry trend is to provide funding for looping systems. In return for funding an induction loop system for a local church or meeting room, you can ask the facility where the loop was installed to provide educational support in the form of lectures or support groups to the members of that facility. The February 2010 issue of *The Hearing Review* provides details on how to administer a PR campaign around loop systems.

TAKE FIVE: Patient Retention Programs are an Investment in Future Growth

Any time or money you spend on increasing office traffic is akin to investing money in the stock market. There is always some risk involved in your investment choice. By allotting time and money toward marketing your existing database, you are minimizing the risk.

Setting aside 30 minutes per day or 2½ hours per week to market to your existing database using the four tactics we described will pay off in more word-of-mouth referrals and greater office traffic for your practice over the long haul.

Finally, a critical part of any patient retention program is reaching out to influencers. An influencer would be defined as anyone who can raise awareness of a condition or assist in the decision making process of the patient. For example, older adults with hearing loss often rely on their children and even grandchildren for advice about their undiagnosed medical condition. You can reach influencers through public relations campaigns. There are several "apps" that can be downloaded onto a tablet computer that can be used as hearing screeners. These applications and devices are ideal ways for "influencers" to have a conversation with their grandparents about hearing loss. These types of devices can even be used as part of a networking or referral campaign with physicians and other medical professionals.

Units Sold

From its birth in the 1920s to its present status as the world's number one manufacturer of work apparel, the Williamson-Dickie Mfg. Co. has earned a reputation for quality workwear that delivers outstanding durability and support. Initially, a small family enterprise focused on producing bib overalls, the company grew rapidly and became a major player in the uniform apparel market and in World War II millions of soldiers wore uniforms bearing the Williamson-Dickie label of quality. Today, the company is committed to producing the most innovative work apparel with the latest in fabric technology. The Working Person's Store offers a wide variety of Dickies products from coats, to coveralls, to scrubs.

—From http://www.dickies.com

Perhaps the single greatest opportunity to increase revenue in your practice is by gaining a buying commitment from just one or two prospects each month. The number of prospects who are motivated to purchase and actually deciding to buy at the time of their consultation appointment is around 40%. This would suggest that over half of all prospects going through a 60- to 90-minute appointment are walking out the door without agreeing to purchase hearing instruments. Clearly, there is an opportunity to increase productivity through better management of the consultation appointment.

If you were a farmer back in 1920, chances were pretty good that you wore a pair of Dickies bib overalls while you sat on your steel wheel tractor. Times have certainly changed. There are many fewer farmers today and the ones that still toil often do it from a temperature-controlled climate of the cab on the tractor, where shorts and a T-shirt are perfectly acceptable attire.

The consultative audiology process is similar. Advances in diagnostic and hearing aid fitting technology has rendered some tests obsolete. Like the popular bib overalls of the 1920s, there are some components of the consultative test battery that have been modernized. Unfortunately, many professionals still rely on outdated testing procedures for making important clinical decisions and establishing relationships with patients.

Based on research findings there are at least two clinical tests that can be used to better understand the impaired auditory system. In addition, because these prefitting speech tests can be designed to simulate real-world listening, they allow the patient to participate in the process in a far more meaningful way. You already know about these tests from our discussion in Chapter 11: the QuickSIN and Acceptable Noise Level (ANL) Test. Both of these measures not only provide important diagnostic information, but they allow the professional to be more persuasive. Why? Because you have considerable more information that directly relates to the patient's problems.

When you boil it all down, professionals who are successful in the commercial hearing aid dispenser sector of the market have two skills that make them persuasive: relationship building skills and technical ability. When both these skills are in abundance, professionals have the innate ability to gain agreement from patients.

For the rest of us who may not be so lucky, we can learn to be more persuasive. Robert Cialdini has written extensively about the "six weapons of influence."

1. Reciprocation:
   All of us are taught we should find some way to repay others for what they do for us. Most people will make an effort to avoid being considered a person that *doesn't* return a favor. Providing patients useful educational information about the consequences of untreated hearing loss is one of the best ways to leverage the concept of reciprocation.

2. Commitment and Consistency:
   Once people have made a choice, they are under both internal and external pressure to behave consistently. No one wants to be labeled a hypocrite. When you get someone to commit verbally to an action, the chances of them actually doing it go up considerably. By breaking the prefitting consultation into a series of next steps in which you ask the patient's permission to move to the next step is a great way to capitalize on the concept of commitment and consistency.

3. Social Proof:
   We decide what is correct by noticing what other people think is correct. Professionals can use testimonials during the consultation as evidence that other like-minded patients are satisfied with their decision to do business with you.

4. Liking:
   People love to do business with people they enjoy being around. Taking the time to flatter your patient during the appointment, referring often to them by their name, and providing a memorable office experience for the patients are examples of the liking principle.

5. Authority:
   Most people have a respect for authority figures. You can put this principle to go use by dressing professionally, maybe wearing a lab coat (implied authority) and by effectively communicating the research that supports your recommendation for the patient (real authority).

6. Scarcity:
   Remember how popular Coors beer was when it only was available in Colorado? Opportunities seem more valuable when they are less available. Things that are hard to get are perceived as having more value. You can leverage the Scarcity principle by referring to the limited resources and time that might be available to help a patient. For example, your receptionist uses the scarcity principle when she mentions to a patient that your schedule is really full and it's best to get some time booked now, rather than waiting.

Average Selling Price

In a high-margin/low-volume business, like hearing aid dispensing, managing your average selling price (ASP) can have a huge impact on business. Rather than thinking about ASP increases as simply 'raising prices on my patients', let's examine how practitioners can add value at specific price points without lowering prices. Figure 12–11 illustrates the value-added concept. No matter

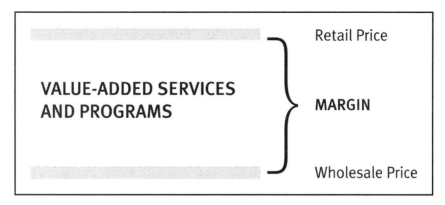

Figure 12–11. An illustration of value in the eyes of the professional.

what your patient mix and price strategy, all managers work with a wholesale and retail price (represented by the floor and ceiling in Figure 12–11, the real opportunity is to maintain a healthy margin and to fill this margin with as much value as possible. Value can take the form or extra time spent with patients or providing additional services.

TAKE FIVE:
What's a "Touchpoint?"

A term that you hear quite a bit these days in the business world is "Touchpoint," or touch point. This could refer to a customer contact or a point of contact. On the other hand, it could be a *brand* touchpoint. In general, this is the interface of a product, a service, or a brand with customers, noncustomers, employees, and other stakeholders—before, during, and after a transaction.

Many professionals make the mistake of equating value with technology. Improved technology has certainly cre-

ated an opportunity for offering products at a higher retail price, but don't be fooled into thinking that all of the value is related to the technology supplied to us by our manufacturing partners. Professionals relentlessly need to be looking for ways to add value by improving service and the overall office experience. There are at least three tactics you can employ that add value and allow you to command a higher ASP:

1. Offer comprehensive follow-up services:
   A good example of a value-added program is LACE offered from Neurotone. For a small investment, which can be bundled into the price of the purchase, patients are able to complete 10 or more training exercises. As the exercises are self-guided, the practice manager does not have to devote staff to the program.

2. Spend more time conducting "Best Practice" testing:
   A recent HIA study shows that patients are more likely to report higher levels of satisfaction when professionals spend more face

time with the patient and use state-of-the-art testing, like probe-microphone speech-mapping analysis, as part of the testing process. These findings were also supported by the latest MarkeTrak VIII data.

3. Add more touchpoints: This simply means that you are giving patients more direct access to your practice. Touchpoints can include annual checkups, follow-up appointments, and visits to your Web site to obtain information and to purchase accessories, like batteries. Another way to add touchpoints is by hiring a hearing aid wearer you fitted to conduct support groups for your practice. The bottom line is that you can add value by making your practice more accessible to your patients.

Avoiding Big Mistakes

In these busy times, there is a real need to prioritize and plan in your clinic or office. All of us are drowning in information from a variety of sources, including social media and the Internet. Studies have shown that when people are given too much information their ability to make good choices becomes extremely slow and sometimes paralyzed. The following section of this chapter aims to help you cut through the clutter by avoiding some common mistakes and offer some suggestions for managing a more successful business.

Big Mistake No. 1: Trying to Be All Things to All People

If you are offering several products to customers at many tiers/prices, using low price point advertising and trying to be known for delivering the highest quality care, chances are you are trying to do too much. To avoid this mistake, ask yourself this question, "What do I want my business to be known for?" Your answer should be one of the five following choices:

1. Low Prices (you are known for having the lowest prices). This means you have the lowest price hearing aids in your marketplace. Given the low number of hearing aid dispensed in a given month or year compared to other products, it is difficult to built a successful practice on being the low price leader.
2. Convenience (you are known for making the hearing aid transaction process as easy as possible). In the hearing aid business this might mean you're delivering your product and services to the customer in their home. It might also mean you're conducting business in a mobile unit that goes to nursing homes, retirement villages and hard to reach rural locations.
3. Technology (you are known for offering the most innovative technology). In the fast changing world of digital electronics it is difficult to offer a product that is clearly superior to a competitor's offering. This is certainly the case with hearing aid devices, as each

of the major manufacturer's launch new and very similar products two to three times per year.

4. Customer Service (you're service is fast, friendly, and reliable). In a hearing aid practice, you and your staff answer the phone within a couple of rings, work patients into the schedule quickly and offer a fast turnaround time on repairs. In short, your work processes are geared to pleasing your customers.

5. Engaging Experience (you're connecting with your customers on a personal level). In a hearing aid dispensing practice, you can create a memorable and emotionally engaging experience by bonding with your customers.

After you have asked the question, "what do you want your practice to be known for? pick one of the five alternatives listed here and begin to build your business around it.

Big Mistake No. 2: Failing to Be Memorable to the Customer

Keeping with the engaging experience concept, it is critical in the hearing aid business to be striving to have as many extremely satisfied customers as possible. There are a couple of reasons for this. One, it is common sense that you want all your customers to be as happy as possible. (Does any business owner want an unhappy one?) But, beyond just having extremely satisfied customers for the sake of it, there's an important business purpose. Extremely satisfied customers are promoters of

your practice. That is, they refer others to your practice. These referred patients cost virtually nothing to obtain and often are easier to work with.

Big Mistake No. 3: Focusing Exclusively on Business Results, Namely, Profit and Revenue

To state the obvious, a business must generate a profit if it is going to remain open. This mistake occurs when owners and managers focus too heavily on the "numbers" that drive their business, such as, net profit and close rate, rather than the core behaviors staff must engage in for the business to perform.

The question you have to ask yourself is, "What actions do I have to take to achieve profitability and revenue standards that are right for my business?" You must consider the actions and behaviors that you and your staff engage in with customers on a daily basis that are important to the sustainability of your practice.

Big Mistake No. 4: Failure to Identify the Strengths and Weaknesses of your Practice

A SWOT analysis can be used to identify strengths and weaknesses of a practice. SWOT is simply an acronym:

S = strengths

W = weaknesses

O = Opportunities

T = Threats

The purpose of a SWOT analysis is to identify areas within your practice that need refinement and clarity. By working with your staff you can conduct a SWOT analysis and identify how your business can be more successful. Table 12–6 shows a sample SWOT analysis for a practice.

Big Mistake No. 5: Failing to Have an Action Plan

Once you've completed your SWOT analysis, the next step is to create goals. Typically in a hearing aid practice your business goals will revolve around patient satisfaction, the number of units dispensed on a monthly basis and margins, which is the difference between what you pay for the hearing aid and what the customer pays for it. A solid action plan is needed to achieve a goal. Once you've established a goal (example: improve your close rate by 15% this year), the next step is to formulate how you plan to achieve this reach. In other words, what measures will your business employ to achieve this goal? It is likely that you will at list a couple of different tactics you will use to achieve it. In this example, it might mean you will execute a best practice process during the pre-fitting appointment, train your front office staff to more effectively book appointments and begin tracking your close rate more carefully. For each of these steps it is also important to designate a person responsible for achieving the goal, along with a time line for completing the task.

Big Mistake No. 6: Not Paying Attention to Margins

In simple terms, margin is the difference between the retail and wholesale cost of hearing aids. Because the hearing aid business is a relatively low volume (the average practice dispenses about 20 hearing aids per month), the margins must be relatively high in order to make a profit. When you begin working in a practice it's critical to pay attention to a couple of things that affect your profit margin, which include: the price you pay the manufacturer for hearing aids, the price you charge the customer, and, finally, the fixed and variable expenses associated with fitting hearing aids. In general terms,

Table 12–6. Example of a SWOT Analysis

Strengths	Weaknesses
Steady referrals from ENT	Turnover at front desk position has been high
Location of practice is excellent	Poor closing rate
Margins are healthy	Too many lost opportunities
Threats	**Opportunities**
Loss of ENT referrals	Improved close rate will result in significant revenue increase
Internet sales	

about one-third of the retail cost goes to pay the manufacturer, one-third goes to cover expenses in your practice (like rent, utilities, payroll, etc.), and the last third goes toward profit, which can be used to pay the manager, owner, and be invested back into the business to pay for marketing or new equipment. Margins and the entire topic of business management are worthy of additional study, more than we can cover in a few pages in this chapter. We recommend you take a couple of business management and operations courses from your local university or community college.

Not only is it important to avoid big mistakes, you also have to devise a great long-range strategic plan for your practice. The ability to prioritize—to know the most important things to get done first in your busy practice to generate more revenue—takes on greater importance in a world drowning in an abundance of information. Your ability to prioritize and simplify is a skill that often times separates a mediocre practice from a successful one. Recall that earlier we talked about the Practice Oriented Scale of Improvement (POSI), which you can use to help target and prioritize the needs of their practice (Figure 12–12).

The main theme of this chapter has been college basketball, and we can think of no better way to end it than by mentioning the legendary UCLA basketball coach John Wooden, who died at the age of 99 in 2010. Mr. Wooden not only won 12 NCAA basketball championships he was a mentor and teacher to his players long after their playing days were over. John Wooden created something called the Pyramid of Success. It summarized 15 essential values and characteristics of a championship team. We taken his idea and adapted it to running a practice. Figure 12–13 shows the 15 essentials values and characteristics of a world-class hearing aid dispensing business.

Your Path to Success

Well, there ain't no shame in a job well done
From driving a nail to driving a truck
As a matter of fact, I'd like to set things
  straight
A few more people should be pullin' their
  weight
If you want a cram course in reality
You get yourself a working man's Ph.D.

—Aaron Tippin

Several ideas for increasing productivity in a practice have been presented here, each of them addressing one of the three parts of the Productivity Trinity: office traffic, units sold, and ASP. Once you have decided you need to increase productivity, you can put this 5-step plan to work for you:

Step 1. Identify the gaps in productivity through benchmarking your practice against some industry averages.

Step 2. Understand how each of the four walls of your practice (people, process, financials, sales/marketing tactics) contribute to current productivity.

Step 3. Uncover the root causes of your productivity gaps by brainstorming all of the causes and effects of the productivity gaps in your practice. Once you have

Practice - Oriented Scale of Improvement*
(POSI)

Over the next 6 to 12 months, what are the most critical needs in your practice?

Name of Practice	
Practice Address	
City, State, Zip Code	
Name of Contact	
Contact Phone Number	
Account Executive	

Ranking Order	Please Rank in order - #1 being the most critical need in your practice.
☐	
☐	
☐	
☐	
☐	
☐	*UNSURE . . . NEEDS OR CONCERNS*

☐ Rank Order	Common Challenges	
1 - MOST critical	Advertising	Personnel / Staffing
2 -	Patient Retention	Keep up w/ Technology
3 -	Salesmanship	Profitability
4 -	Pricing	Cost Containment
5 - Least Critical	Time Management	

Would you like to be contacted by a Unitron Practice Development Specialist?	☐ YES ☐ NO
When is the best time to contact you?	☐ Morning ☐ Afternoon
How would you prefer to be contacted?	☐ In Person ☐ Call Before Stopping By
- If you would like to be called first please identify the best number to reach you:	( ) -

Figure 12–12. The Practice Oriented Scale of Improvement. Reprinted with permission from Unitron, all rights reserved.

listed all the possible causes of a productivity gap, you can prioritize them.

Step 4. Conduct a POSI and develop clear goals and an action plan that addresses each of the causes of the productivity gap.

Step 5. Execute the plan and monitor results on a weekly or biweekly basis

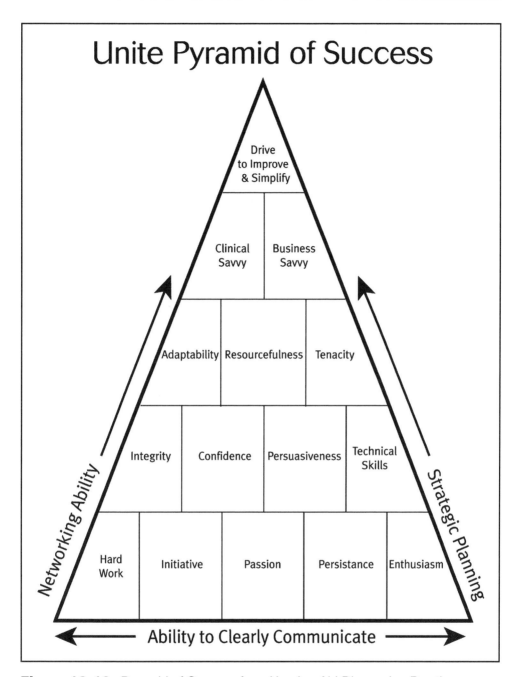

Figure 12–13. Pyramid of Success for a Hearing Aid Dispensing Practice.

This 5-step process is commonly known as "deep dive business review," and it allows the busy practice owner or manager to maintain a laserlike focus on seeing patients while managing their business.

In Closing

Although most audiologists and hearing instruments specialists have all the essential technical and interpersonal skills to excel in clinical practice, there is a need for both a consultative sales system to improve face-to-face communication with patients in a competitive commercial environment and a structure to improve quality and productivity within a practice. When the 2-step Discovery-Fulfillment consultative selling model outlined here is implemented, professionals will become more proficient at building relationships with patients and asking for the business at the end of the communication assessment appointment.

You don't have to be a college basketball fan or even a sports fan to appreciate the effectiveness of a well executed system. With some extra reading and a bit of practice you can take all the technical skills you learned in the first 11 chapters of this book and apply them to your interaction with patients by using the techniques and tactics outlined in this chapter.

And how about quality and productivity? It all starts with putting on your Carhartt jacket, Dickie's bib overalls, and bringing your lunch pail to work. And then getting busy taking care of business. In a competitive business situation, executing many of the tactics described here can be the difference in helping more patients embrace your mission of providing improved communication through amplification and counseling.

Appendix

As an old buddy of ours, Sam Johnson once said back in 1775:

"Knowledge is of two kinds: we know a subject ourselves, or we know where we can find information upon it."

Like the many of our Tips and Tricks and Take Five sections in this book, the appendix is the latter type of knowledge. We hope that you will refer to it when you are looking for an important tidbit of clinical information.

One of the keys to learning, of course, is reading. Keeping up with the literature is tough—there are about 12 audiology journals to read, with many more hearing science and otolaryngology journals with related important information. But, you know, keeping up is just something that professionals do. It's one of the many things that will separate you from the rest of the pack.

So, we're here to help: The following journals are available FREE of charge. There is a subscription form in most every journal (and you probably can sign up by phone or online). *IMPORTANTLY*, you can read recent articles online at these sites.

- *The Hearing Journal*,
  http//www.thehearingjournal.com

- *The Hearing Review,*
  http://www.hearingreview.com
- *Advance For Audiologists*,
  http://www.advanceforaud.com
- AudiologyOnline,
  http://www.audiologyonline.com

Audiology Online is not really a journal per se, but they post many excellent articles, along with live and recorded seminars. We're especially fond of the 20Q feature. It's an outstanding resource for all things related to dispensing hearing aids—the Ask the Expert series has a ton of questions that will relate directly to your daily practice. It's a Web site worth checking on a daily basis.

You can find articles easily on PUBMED (http; //www.pubmed.com) or even on Google Scholar. In fact, sometimes Google is better as it will have articles PUBMED doesn't (e.g., ones that are not from peer-reviewed journals). Just for practice: Type into Google "beer + audiology" and see what article you get!

There are many peer-reviewed journals available that usually have at least one hearing aid article each month. For audiologists, these journals are more or less mandatory reading. For nonaudiologists dispensing hearing aids, it's good to know they exist. You might even want to subscribe to one or two and read them. You can read to abstract for no charge at PUBMED.

The following journals are provided to the membership of the American Academy of Audiology (AAA)—go to http://www.audiology.org .

■ *JAAA*
■ *Audiology Today*

The following journal is provided to members of the American Auditory Society (AAS). Dues are cheap and the journal is free! You do not have to be an audiologist to become a member.

■ *Ear and Hearing,* e-mail: amaudsoc@aol.com or http://www.ear-hearing.com

The following journals are provided to members of the ASHA (although there's an extra fee to obtain both). If you're not already a member, it may not be worth joining just to obtain the journals—you can read the abstracts (JSLHR) or articles (AJA) at http://www.professional.asha.org .

■ *JSLHR*
■ *AJA*

The Academy of Doctors of Audiology (ADA) publishes a quarterly journal called *Audiology Practice*. Their Web site (http://www.audiologist.org) is also a great resource for private practice owners and manager.

The *International Journal of Audiology* is provided to members of the International Society of Audiology. Another good organization with very reasonable annual dues.

■ For membership: http:// www.eur.nl/fgg/kno/isa/isa.htm

Two good quarterly journals that publish review articles:

■ *Trends in Amplification* http://www.tia.sagepub.com
■ *Seminars in Hearing* http://www.thieme.com (To view articles online go to http://www.thieme-connect.com)

For many years, *The Hearing Journal* reviewed all the good hearing aid articles of the previous year. Pull these issues from last four to five years off your shelf and you can catch up in a hurry. Or, guess what: they are all posted at the journal's Web site! Search under "Mueller," as they don't always appear in the same month.

For nonaudiologists, the *International Hearing Society* (http://www.ihs info.org) IHS publishes a trade journal called *Hearing Professional*. It has plenty of pragmatic articles related to dispensing practices around the globe.

There are also many great textbooks (some of them we mentioned in the book) Plural Publishing (http://www .pluralpublishing.com), the publisher of this book, is continually adding selections to its online library. You can peruse its list and maybe order one or two by visiting its Web site.

Speech Tests

■ Auditec of St. Louis (http://www.auditec.com), Dr. Bill Carver at Auditec is the go-to guy, and has been supplying recorded speech testing to audiologists and dispensers for decades. Check out the wide range of speech testing available to you at its Web site.

■ Etymotic Research (http://www.eytymoticresearch.com), To obtain a copy of the Quick SIN or a nice set of high fidelity ear phones for your iPod check out this great site.

■ Frye Electronics (http://www.frye.com) distributes the Acceptable Noise Level test

Hearing Aid Programming Software

Just about every manufacturer in the hearing aid industry is part of a consortium called the Hearing Instrument Manufacturer's Software Association or HIMSA. HIMSA. NOAH 3 and NOAH-Link are current products developed and supported by HIMSA. Usually, clinicians don't deal directly with HIMSA (the hearing aid manufacturer sells these products to you), nevertheless it helps to know their Web site. To see the latest news in the programming software world and to subscribe to their newsletter go to http://www.himsa.com.

Supplies

Anything from ear impression material to telephone amplifiers to infection control equipment can be obtained from the companies listed below.

■ Oaktree Products (http://www.oaktreeproducts.com)

■ Hal Hen Company (http://www.halhen.com)
■ Warner Tech Care (http://www.warnertechcare.com)

Hearing Aid Fitting Formula Software and Other Great Tools

Several hearing aid research labs from around the world have fantastic Web sites with tons of useful information. There are different hearing aid fitting software packages than can be obtained from these Web sites. The fitting formula and the Web site are listed below. In additional to the fitting formula check out the questionnaires and other clinical tools they may have to offer.

■ DSLv5.0a—http://www.dslio.com: Up north in Canada, the folks at the University of Western Canada are continuing to pioneer pediatric audiology fitting protocols. The big news is the DSL works equally well for adults, too! Read the latest about their fitting algorithm at the Web site.

■ NAL-NL2—http://www.nal.gov.au: Our mates in Australia have finally launched the much anticipated NL2 version. The COSI also can be downloaded from this site. And while you're there, check out all the great presentations that they have posted.

■ CAMEQ: Across the pond, Brian Moore continues to do work on his fitting formulae (http://www.hearing.psychol.cam.ac.uk). This is also the home of the Ten Test.

■ VIOLA for Windows—http://www.memphis.edu/ausp/harl:

In addition to the IHAFF fitting formula (and the related Cox Contour Test), there are several questionnaires at this site available for download. Recall that throughout the book we talk about the ECHO, APHAB, IOI-HA and the SADL—they all live here (happily)!

Licensing and State Regulations

Information on the International Institute for Hearing Instrument Studies and the American College of Audioprosthology is also found at this Web site. If you are interested in becoming board certified as a hearing instrument specialist this site is useful. (http://www.ihsinfo.org)

American Speech and Hearing Association (http://www.asha.org): ASHA has a booklet called "State Regulation of Audiology and Speech-Language Pathology that is very helpful for finding out how to become licensed in each state.

American Academy of Audiology (http://www.audiology.org): Licensing and other credentialing material for both audiologists and audiology assistants can be found here: Your state licensing board. Your local state is the entity that has the ability to grant you a hearing aid dispensing license. Each state has a slightly different set of requirements to obtain a license. In some states, you need to have a Bachelor's degree and pass a test, whereas in other states you simply have to pass a written and practical test. You can Google "license requirement to dispense hearing aids in (name of state)" to find the requirements in your state. ASHA (http://www.asha.org) also maintains a summary of requirements at its Web site.

References

Berger, K. W. (1984). *The hearing aid: Its operation and development*. Livonia, MI: National Hearing Aid Society.

Bess, F. H., & Humes, L. E. (1995). *Audiology: The fundamentals* (2nd ed.). Baltimore, MD: Lippincott Williams & Wilkins.

Cox, R. M. (1995). Using loudness data for hearing aid selection: The IHAFF approach. *Hearing Journal, 48*(2), 39–44.

Cranford, J. (2008). *Basics of audiology: From vibrations to sounds*. San Diego, CA: Plural Publishing.

Dillon, H. (2001). *Hearing aids: A comprehensive text*. New York, NY: Thieme.

Hammill, T. A., & Price, L. L. (2008). *The hearing sciences*. San Diego, CA: Plural Publishing.

Hear well in a noisy world. (2009, July). *Consumer Reports*, pp. 32–37.

Hirsh, I. J. (1952). *Measurement of hearing*. New York, NY: McGraw-Hill.

Kates, J. M. *Digital hearing aids*. (2008). San Diego, CA: Plural Publishing.

Kochkin, S. (2003). MarkeTrak VI: On the issue of value: Hearing aid benefit, price, satisfaction and brand repurchase rates. *Hearing Review, 10*(2), 12–25.

Kochkin, S., Beck, D., Christensen, L., Compton-Conley, C., Fligor, B., Kricos, P., . . . Turner, R. (2010). MarkeTrak VIII: The impact of the hearing healthcare professional on hearing aid user success. *Hearing Review, 17*(4), 12–34.

Kramer, S. *Audiology: Science to practice*. (2008). San Diego, CA: Plural Publishing.

Larson-Donaldson, L. L. (1988). *Masking: Practical applications of masking principles and procedures* (2nd ed.). Livonia, MI: National Institute for Hearing Instruments Studies.

Mueller, H. G., & Hall, J, W., III. (1998). *Audiologists' desk reference, Vol. II*. San Diego, CA: Singular Publishing Group.

Mueller, H. G., Hawkins, D. B., & Northern, J. L. (1992) *Probe microphone measurements: Hearing aid selection and assessment*. San Diego, CA: Singular Publishing Group.

Newman, C. W., Weinstein, B. E., Jacobson, G. P., & Hug, G. A. (1990). The Hearing Handicap Inventory for Adults: Psychometric adequacy and audiometric correlates. *Ear and Hearing, 11*, 430–433.

Northern, J. (1995.) *Hearing disorders* (3rd ed.). Boston, MA: Allyn & Bacon.

Palmer, C. P., Mueller, H. G., & Moriarty, M. (1999). Profile of aided loudness: A validation procedure. *Hearing Journal, 52*(6), 3–42.

Palmer, C. V., Solodar, H. S., Hurley, W. R., Byrne, D. C., Williams, K. O. (2009). Self-perception of hearing ability as a strong predictor of hearing aid purchase. *Journal of the American Academy of Audiology, 20*, 341–347.

Pickles, J. O. (2008). *An introduction to the physiology of hearing* (3rd ed.). New York, NY: Academic Press.

Rees, Peter. (2003). Escape from Alcatraz, duck quack, stud finder. In *Mythbusters*. San Francisco, CA: Discovery Channel.

Robb, M. P. (2010). *INTRO: A guide to communication sciences and disorders*. San Diego, CA: Plural Publishing.

Sandridge, S. A., & Newman, C. W. (2006). Improving the efficiency and accountability of the hearing aid selection process —use of the COAT. Audiology Online, Article 1541. Retrieved March 6, 2006 from the Article Archives on http://www.audiologyonline.com .

Thibodeau, L. M. (2004). Plotting beyond the audiogram to the TELEGRAM, a new assessment tool. *Hearing Journal*, *57*(11), 46–51. Retrieved May 31, 2006 from http://www.audiologyonline.com.

Venema, T. (1998). *Compression for clinicians*. San Diego, CA: Singular Publishing Group.

Wu Y. H., & Bentler, R. A. (2010a). Impact of visual cues on directional benefit and preference: Part I—laboratory tests. *Ear and Hearing, 31*(1), 22–34.

Wu Y. H., & Bentler, R.A. (2010b). Impact of visual cues on directional benefit and preference: Part II—field tests. *Ear and Hearing, 31*(1), 35–46.

Zemlin, W. R. (1997.) *Speech and hearing science: Anatomy and physiology* (4th ed.). Boston, MA: Allyn & Bacon.

Index

A

Abbreviated Profile of Hearing Aid
    Benefit (APHAB), 352–355, 368
Acceptable noise level (ANL), 154, 176,
    319, 349, 373, 377, 383, 395, 401,
    407
Acclimatization defined, 166
Acoustic reflex, 53–54
Acoustics
  absorption, 23
  amplitude, 33
  auditory area for listening, 33, 34
  compression/rarefaction, 18–20
  dB (decibel), 35
  dB HL (hearing level), 38–39
  dB SL (sensation level), 39–40
  dB SPL (sound pressure level), 36,
    37–38
  diffraction of sound, 23–24
  echoes, 22–23
  filtering, 42, 43
  frequency, 25–26
    versus pitch, 29–30
  fundamental frequency, 26–27
  harmonic, first, 27
  hearing threshold levels, 38–39,
    146–147
  Hertz (Hz), 19, 20
  intensity *versus* loudness, 32–34
  lightning/thunder sound, 20–21
  loudness *versus* intensity, 32–34
  LTASS (long-term average speech
    spectrum), 40–42
  melees, 30
  military sounds dB SPL, 38

  narrowband noise, 31
  noise, 30–31
  nonperiodic sounds/noise, 30–32
  phase(s), 20, 21
  pink noise, 31
  pitch *versus* frequency, 29–30
  rarefaction/compression, 18–20
  reflection, 22–23
  refraction of sound, 24
  resonance, 29
  reverberation, 22
    details, 24
    listening fields: near and far, 24–25
  sensation level (dB SL), 39–40
  sound elements, 18
  sound waves
    wave defined, 18
  speech dynamic range, 41–42
  speech-shaped noise, 31
  timbre, 28
  white noise, 31
Acquired, or postnatal, hearing loss, 134
Adaptation defined, 166
Adjustment defined, 166
Advanced features of hearing aids
  achieving directionality with
    microphone methods, 247–249
  activation time (onset/offset
    times)/DNR parameters, 244
  adaptive feedback suppression
    narrowband notch filters, 238
  adaptive polar pattern in directional
    hearing aids, 253–254
  automatic acclimatizaton, 271
  automatic switching in directional
    hearing aids, 253

Advanced features of hearing aids
(*continued*)
  background noise: listening comfort
    activation time (onset/offset
      times)/DNR parameters, 244
    cognitive issues, 246–247
    DNR: how it works, 241–243
    and DNR parameter selection,
      243–245
    filtering and substraction noise
      reduction, 243
    gain enhancement/DNR
      parameters, 244
    gain reduction/DNR parameters,
      244
    impulse noise reduction, 243
    modulation-based noise reduction,
      241–243
    and noise reduction history, 240–241
    SNR and level effects/DNR
      parameters, 244
    sound smoothing, 243
  background noise: listening comfort
    in, 240
  Bluetooth applications, 273–274
  building blocks, 233–275
  cognitive issues, 246–247
  common directional hearing aid
    features, 253–254
  compression effects on directivity,
    258–259
  convenience/ease of use
    enhancement, 263–275
    automatic acclimatizaton, 271
    Bluetooth applications, 273–274
    data logging, 266–269
    hearing aid to hearing aid
      communication, 273
    multiple memory capacity, 264–266
    signal classification, 263–264
    in situ testing, 274–275
    trainable hearing aids, 269–271
    wireless connectivity, 271–274
  data logging, 266–269
    changing the fitting, 268
    for data training, 268–269
    day of fitting, 266
    follow-up counseling, 266–267

  troubleshooting, 267–268
  digital thinking overview, 231–232
  directional microphone technology,
    247–263
  directivity index (DI) of aids, 253
  DI/speech understanding
    relationship, 255
  distance and reverberation effects on
    directionality, 257–258
  DNR: how it works, 241–243
  and DNR parameter selection,
    243–245
  factors affecting directional
    microphone performance,
    255–260
  filtering and substraction noise
    reduction, 243
  frequency lowering, 237
  frequency response equalization,
    249–250
  and fundamental acoustic standards
    frequency response: smooth and
      undistorted, 232
  gain enhancement/DNR parameters,
    244
  gain reduction/DNR parameters, 244
  good feedback reduction algorithm
    downsides, 239–240
  hearing aid to hearing aid
    communication, 273
  impulse noise reduction, 243
  and low-frequency gain, 258
  microphone port alignment effects
    and directional microphone
    performance, 256–257
  modulation-based noise reduction,
    241–243
  multichannel processing, 235–237
  multiple memory capacity, 264–266
  narrowband notch filters, 238
  overview, 234–235
  phase cancellation, 238
  and polar plots (patterns) for
    microphones, 250–255
  popular opinion on noise-reduction
    schemes potential
    listening comfort in noise
      improvement, 246

reduction of loud sound
    annoyance, 245–246
speech intelligibility improvement,
    245
quiet listening: audibility,
    intelligibility, loudness comfort
adaptive feedback suppression,
    237–239
    narrowband notch filters, 238
    phase cancellation, 238
frequency lowering, 237
multichannel processing, 235–237
and OC fittings, 239
real-world directional hearing aid
    benefit, 260–261
sensorineural hearing aid priorities in
    order, 234–235
signal classification, 263–264
in situ testing, 274–275
SNR and level effects/DNR
    parameters, 244
sound smoothing, 243
speech intelligibility in noise
    achieving directionality with
        microphone methods, 247–249
    adaptive polar pattern in
        directional hearing aids,
        253–254
    automatic switching in directional
        hearing aids, 253
    common directional hearing aid
        features, 253–254
    directional microphone technology,
        247–263
    DI/speech understanding
        relationship, 255
    distance and reverberation effects
        on directionality, 257–258
    factors affecting directional
        microphone performance,
        255–260
    frequency response equalization,
        249–250
    low-frequency gain, 258
    microphone port alignment effects
        and directional microphone
        performance, 256–257
    overview, 247

and polar plots (patterns) for
    microphones, 250–255
real-world directional hearing aid
    benefit, 260–261
venting effects and directional
    microphone performance, 256
trainable hearing aids, 269–271
true patient benefit assessment,
    245–246
venting effects and directional
    microphone performance, 256
wireless connectivity, 271–274
Air conduction testing, 79, 80
Aminoglycoside antibiotics, ototoxicity,
    126
Anatomy
    auditory transduction processes
        summary, 68
    balance nerve illustrated, 47
    cochlear nerve illustrated, 47
    cochlea
        auditory nerve, 57
        basilar membrane, 57
        illustrated, 57
        organ of Corti, 57
        perilymph, 57
        role of, 55–59
        scala vestibuli, 57
    cochlea illustrated, 47
    cochlear partition, 58
    ear canal (external auditory
        canal/meatus)
        and earmold fitting, 48
        illustrated, 47
        overview, 48
    ear canal (external auditory
        canal/meatus) illustrated, 47
    earlobe illustrated, 47
    eighth cranial nerve, 59–60
    eustachian tube illustrated, 47
    external ear illustrated, 47
    facial nerve illustrated, 47
    hair cells, 58
    incus (anvil), 50
        illustrated, 47, 51
    inner ear, 55
        central auditory pathways, 59–60
        cochlea, 55

Anatomy; inner ear *(continued)*
   cohelear artery, 59
   eighth cranial nerve, 59–60
   energy supply, 59
   spiral ligament, 59
   stria vascularis, 59
  inner hair cells (IHC), 58
  internal auditory canal illustrated, 47
  malleus, 50
   illustrated, 47, 51
  organ of Corti, 58
   hair cells, 58
  ossicular chain, 50
   incus (anvil), 50
   malleus, 50
   stapes (stirrup), 50
  outer ear, 47–49
  outer hair cells (OHC), 58
  oval window illustrated, 47
  overview, 69
  pinna
   illustrated, 47
   landmarks illustrated, 48
   overview, 46
  round window illustrated, 47
  semicircular canals illustrated, 47
  stapes (stirrup), 50
  stapes (stirrup) illustrated, 47
  tectorial membrane, 59
  temporal nerve illustrated, 47
  tympanic membrane (TM), or
   eardrum, 50
   illustrated, 47, 51
  utricle illustrated, 47
  vestibular nerve illustrated, 47
ANSI (American National Standards
  Institute) dB Hl scale, 39
ASHA (American-Speech-Language-
  Hearing Association) chart of
  standard audiogram symbols,
  82
Aspirin, ototoxicity, 126
Audiograms
  ASHA (American-Speech-Language-
  Hearing Association) chart of
  standard audiometer symbols,
  82
  asymmetric hearing loss, 85

  cookie-bite shape, 85
  corner audiogram shape, 85
  flat shape, 85
  gradually sloping shape, 85
  noise notch, 85
  "normal," 82–84
  overview, 81
  precipitously sloping (ski slope)
   shape, 85
  presbycusic shape, 85
  reverse slope shape, 85
  shapes, 84–85
  symbols of, 81–82
  symmetric hearing loss, 85
Auditory learning defined, 166
Auditory training
  Computer-Assisted Speech Perception
   Testing and Training at the
   Sentence Level (CASPERSent),
   370–371
  Computer-Assisted Speech Training
   (CAST), 371
  Computer-Assisted Tracking
   Simulation (CATS), 371
  eARena, 371
  future of, 372
  Listening and Communication
   Enhancement (LACE), 371
Auditory transduction processes
  summary, 68

B

Background noise level (BCL), 154
*Basics of Audiology: From Vibrations to
  Sounds* (Cranford), 69
Von Békésy, Georg (1899–1972), 62–63
Bell, Alexander Graham, 35
Benefit defined, 333
BiCROS (bilateral contralateral routing
  of signal)/CROS (contralateral
  routing of signal) designs,
  178–180
Bony labyrinth. *See* Inner ear *main entry*
Boothroyd, Arthur, 25, 370
Boyle, Robert (1627–1691; Scottish
  scientist known for gas laws),
  82

Boyle, Robert (1627–1691; Scottish scientist known for gas laws), 71
Boyle's law, 107
Bumax, ototoxicity, 126

C

Cancer chemotherapeutics, ototoxicity, 126
Carboplatin, ototoxicity, 126, 127
Carhart, Raymond, 118
Case history taking
 overview, 110
 symptoms, common
  aural fullness, 111
  hyperacusis, 111
  otalgia, 111
  tinnitus, 110–111
  vertigo/dizziness, 111
CASPA (Computer-Assisted Speech Perception Assessment), 340
CCT (California Consonant Test), 339
Central auditory disorders, 130
Characteristics of Amplification (COAT), 141, 142, 176
CID W22 test, 338–339
Cisplatin, ototoxicity, 126, 127
Client Oriented Scale of Improvement (COSI), 143, 144, 266, 350–351, 352, 368, 389
 completing a detailed COSI postfitting
  establish realistic expectations for the two selected areas, 381–383
  pick two specific areas among five most important, 381
  get the details, 381
  list and target, 380
  overview, 379–380
Clinical outcome measures
 audibility measures, 336–337
 speech audiometry
  CASPA: monosyllabic speech tests, 340
  CCT: monosyllabic speech tests, 339
  CID W22: monosyllabic speech tests, 338–339
  CST: sentence-length speech tests, 340–341

  monosyllabic speech tests, 338–340
  NU-6: monosyllabic speech tests, 339
  overview, 337–338
  PBK-50: monosyllabic speech tests, 340
  QuickSIN: sentence-length speech tests, 341
  selecting test to use, 341–342
  sentence-length speech tests for validation, 340–341
  speech validation childhood tests: monosyllabic speech tests, 340
  SPIN: sentence-length speech tests, 340
  WIPI: monosyllabic speech tests, 340
Cochlea
 anatomy
  auditory nerve, 57
  basilar membrane, 57
  illustrated, 57
  organ of Corti, 57
  perilymph, 57
  scala vestibuli, 57
 auditory nerve
  illustrated, 57
 basilar membrane
  illustrated, 57
 channels, 56–57
 design intricacy, 56
 engineering of, 55–56
 illustrated, 55
 organ of Corti
  illustrated, 57
 perilymph
  illustrated, 57
 role of, 55–59
 scala tympani
  illustrated, 57
 scala vestibuli
  illustrated, 57
Cochlear partition
 anatomy, 58
Components of hearing aids, basic
 amplifiers, 209–210
 batteries, 204
 illustrated, 202

Components of hearing aids, basic (*continued*)
    microphones, 205–206
    receivers
        aspects of, 208–209
        styles, 208
    telecoils
        disadvantage, 208
        nontelephone uses, 207–208
    transducers, 204–209
Compression for Clinicians (Venema), 222
Computer-Assisted Speech Perception Testing and Training at the Sentence Level (CASPERSent), 370–371
Computer-Assisted Speech Training (CAST), 371
Computer-Assisted Tracking Simulation (CATS), 371
Congenital hearing loss, 134
Consumer's Report (probe-microphone measures), 297
Count-the-dots audiograms
    measure of audibilty outcome, 336–337
    prefitting hearing assessment, 150
Cox contour loudness anchors, 148, 344, 347
Cox Contour Test, 148, 344
CROS (contralateral routing of signal)/BiCROS (bilateral contralateral routing of signal) designs, 178–180
CST (Connected Speech Test), 340–341
Cytomegalovirus (CMV), 128

D
DeSogra, Robert, 127
Digital Hearing Aids (Kate), 243
Digital hearing instruments
    and outer hair cell damage, 58–59
    wide dynamic range processing, 59
Disorders of inner ear
    cholesteatoma, 120
    eustachian tube, patulous, 121
    middle ear effusion/negative middle ear effusion, 118–119

negative middle ear pressure/middle ear effusion, 118–119
    ossicular disarticulation, 120–121
    otitis media, 119–120
    otosclerosis, 117–118
    overview, 117
    tympanosclerosis, 120
Disorders of outer ear
    cerumen impaction, 114–115
    ear canal collapse, 113–114
    otitis externa, 115–116
    tumors of external ear canal, 116
    tympanic membrane perforation, 116–117
Disorders of the cochlea
    overview, 121–122
    presbycusis, 122
Dizziness, 61. *See also* Vertigo *main entry*
DSI (Dichotic Sentence Identification), 163–164, 164

E

Ear balance system
    physiology, 61
Ear canal (external auditory canal/meatus)
    anatomy
        and earmold fitting, 48
        overview, 48
    physiology
        resonance, 48–49
eARena, 371
Ear impressions (EI). *See also* Earmolds
    importance of, 181
    impression gun with silicone method, 185
    process
        explaining to patient, 185
        infection control, 182–183
        inspect ear canal/EI, 186
        materials, 182
        mixing impression material, 184
        open or closed jaw?, 184, 186
        otoblock/ear dam placement, 183
        otoscopic examination, 183
        otoscopic examination/bracing otoscope, 183

procedures, 182–187
  removing the finished EI, 186
  sending impression/information to
    manufacturer, 187
  syringe with silicone method, 185
Earmolds. *See also* Ear impressions (EI)
  bore modifications, 196, 197
  finishes/color, 193–194
  horn effect, 195–196
  illustrated, 189
  materials, 193
  NAEL (National Association of
    Earmold Labs), 188
  overview, 187
  style, 188
  tubing modifications, 193–194, 194–195
  venting
    and gain, 192
    size, 190–192
ECHO (expected consequences of
    hearing aid ownership), 145
Eighth cranial nerve
  anatomy, 59–60
  and neural transduction process, 60
Eloxtin, ototoxicity, 127
Endocochlear potential, 59
Endolymphatic hydrops, 128
Etiology *versus* symptoms, 110
Eustachian tube
  middle ear effusion, 54, 118–119
  patulous, 121
  physiology, 54
  Toynbee maneuver, 119
Eustachius, Artolomeo 1500/1514–1574,
    54
Expected Consequences of Hearing Aid
    Ownership (ECHO)
    questionnaire, 357

F

Fletcher, Harvey, 165
Form factor. *See* Hearing aid styles
Forms
  Characteristics of Amplification
    (COAT), 141
  sample case history form, 139
Furosemide, ototoxicity, 126

G

Gentamycin, ototoxicity, 126

H

Hair cell anatomy, 58. *See also* Inner hair
    cells (IHC); Outer hair cells
    (OHC)
Health-related quality of life (HRQoL),
    332
Hearing Aid Checklist example, 400
Hearing aid fitting procedures, 65–66.
    See also Hearing aid fitting
    procedures; Hearing aid fitting
    process
  coupler measures and the real ear,
    281–282
  different from fitting eye glasses, 67–68
  hearing aid orientation
    checklist use/contents, 318
    follow-up: short-term, 318–319
    informational counseling facts,
      317–318
    three steps of, 316–317
  hearing aid specification sheets,
    282–287
  overview, 137–138, 277–278
  prefitting considerations
    acclimatization underlying
      mechanisms, 167
    amplification and suspected
      cochlear dead region, 162
    auditory acclimatization, 164–167
    auditory deprivation prevention, 159
    auditory processing disorder
      (APD), 163–164
    bilateral *versus* unilateral fitting,
      156–160
    binaural interference, 160
    cochlear dead regions, 160–162
    DSI (Dichotic Sentence
      Identification), 163–164
    loudness summation, 157–158
    speech understanding in noise
      improvement, 157–158
    TEN (HL) Test, 162
    unilateral rationale, 159–160

Hearing aid fitting procedures
(continued)
  prefitting hearing assessment
    acceptable noise level (ANL) test,
      154, 176
    audibility/articulation index, 150,
      151
    background noise level (BCL), 154
    case history, 138–140
    Characteristics of Amplification
      (COAT), 140, 141, 176
    Client Oriented Scale of
      Improvement (COSI), 143, 144
    count-the-dots audiogram, 150
    ECHO (expected consequences of
      hearing aid ownership), 145
    explanation of results, 155–156
    Hearing Handicap Inventory for
      the Elderly-Screening Version
      (HHIE-S), 140, 142–143, 176
    Hearing-in-Noise Test (HINT), 152
    hearing test battery, 145–154
    hearing threshold levels, 38–39,
      146–147
    Independent Hearing Aid Fitting
      Forum (IHAFF) loudness
      anchors, 148
    loudness discomfort level (LDL),
      146, 147–148
    most comfortable listening level
      (MCL), 152, 154, 160
    patient expectations questionnaire,
      143, 144
    QuickSIN (speech-in-noise),
      152–154, 176
    red flags, 138
    sample case history form, 139
    speech audiometry, 148–149
    Speech Intelligibility Index (SII), 150
    WIN (Words in Noise), 152
  prescriptive fitting methods
    DSL and NAL, 295–298
    equalization/normalization, 294
    NAL-NL2 *versus* DSL, 296
    overview, 293–294
    verification need, 296–298
  prescriptive target matching, 306–315
    REAR for verification (probe-
      microphone), 307–308

REIG for verification (probe-
  microphone), 306–307
Step 1: use 2-cc coupler to test aids,
  313
Step 2: preprogram aids, 313
Step 3: on patient arrival, insert
  aids into ear, checking fit, 313
Step 4: establish realistic
  expectations with patient, 314
Step 5: run probe-microphone
  REOR test, 314
Step 6: verify aids performances
  with REAR mapping or REIG
  calculations, 314
Step 7: counsel patient on
  expectations, limitations,
  insertion, removal, care, and
  use, 314
Step 8: schedule a one-week
  followup appointment, 314
Step 9: call patient 24 to 48 hours
  postfitting to check status, 314
targets/target matching (probe-
  microphone), 308–313
programming of hearing aids
  (hardware/software), 287–291
  automated programming to "first-
    fit" system, 289–290
  Hi-Pro linkage for hearing aids to
    office NOAH system, 288–289
  iCube (Phonak) wireless
    programming system, 289
  NOAH software umbrella allowing
    common patient data saving
    and retrieval from any
    manufacturer, 288–289
  terms, 290–291
  validated prescriptive method
    (NAL-NL2 or DSL 5.0), 289, 290
  wireless programming systems, 289
selection recipe, 176
troubleshooting common problems,
  322–324
  acoustic feedback, 321–322
  adjustment guidelines for patient
    complaints for soft, afvera, and
    loud inputs, 325
  counseling patient to have patience
    with hearing aid, 324, 326

loud sounds are too loud, 322–324
occlusion effect: fixes, 319–320
occlusion effect: what doesn't work well, 320–321
problems talking on telephone, 326–327
2-cc coupler measures quality control
examples of hearing aid information from measures, 286–287
overview, 278
test equipment for, 278–281
verification process
acronyms explained simply: probe-microphones, 305
non-ANSI terms: probe-microphones, 304
audibility, 292
equipment: probe-microphones, 298
functional gain, 291–292
loudness ratings, 292
patient positioning: probe-microphones, 298
probe-microphone equipment/procedures, 298–305
probe-microphone measures, 291, 297
probe tube: probe-microphones, 299–300
speech intelligibility measures, 292
speech quality judgments, 293
Hearing aid follow-up appointments, 372–373
Hearing aid form factor. See Hearing aid styles
Hearing aid history, 203
Hearing aid mechanics
amplification defined, 202
attack and release times, 224–227
audio expansion, 227–229
components of hearing aids, basic, 202–210. *See also* Components of hearing aids, basic *main entry*
compression adjustment variability, 224
compression basics
ACGo compression clinical applications, 221–222
input/output functions, 217

input *versus* output compression, 218–222
like driving a car, 215–217
wide dynamic range compression (WDRC) clinical applications, 221–222
wide dynamic range compression (WDRC) *versus* ACGO compression (output-limiting compression), 220–221
compression kneepoint, 222, 223
contrasting key elements
channels *versus* bands *versus* handles, 213–214
frequency response: smooth *versus* distorted, 212–213
linear aids *versus* compression aids, 214–215
output *versus* gains, 212, 213
multiple channels
for AGCo, 227
overview, 227
overview, 201–202
performance descriptors
frequency response, 211–212
gain, 210–211
output, 211
Hearing aid orientation
during postfitting outcome measure taking, 366–367. *See also* Hearing aid fitting procedures *main entry for details*
Hearing aids
selection recipe, 176
wide dynamic-range multiband compression (WDRC), 167
Hearing aid styles
Baha implantable bone conduction design, 180
behind-the-ear (BTE) models
advantages, 170, 172
for children, 171
damping, 196
detailed, 170–171
indications for, 172
return rate, 170–171
size of, 171
tone hooks, 196
tubing, 194

Hearing aid styles *(continued)*
  BiCROS (bilateral contralateral
    routing of signal)/CROS
    (contralateral routing of signal)
    designs, 178–180
  body aids, 176–177
  completely in-the-canal (CIC)
    detailed, 172, 175–176
  CROS (contralateral routing of
    signal)/BiCROS (bilateral
    contralateral routing of signal)
    designs, 178–180
  damping, 196
  eyeglass hearing aids, 177–178
  in-the-ear (ITE) detailed, 174–175
  open canal (OC) fittings. *See also*
    receiver in the canal (RIC)
    instruments *in this section*
    detailed, 171–174
    effects *versus* closed system,
      198–200
    as mini-BTEs, 173–174
    receiver-in-the-aid (RITA) device,
      173, 195
    tubing, 195
  overall: venting, damping, horn
    effects, 197–198
  overview, 169–170
  receiver in the canal (RIC)
    instruments, 171
    detailed, 164, 171, 172, 173, 174
    tubing, 195
  RITE device. *See* receiver in the canal
    (RIC) instruments *in this section*
  selection process, 180
  tone hooks, 196
  Trans Ear bone conduction design,
    180
Hearing disorders, common
  and balance, 61
  central auditory disorders, 130
  classification by onset age
    acquired, or postnatal, hearing loss,
      134
    congenital hearing loss, 134
    overview, 133–134
    perinatal hearing loss, 134
    prenatal hearing loss, 134
  cochlear disorders, 121–122

congenital hearing loss, 128
diseases acquired after birth, 128
hereditary hearing loss
  Mendelian laws, 132–133
  transmission modes, 133
Ménière disease, 128–129
middle ear disorders, 117–121. *See also*
  Disorders of middle ear *main*
  entry for details
noise-induced hearing loss (NIHL),
  123–126. *See also* Noise-induced
  hearing loss (NIHL) *main entry*
nonorganic hearing loss, 130–132
ototoxicity, 126–127
  and medication duration, 127. *See*
    listings for ototoxic drugs
  summary of common drugs
    harming hearing, 126
outer ear disorders, 113–117. *See also*
  Disorders of outer ear *main*
  entry for details
overview, 113
retrocochlear disorders, 129–130
viral/bacterial diseases, 128
Hearing Handicap Inventory for Adults
  (HHIA), 356–357
Hearing Handicap Inventory for the
  Elderly (HHIE), 356–357
Hearing Handicap Inventory for the
  Elderly-Screening Version
  (HHIE-S), 140, 142–143, 176
Hearing-in-Noise Test (HINT), 152
Hearing loss
  asymmetric, 85
  and hearing in noise, 66–67
  mild-to-moderate, 65
  presbycusic, 85
  process, physiological, 63–65
  sensorineural, 65, 126
    outer hair cells (OHC), 58–59, 65
  symmetric, 85
Hearing measurement. *See*
  Measurement of hearing
Hearing test battery
  audiometer/pure-tone audiogram,
    76–77
  and earphones, 77–79
  insert earphones, 78–79
Helmholz resonators, 29

Hereditary hearing loss
    Mendelian laws, 132–133
    transmission modes, 133
Herpes simplex disease, 128
Herpes zoster oticus, 128
Hertz, Heinrich Rudolf, 19
HIMSA (Hearing Instrument
        Manufacturer's Association)
    hearing aid software certification, 289
    NOAH software umbrella allowing
        common patient data saving
        and retrieval from any
        manufacturer, 288–289
History of hearing aids, 203
HLAA (Hearing Loss Association of
        America) checklist for hearing
        aid dispensing office
        consumers, 391
Hughson-Westlake procedure. *See*
        Pure-tone air conduction
        audiometry

I

Immitance audiometry, 118
Immittance meters, 53–54
Incus (anvil) anatomy, 50
Independent Hearing Aid Fitting Forum
        (IHAFF) loudness anchors, 148
Inner ear
    anatomy, 55
        central auditory pathways, 59–60
        cochlea, 55
        cohelear artery, 59
        eighth cranial nerve, 59–60
        energy supply, 59
        spiral ligament, 59
        stria vascularis, 59
    cochlea
        illustrated, 55
    endocochlear potential, 59
    physiology, 55–66
        endocochlear potential, 59
    semicircular canals
        illustrated, 55
    vestibule
        illustrated, 55
Inner hair cells (IHC)
    anatomy, 58

    damage results, 64–65
    innervation, 60
    neural transduction process, 60
    quick guide, 64
International Outcome Inventory—
        Hearing Aids (IOI-HA), 357,
        361, 362
*An Introduction to the Physiology of
        Hearing* (Pickles), 69

J

Jackson, Phil, 390

K

Kanamycin, ototoxicity, 126
Killion, Mead, 165, 195, 233, 281

L

Lasix, ototoxicity, 126
Levitt, Harry, 371
Libby, Cy, 195, 198
Listening and Communicaton
        Enhancement (LACE), 371
Loop diuretics, ototoxicity, 126
Loudness discomfort level (LDL), 100,
        101, 112, 146, 147–148, 176

M

Malleus (hammer)
    anatomy, 50
        illustrated, 47, 51
    physiology, 53, 56
        sound magnification, 52
Margolis, Bob, 317
Marketing. *See* Sales *main entry*
Masking: air conduction
    equipment preparation, 95–96
    procedure, 96
    purpose of, 95
    timing of, 95
Masking: bone conduction
    equipment preparation, 94
    overview, 93–94
    patient instruction script, 94
    plateau method, 94–95
    procedure, 94

Masking, effective
interaural attenuation, 93
occlusion effect, 92–93
overview, 91
patient instruction script, 92
procedure, 92
settings for equipment, 91–92
Masking: Practical Applications (Linda
Donaldson), 95
Measles, 128
Measurement of hearing
air conduction testing, 80
and audiograms, 81–85. *See also*
Audiograms *main entry for
details*
bone conduction testing, 79–80
effective masking, 91–93. *See also*
Masking, effective *main entry
for details*
hearing test battery, 76–79. *See also*
Hearing test battery *main entry
for details*
masking for bone conduction, 93–95.
See also Masking: bone
conduction *main entry for details*
most comfortable and uncomfortable
loudness levels, 106–107
otoscopy, 72–76. *See also* Otoscopy
main entry for details
overview, 71
pure-tone air conduction audiometry,
85–88. *See also* Pure-tone air
conduction audiometry *main
entry for details*
pure-tone bone conduction
audiometry, 88–91. *See also*
Pure-tone bone conduction
audiometry *main entry for
details*
speech audiometry, 96, 148–149
speech recognition testing (SRT),
96–99. *See also* Speech
recognition testing (SRT) *main
entry for details*
word recognition testing, 99–106. *See
also* Word recognition testing
main entry for details
Ménière disease, 128–129
Meningitis, bacterial, 128

Middle ear effusion, eustachian tube, 54,
118–119
Moore, Brian C. J., 162
Most comfortable and uncomfortable
loudness levels, 106–107
Most comfortable listening level (MCL),
152, 154, 160
Mumps, 128

N

NOAHLink, Bluetooth transmission
process, 288–289
NOAH software umbrella allowing
common patient data saving
and retrieval from any
manufacturer, 288–289
Noise-induced hearing loss (NIHL)
maximum permissible noise levels,
125
noise notch audiogram pattern, 124
onset characteristics, 125
and OSHA (Occupational Health and
Safety Agency), 125, 126
overview, 123–124
Nonorganic hearing loss, 130–132
NU-6 test, 339

O

Organ of Corti
anatomy, 58
hair cells, 58
Ossicular chain
anatomy, 50
and incus (anvil), 50
and malleus, 50
and stapes (stirrup), 50
physiology, 50–51
Otoscopy
equipment
video otoscopy advantage, 73–74
examination process (step-by-step),
74–75
general purpose of, 74
Outcome measures
acclimatization, 361
and improvements in speech
understanding, 365–366

aided measures of sound quality, 343–344, 345–346
background, 330
benefit defined, 333
benefit measurement, 333–334
benefit *versus* satisfaction, 333
clinical, 336–347. *See also* Clinical outcome measures *main entry for details*
clinic *versus* real world, 334–336
hearing aid orientation, 366–367
HIO Basics (hearing instrument orientation BASICS), 366–367
measurement parameter, 333
measures of directional microphone benefit, 334–346
measures of loudness discomfort, 346–347
QuickSIN: aided measures of sound quality, 345–346
satisfaction defined, 334
satisfaction measurement, 334
self-reports, 347–366. *See also* Self-reports of hearing aid outcome *main entry for details*
treatment assessment, 330–331
types, 332–333
validation defined, 330
WHO (World Health Organization) guidance, 331–332
Outer ear anatomy, 46–47
Outer hair cells (OHC)
  anatomy, 58
  and cochlear amplification, 63
  damage, 58–59, 64
  and digital hearing instruments, 58–59
  innervation, 60
  quick guide, 64
  sensorineural hearing loss, 58–59, 65
  and tectorial membrane, 59

P

Palmer, Catherine, 167, 269
PBK-50 (Phonetically Balanced Kindergarten) test, 340
Perinatal hearing loss, 134
Physiology
  acoustic reflex, 53–54

auditory transduction processes summary, 68
cochlea, sound analysis of, 62–63
ear balance system, 61
ear canal (external auditory canal/meatus), 48
  resonance, 48–49
eustachian tube, 54
impedance mismatch solution, 51–52
inner ear, 55–66
  endocochlear potential, 59
malleus, 53
  sound magnification, 52
malleus (hammer), 56
middle ear mechanics, 50–52, 54
ossicular chain, 50–51
outer hair cells (OHC)
  and cochlear amplification, 63
overview, 69
pinna
  shaping of sounds, 48
stapedius muscle, 53
stapes (stirrup), 53
  pushing on cochlear oval window, 51
tensor tympani muscle, 53
traveling wave, 63
tympanic membrane (TM), or eardrum,
  overcoming impedance mismatch, 52–53
  pushing on ossicles, 51
vibratory-to-mechanical sound transmission, 51
Pinna
  anatomy
    illustrated, 47
    landmarks illustrated, 48
    overview, 46
Platinum-based chemotherapy agents, ototoxicity, 127
POSI (Practice-Oriented Scale of Improvement), 394, 413, 414
Postfitting follow-up
  auditory training, 370–372
    future of, 372
  and aural rehabilitation, 368–369
    for New Age patients, 369–370
  family counseling, 368
  overview, 368

Prefitting Clinical Protocol Checklist
example, 399
Prenatal hearing loss, 134
Profile of Aided Loudness (PAL),
355–356, 358–360
Psychology of hearing loss
anger of loss grief, 6–7
audiologic variable, 3
avoidance in loss grief, 6
counseling strategies, 9–10
counseling types, 8–9
dealing with individuality of patients,
1–2
foundation for informed buying
decision, 14
gradual *versus* rapid hearing loss, 3
grief of loss, 3–4, 5–8
hearing loss stages of grieving, 4
hostility in loss grief, 6–7
informational counseling, 8
informed buying decision, 14–15
Kübler-Ross stages of grieving, 4
late *versus* early onset loss, 3
maximizing patient interaction,
11–15
overview, 1, 15
patient ownership, 9, 11
patient-to-professional
communication flow, 13
personal adjustment counseling, 9
professional learning stance, 12–13
professional teaching stance, 13–14
self-esteem, 4–5
selfishness of loss grief, 8
stigma of loss, 2–3
suspicion in loss grief, 8
withdrawal in loss grief, 6
Pure-tone air conduction audiometry
equipment preparation, 86
Hughson-Westlake procedure, 85
interpretation, 88
overview, 85
patient instruction script, 86
pure-tone average (PTA),
three-frequency, 88
purpose of, 85
recording of results, 88
standard procedure, 86–88

Pure-tone bone conduction audiometry
equipment preparation, 88–89
interpretation, 90–91
overview, 88–89
patient instruction script, 89–90
procedure, 90
purpose of, 88–89, 89

Q

QuickSIN (speech-in-noise), 152–154,
176, 334, 341, 342, 343, 345–346
Quinine, ototoxicity, 126

R

Reagan, President Ronald, personal
hearing aid feature, 240
Retrocochlear disorders, 129–130
Rubella, 128

S

Sales
average selling price, 408–409
average selling price: 3 adding
touchpoints, 410
average selling price: 2 "best practice"
testing, 409–410
average selling price: 1 follow-up
services, 409
avoiding big mistakes
of exclusive focus on profit and
revenue, 411
of failing to be memorable to
customer, 411
of failing to have an action plan, 412
of not identifying practice strengths
and weaknesses, 411–412
of not paying attention to margins,
412–413
of trying to be all things to all
people, 410–411
based on practice quality and
productivity, 391–392
consultative selling phase 1:
discovery, 376–377
step 1: rapport/trust, 377–379

step 2: assessing communication needs, 379–383. *See also* completing a detailed COSI postfitting *under* Client Oriented Scale of Improvement (COSI)

step 3: audiologic assessment, 383–384

consultative selling phase 2: fulfillment RED DOOR (*r*eview, *e*ducate, *d*emonstrate, *d*iscuss options, *o*ffer choices, *o*vercome objections, *r*eassure), 384

step 1: review results, 385–386

step 2: educate (discuss consequence of untreated hearing loss), 386–388

step 4: discuss options, 388–389

step 5: offer choices, 389–390

step 6: overcome objections/ask for business, 390

step 6: reassurance, 390–391

consultative selling rationale, 376

Hearing Aid Checklist example, 400

overview, 375–376

path to success 5-step plan, 413–414

patient comment card to assess relationship-building skills, 399

POSI (Practice-Oriented Scale of Improvement), 394, 413, 414

practice productivity

office traffic: 1. incentivize word-of-mouth referrals, 404–405

office traffic: 3. mine existing database, 405

office traffic: 3. reach out to patients and influencers, 405–406

overview, 401–403

units sold, 407–408

units sold: 5 authority, 408

units sold: 3 likeability, 408

units sold: 4 likeability, 408

units sold: 1 reciprocation, 408

units sold: 6 scarcity, 408

units sold: 3 social proof, 408

practice quality gap caveat, 392–393

practice quality measures, 395–396

Pyramid of Success, 415

quality elements

appearance of physical location, 398

interpersonal communication skills, 398

laboratory/self-reports of hearing aid benefit, 401

patient device use time, 401

patient wait time/initial greeting, 396–397

product quality, 400–401

technical skills, 398–400

technical skills of staff, 398–400

3-E's of quality, 393–395

Salicylates, ototoxicity, 126

Satisfaction defined, 334

Satisfaction with Amplification in Daily Life (SADL), 357. *See also* Expected Consequences of Hearing Aid Ownership (ECHO) questionnaire

Self-reports of hearing aid outcome

closed-ended self-report measures

Abbreviated Profile of Hearing Aid Benefit (APHAB), 352–355

Hearing Handicap Inventory for Adults (HHIA), 356–357

Hearing Handicap Inventory for the Elderly (HHIE), 356–357

International Outcome Inventory—Hearing Aids (IOI-HA), 357, 361, 362

overview, 352

Profile of Aided Loudness (PAL), 355–356, 358–360

Satisfaction with Amplification in Daily Life (SADL), 357

TELEGRAM (*t*elephone, *e*mployment, *l*egislation [such as ADA], *e*ntertainment, *g*roups [church, parties, meetings], *r*ecreation, *a*larms [doorbell, smoke, clock], *m*embers of family), 361, 363

open-ended self-report measures

Client Oriented Scale of Improvement (COSI), 350–351, 352

Glasgow Hearing Aid Benefit Profile (GHABP), 351

Self-reports of hearing aid outcome
(*continued*)
    overview, 347–348
    rationales for, 348–350
Shearing aid fitting procedures
    verification process
        real-ear terminology:
            probe-microphones, 301
SNR (signal-to-noise ratio), 150–152
Speech and Hearing Science (Zemlin), 69
Speech audiometry, 96, 148–149
    clinical outcomes measures, 337–343.
        See also Clinical outcomes
        measure *main entry for details*
    prefitting hearing assessment,
        148–149
Speech-in-noise testing, 149–154
Speech Intelligibility Index (SII), 150
Speech recognition testing (SRT)
    equipment preparation, 97
    interpretation, 99
    overview, 96–97
    patient instructions, script, 97
    procedure, 97–98
    results, 98
SPIN (Speech Perception in Noise) test,
    340
Stapedius muscle physiology, 53
Stapes (stirrup)
    anatomy, 50
    illustrated, 45
    physiology
        pushing on cochlear oval window,
        51, 56
Streptomycin, ototoxicity, 126
Sullivan, Roy (video otoscopy pioneer),
    73
Symptoms *versus* etiology, 110
Syphilis, 128

T

Take Five
    and acclimatization term for speech
        processing, 166
    adaptive directional hearing aid
        testimonial, 254
    attacking and releasing for aided
        "woof" intelligibility, 225

audibility/articulation index, 150
audiogram anecdote, 82
audiologic reactions to medications,
    127
auditory acclimatization anecdote, 165
aural rehabilitation, 368
behavioral shapes of hearing
    impairment, 12
benefit/satisfaction quiz, 335
binaural or bilateral?, 157
binaural preference demonstration,
    160
the black box, 241
Bluetooth probe-microphone
    transmission, 298
caveat on hearing aid verification
    survey, 297
checking out volunteers' ear canals,
    76
classroom reverberation computer
    simulation, 25
cochlear anatomy/physiology quick
    guide, 64
compression sense, 222
computer-based auditory training
    programs, 372
contemporary audio expansion
    programming, 229
CounselEar to design patient
    counseling material, 318
data logging and females, 269
dB and dB SPL relativity, 38
Device-Oriented Subjective Outcome
    Scale (DOSO), 363
DNR +, 245
DNR extras, 243
duck quack echo, 23
Earmold resources, 187
earmold video, 187
environmental influence on hearing,
    21
eustachian tube, 119
females and data logging, 269
gain and output "first-fit" pointers,
    290
guided Internet ear tour, 54
hearing aid market statistics, 162
hearing aid measurement exercises,
    286

hearing aid orientation DVD for patients, 367

hearing aids: quality of life, 332

hearing aid signal classification, 264

hearing aid tubing for custom products, 195

honing masking understanding, 95

informational counseling: sales, 385

medical terminology, 111

negative middle ear pressure relief, 54

NFMI (near-field magnetic induction) for wireless, 273

NOAH-compliant computers, 289

patient retention programs, 406

PBmax explained, 102

personal stereo systems/NIHL, 125

presbycusis social engineering, 123

prescriptive targets: infants/toddlers, 295

proprietary hearing aid algorithms, 296

"response" *versus* "gain," 301–302

rollover ratio formula, 102

self-hearing ability rating/purchase decision, 10

significant others and prefitting appointments, 145

simulate personal hearing loss, 5

single-sided deafness treatment options, 180

smaller CICs, 176

Speech Intelligibility Index (SII), 150

strategic practice quality execution, 396

tactic to address most objections in marketing, 391

taking action to meet practice quality goals, 395

timbre/hearing pleasure, 28

Touchpoints of sales, 409

Toynbee maneuver, 119

Transducers 101, 209

types of audiometers, 77

unaided ear effect, 159

unique polar patterns of microphones, 253

Valsalva procedure, 119

verification *versus* validation, 330

video-otoscopy, 184

virtual audiometer simulation on Internet, 79

virtual tour of outer, middle, and inner ear, 56

what is AI-DI?, 255

wireless communication between hearing aids, 273

Technique importance, 72

TELEGRAM (*t*elephone, *e*mployment, *l*egislation [such as ADA], *e*ntertainment, *g*roups [church, parties, meetings], *r*ecreation, *a*larms [doorbell, smoke, clock], *m*embers of family), 361, 363

TEN (HL) Test, 162, 274

Tensor tympani muscle physiology, 53

Tesla effect (Nicola Tesla), 271–272

Thibodeau, Linda, 361

Tillman, Tom, 233

Tips and Tricks

acclimatization: practical issues, 365

advances in wireless transmission signals, 274

anger of acquiring hearing loss, 7

APHAB use, 354

ASG/ear canal variation, 238

on audiograms: when to test extra frequencies, 83

audiometer calibration standards, 78

auditory landmarks, 61

better speech understanding in background noise, 158

BTE spec sheets, 285

Carhart notch, 118

cerumen management, 115

channels/prescriptive fitting targets, 236

checking out ear internal photos, 75

clean hearing aid ports are critical, 249

compression terms: beyond basic, 226

coupler/hearing aid pairings, 280

directionality tweaks by hearing aid manufacturers, 260

ear impression (EI) blow-by problem, 183

ear impression methods, 185

ear impressions/PE tubes, 120

Tips and Tricks *(continued)*
  effective information provision, 7
  external otitis/hearing loss, 115
  getting started with QuickSIN, 154
  good question examples, 10
  hearing aid alignment, 257
  hearing aid battery life, 205
  hearing aid 3 dB SNR advantage, 261
  hearing instrument troubleshooting, 32
  HHIE versions, 142
  human ear canal resonance, 29
  insider bone conduction testing information, 91
  is negative DI possible?, 256
  loudness perception, 112
  measuring outcome with the COSI, 351
  memorable reporting to patients, 156, 158
  monosyllabic speech tests, hearing aid validation, 339
  multifrequency directionality, 254
  open fittings pluses and minuses, 199
  outcome measures: practical issues, 364
  outer hair cell damage, 59
  Patient "Need to Know" about directional microphone products, 262–263
  patient with APD, 163
  pitch for counseling communication, 30
  practical uses of outcome measures, 331
  practical uses of self-report outcome measures, 349
  presbycusis etiology, 122
  QuickSIN/audibility validation, 342
  recruitment, 112
  REUG stored average for probe microphone verification, 307
  RIC myths?, 173
  signal-to-noise ratio (SNR), 242
  speech understanding and reverberation, 258
  SRT measurement, 98
  "stable gain" meaning, 239
  10 best words, 100
  testing hearing aids, 22
  tinnitus, 112
  "trial closing" in sales, 389
  validation of maximum loudness, 347
  when an omni-directional hearing aid is the solution, 265
  zero dB HL, 39
Toxoplasmosis, 128
Tympanic membrane (TM), or eardrum, anatomy, 50
  illustrated, 47
  physiology
    overcoming impedance mismatch, 52–53
    pushing on ossicles, 51

V

Valsalva, Antonio Maria (1666–1723), 54
Vancomycin, ototoxicity, 126
Venema, Ted, 222
Vertigo defined, 61. *See also* Dizziness *main entry*
Vincristine, ototoxicity, 127
Von Békésy, Georg (1899–1972), 62–63

W

Web sites
  acoustics, 18
  American Tinnitus Association, 112
  ASHA (American-Speech-Language-Hearing Association) chart of standard audiogram symbols, 82
  audiologic reactions to medications, 127
  Audiology Online, 165, 173
  audiometer simulators, 79
  Augustana College, Sioux Falls, SD, 56
  behavioral shapes of hearing impairment, 12
  Better Hearing Institute, 162
  Boothroyd, Arthur, 25
  classroom reverberation computer simulation, 25

Computer-Assisted Speech Perception Testing and Training at the Sentence Level (CASPERSent), 370–371

CounselEAR customized reports, 155

CounselEar for designing patient materials, 318

DSI (Dichotic Sentence Identification), 164

eARena, 371

earmold instructional information, 187

earmold video, 186

Etymotic Research insert earphones, 78

on excellent worksites, 405

hand-held audiometer, 77

hearing aids and cell phones, 327

hearing disorders/emedicine, 113

Hearing Journal, 165, 173

and hearing loss stigma, 3

Hertz (Hz), 19, 20

HIMSA (Hearing Instrument Manufacturer's Association), 289

HLAA (Hearing Loss Association of America) checklist for hearing aid dispensing office consumers, 391

interactive audiogram exercises, 84

International Hearing Society, 95

Knowles Electronics, 209

"looping" spaces for telecoil reception, 208

masking, 95

medical dictionary, 111

QuickSIN (Etymotic), 154

Robyn Cox's Hearing Aid Research Laboratory, 341

Roy Sullivan on video otoscopy use, 73

SADL, 357

Sonion, 209

sound elements, 18

Tinnitus Retraining Therapy (TRT), 112

tour of outer, middle, and inner ear, 56

video otoscopes' comparisons, 74

WHO (World Health Organization) outcome measures guidance, 331–332

terms employed by, 332

WIN (Words in Noise), 152

WIPI (Word Intelligibility by Picture Identification), 340

Word recognition testing

equipment preparation, 101

number of words presented, 100

patient instructions, script, 101

presentation level, 100

presentation mode, 101

purpose, 99

score interpretation, 102, 103

scoring, 102, 103

significant differences/changes in scores, 104, 105–106

test procedure, 101

word lists, 99